SENSORY PERCEPTION IN THE MEDIEVAL WEST

UTRECHT STUDIES IN MEDIEVAL LITERACY

34

UTRECHT STUDIES IN MEDIEVAL LITERACY

SENSORY PERCEPTION

IN THE MEDIEVAL WEST

Edited by

Simon C. Thomson and Michael D. J. Bintley

BREPOLS

British Library Cataloguing in Publication Data

A catalogue record for this book is available from the British Library

D/2016/0095/26

ISBN 978-2-503-56714-3

e-ISBN 978-2-503-56717-4

DOI: 10.1484/M.USML-EB.5.109361

Printed in the EU on acid-free paper

Contents

Abbreviations vii
Acknowledgements ix

Sensory Perception in the Medieval West: Introduction
SIMON C. THOMSON 1
Heaven Ahoy! Sensory Perception in *The Seafarer*
RICHARD NORTH 7
The Sensory Cost of Remediation; or, Sniffing in the Gutter of Anglo-Saxon Manuscripts
JONATHAN WILCOX 27
The *York Mystery Plays*: Exploring Sound and Hearing in Medieval Vernacular Drama
MARIANA LOPEZ 53
Birds and Words: Aurality, Semantics and Species in Anglo-Saxon England
ERIC LACEY 75
"Whistle While You Work": Scribal Engagement with Old English Poetic Texts
SIMON C. THOMSON 99
Doing Things with Words: Language and Perception in Old English Riddles and Charms
VICTORIA SYMONS 123
Sight, Sound, and the Perception of the Anglo-Saxon Liturgy in Exeter Book *Riddles 48* and *59*
FRANCESCA BROOKS 141
All that Glitters: The Role of Pattern, Reflection, and Visual Perception in Early Anglo-Saxon Art
MELISSA HERMAN 159

Taking Out the Eye of a One-Eyed Man and Other Hypothetical Moments of Sensory Impairment in Early Medieval Law
PATRICIA SKINNER 181

Dis-embodied Cognition and Sensory Perception in *Sólarljóð*
PETE SANDBERG 195

(Re-) Viewing "*Iuxta Morem Romanorum*": Considering Perception, Phenomenology, and Anglo-Saxon Ecclesiastical Art and Architecture
MEG BOULTON 207

Plant Life in the *Poetic Edda*
MICHAEL D.J. BINTLEY 227

Index 245

Abbreviations

ASPR	*The Anglo-Saxon Poetic Records*, ed. G.P. KNAPP and E.V.K. DOBBIE, 6 vols. (New York, 1931-1942).
BHL	*Bibliotheca Hagiographica Latina*, 2 vols. (Brussels, 1899-1901), with *Supplementum* by H. FROS (Brussels, 1986).
DOEC	*Dictionary of the Old English Corpus* <http://tapor.library.utoronto.ca.libproxy.ucl.ac.uk/doecorpus/simple.html>.
MGH	*Monumenta Germaniae Historica.*
LL Nat. Germ.	*Leges nationum Germanicarum*, 1- (Hanover, 1892-).
SRG	*Scriptores rerum Germanicarum: Nova Series*, 1- (Munich, 1922-).
SRM	*Scriptores rerum Merovingicarum*, 7 vols. (Hanover and Leipzig, 1884-1951).
SS	*Scriptores (in Folio)*, 30 vols; *(in Quarto)*, vols. 31-34 (Hanover, 1826-1980).
PL	*Patrologiae cursus completus ... Series Latina*, ed. J.P. MIGNE, 221 vols. (Paris, 1841-1864).

Acknowledgements

This volume was inspired by a conference held at University College London on 12th and 13th April 2014. The event was the eighth in what is now the Northern / Early Medieval Interdisciplinary Conference Series, founded at UCL and the University of York, and this is the fourth volume to be published as a result of the productive and challenging dialogues held within that series. All of the contributors and attendees at that conference generated thought-provoking debate in a warm and scholarly atmosphere characteristic of the series' events. The conference itself could not have taken place without the support of UCL's Faculty Institute of Graduate Studies, Department of English Language and Literature, and Institute of Archaeology, for whose generosity and long-standing support we are also grateful. The editors would like to thank the contributors for their patience, persistence, and perspicacity throughout the project. Special thanks are due to Guy Carney at Brepols for his smooth management of the process, and to the Series Editor Marco Mostert for his encouragement, oversight, and swift work. Simon would particularly like to thank Mike for his guidance and advice from inception to completion of the volume, and Mike would similarly like to thank Simon for his invulnerable energy and enthusiasm.

Sensory Perception in the Medieval West: Introduction

SIMON C. THOMSON

It is many years since I first visited the Jorvik Viking Centre as a nine year old. It remains etched in my memory, not for archaeological discoveries or exciting facts learned about the Scandinavian kingdom at York – but for the smells that surrounded the snuffling plastic pigs. It has long been known that olfactory perception is more keenly associated with memory than other senses.[1] It is a truth so self-evident as to be clichéd that seeing, hearing, smelling, touching, and tasting enable us to engage with the world in ways different from one another and different again from intellectual engagement. And it is clear to the most casual of observers that the modern deodorised world is some distance removed from medieval experience; that a cleanly printed text is not the same as the ink marks on a unique piece of animal skin; that artefacts pinned beneath glass and bathed in halogen lighting are a world apart from objects handled and used by the light of fires or the sun. The chapters in this volume explore these two cruxes: how an audience's sensory perception could be exploited or piqued

[1] See e.g. R.S. HERZ, "A comparison of olfactory, visual and tactile cues for emotional and non-emotional associated memories", *Chemical Senses* 21 (1996), pp. 614-615, and much of Herz's work.

Sensory Perception in the Medieval West, ed. Simon C. THOMSON and Michael D.J. BINTLEY, *Utrecht Studies in Medieval Literacy*, 34 (Turnhout: Brepols, 2016), pp. 1-5.

BREPOLS PUBLISHERS DOI 10.1484/M.USML-EB.5.109501

by objects and experiences in the medieval world; how scholars can attempt to bridge the gap between present and past sensory engagements. Some chapters explore the underlying and more demanding question of how the medieval world understood sensory perception to function.

These broad areas of interest have become of increasing interest to students of different periods and disciplines over the past thirty years or so. The principle, *contra* Descartes' disembodied conscious mind, that human bodies form a key element in intellectual understanding, is an old one: even in the modern world it is embedded in the work of thinkers such as Heidegger and Merleau-Ponty,[2] and has formed a key element in understanding of human growth and development in work that builds most obviously on Piaget's identification, built upon by Vygotsky, of the interdependence between children's physical and mental capacities.[3] The basic principle of this interest in 'embodied cognition' is that

> [o]ur bodies and their perceptually guided motions through the world do much of the work required to achieve our goals, *replacing* the need for complex internal mental representations. This simple fact utterly changes our idea of what 'cognition' involves, and thus embodiment is not simply another factor acting on an otherwise disembodied cognitive processes [*sic*].[4]

Other well-known work has explored how this theory of perception as embodied can explain such fundamental ideas as linguistic structures and how we use figurative language.[5] And a forthcoming volume edited by Eleanor Betts could

[2] M. HEIDEGGER, *Sein und Zeit* (Halle a. S., 1927), English trans.: *Being and Time*, trans. J.M. MACQUARRIE and E. ROBINSON (Oxford, 1962); M. MERLEAU-PONTY, *Phénoménologie de la perception* (Paris, 1945), English trans.: *Phenomenology of Perception* (London and New York, 1962), e.g. p. 273; Cf. the general discussion in G. LAKOFF and M. JOHNSON, *Philosophy in the Flesh: The Embodied Mind and Its Challenge to Western Thought* (New York, 1999).

[3] J. PIAGET, *The Origins of Intelligence in Children* (New York, 1952); L. VYGOTSKY, *Interaction Between Learning and Development* (Cambridge, MA, 1978).

[4] A.D. WILSON and S. GOLONKA, "Embodied cognition is not what you think it is", *Frontiers in Psychology* 4.58 (2013), <http://journal.frontiersin.org/article/10.3389/fpsyg.2013.00058/full> (emphasis theirs) [accessed 23 July 2015]; Cf. A. BAILEY, "Consciousness and the embodied self", unpublished, available online <https://www.academia.edu/14194800/Consciousness_and_the_Embodied_Self> [accessed 25 July 2015].

[5] G. LAKOFF and M. JOHNSON, *Metaphors We Live By* (Chicago, 2003); *Grounding Cognition: The Role of Perception and Action in Memory, Language, and Thinking*, ed. D. PECHER and R.A. ZWAAN (Cambridge, 2005).

be read in parallel to this one, exploring as it does the value of applying a sensory approach to the archaeology of the ancient world.[6]

This movement away from perception as a purely mental process and engagement with individuals' sensory experiences of specific environments makes engaging with historical perception significantly more challenging than simpler descriptions of understanding or interpretation. This challenge perhaps explains why medieval scholarship has arrived at the party of sensory perception a little late in the day. Manuscript scholarship has, nonetheless, become increasingly interested in how medieval audiences and producers experienced their work. Benjamin Withers' major study of the Old English Hexateuch sought to see that document as "a material thing activated by the body" and to engage with the "sensory environment" that it creates.[7] Thomas Bredehoft has recently considered how the "visible text" functions, considering medieval manuscripts as graphic constructions fully engaged with the spaces and shapes they occupy and create.[8] Perhaps most significantly for this volume, Jonathan Wilcox edited a volume for the same series which sought to provide different scholars' "materially engaged readings of medieval manuscripts".[9] Collectively, this forms a part of what Michelle Brown has called "the New Materiality".[10] Where Malcolm Parkes challenges us to see "[t]hrough the eyes of scribes and readers",[11] this wider interest in sensory experience demands that we also smell with their noses, hear with their ears, taste with their mouths: experience, in other words, with their full bodies. Which in turn demands that our own bodies are fully engaged with the evidence we consider.

However, far from all of the chapters in this volume are focussed on the study of literature and it is perhaps inevitable that other material matters led the way in past discussions of how physical and sensory experiences are exploited

6 *Senses of Empire: Multisensory Approaches to Roman Culture*, ed. E. BETTS (Farnham, 2016).

7 B.C. WITHERS, *The Illustrated Old English Hexateuch, Cotton Claudius B. IV: The Frontier of Seeing and Reading in Anglo-Saxon England* (Toronto and London, 2007), p. 4.

8 T.A. BREDEHOFT, *The Visible Text: Textual Production and Reproduction from 'Beowulf' to 'Maus'* (Oxford, 2014).

9 *Scraped, Stroked, and Bound: Materially Engaged Readings of Medieval Manuscripts*, ed. J. WILCOX (Turnhout, 2013: *Utrecht Studies in Medieval Literacy* 23).

10 M.L. BROWN, "Mercian manuscripts: The implications of the Staffordshire Hoard, other recent discoveries, and the 'New Materiality'", in: *Writing in Context: Insular Manuscript Culture 500-1200*, ed. E. KWAKKEL (Leiden, 2013), pp. 23-64.

11 M.B. PARKES, *Their Hands Before Our Eyes: A Closer Look at Scribes: The Lyell Lectures Delivered in the University of Oxford 1999* (Aldershot, 2008), title to chapter 8, pp. 127-145.

or engaged with. As Nicholas Howe has suggested, art historians are often more engaged with the interactions of context and style.[12] Analyses of architecture and artwork have for some time considered the experience of viewers and users of spaces and objects as well as the appearance and design of the objects themselves.[13] Discussions of medieval dramatic performance have similarly long engaged with the contexts of performance and the impact on textual meaning of audiences' extra-textual and sensory experiences.[14]

Such variance in levels of understanding in different disciplines make an interdisciplinary volume doubly useful. Not only do the chapters in this book explore a wide range of aspects of a broad and challenging theme; they also use a wide range of methodologies to approach that theme. Approaches range from linguistic detective work to broad surveys of resources and their implications for our study; from acoustic technology to statistical analysis; from traditional considerations of texts, objects and contexts to close engagement with theoretical models. We hope, therefore, that these chapters contribute to ongoing considerations of both how meaning was made in the medieval world, and how we can seek to apprehend it.

The first two chapters together illustrate the double focus of the book. Richard North uses vocabulary in *The Seafarer* to disentangle how Anglo-Saxons constructed their own sensory perception in fractured and sometimes opposing elements, before Jonathan Wilcox raises the challenge of our own "bodily engagement with medieval sources". In some senses, Wilcox ends where North begins, inviting us to develop a language for sensory perception: a "philology of smell". Where Wilcox explores "the sensory cost of remediation" through digital technology, Mariana López employs technology to recover sensory experience, examining how the performance of the York Mystery Plays may have been designed to provide the richest possible aural experience. Aurality remains the focus in Eric Lacey's consideration of the significance of sound in the naming of birds in Old English, demonstrating the ele-

[12] N. HOWE, "What we talk about when we talk about style", in: *Anglo-Saxon Styles*, ed. C.E. KARKOV and G. HARDIN BROWN (New York, 2003), pp. 169-178, at p. 176.

[13] R. ARNHEIM, *Art and Visual Perception: A Psychology of the Creative Eye* (Berkeley, CA, 1954; rev. edn. 1974); J. BERGER, *Ways of Seeing* (London, 1972); *Reading Medieval Images: The Art Historian and the Object*, ed. E. SEARS and T.K. THOMAS (Ann Arbor, MI, 2002); J. HAWKES, "*Iuxta morem Romanorum:* Stone and sculpture in Anglo-Saxon England", in: *Anglo-Saxon Styles*, pp. 66-99.

[14] The literature on this subject is vast; for overviews, see J.W. HARRIS, *The Medieval Theatre in Context: An Introduction* (London, 1992), and J. STEYN, *The English Stage: A History of Drama and Performance* (Cambridge, 1996).

vated importance of hearing in Anglo-Saxon environmental perception. Simon Thomson argues that scribes of Old English poetry participated in this focus on sound, hearing the poems they copied and creatively reshaping them in the process. Victoria Symons goes on to demonstrate that sound and language were not solely significant in perception, but were deployed to define and shape the world in Old English riddles and charms. Francesca Brooks also explores Anglo-Saxon riddles, finding that the games played by two riddles with the sensory experiences of chalices could develop an audience's spiritual perception and draw closer to the larger world of liturgical performance. Like Symons and Brooks, Melissa Herman finds that patterning and playfulness have meaning beyond their aesthetic interest. Moving the attention of the volume onto sight, Herman argues that Anglo-Saxon metalwork uses its material and design to manipulate an audience's visual perception. Given this focus of medieval culture on the senses of hearing and sight, Patricia Skinner gives an important analysis of provisions made for those deprived of full sensory perception, including an exploration of cases of impairment and how they impacted upon the lives of those whose senses had been damaged.

The final three chapters broaden the focus to multiple forms of perception. Pete Sandberg returns us to North's consideration of how a text represents perception, analysing the sensory language used in *Sólarljóð* and the challenge implied by the language to the poem's project of presenting a disembodied mind. Meg Boulton argues that employing a phenomenological consideration of Anglo-Saxon structures and spaces enables comprehension of the distance between modern and medieval concepts of perception, and that spatial manipulation of sensory experience could shift understanding beyond the human and towards the divine. Finally, Michael Bintley maintains this movement beyond the human, exploring the sensory world of trees as represented by the *Poetic Edda* and demonstrating the sophistication of thinking about and use of sensory perception in the medieval world.

Heaven Ahoy! Sensory Perception in *The Seafarer*

RICHARD NORTH

In 1806, less than a year after Admiral Nelson's death at Trafalgar, a poster was printed in High Holborn, London, with words which it attributed to him and Admirals Duncan and Howe: 'Britons! Fear GOD, Fear SIN, And Then Fear Nothing!'[1] It does not seem too wild to say that *The Seafarer*, though some years older, proceeds in the same way.[2] To most readers it is clear that the seafaring persona of the poet of this work slowly stokes up a landlubber's fear of voyaging at sea, of being surprised and swallowed by the same dark immensity, in order to suggest a more general and non-maritime fear of dying. Gradually, however, he removes this fear by substituting one more pro-

[1] R. BLAKE, *Evangelicals in the Royal Navy, 1775-1815: Blue Lights and Psalm-Singers* (Woodbridge, 2008), pp. 151-152.

[2] Text of *The Seafarer* based on *A Guide to Old English*, ed. B. MITCHELL and F.C. ROBINSON, 6th edn. (Oxford, 2001), pp. 276-282. See also: *The Seafarer*, ed. I.L. GORDON (London, 1960); A.L. KLINCK, *The Old English Elegies: A Critical Edition and Genre Study* (Montreal and Kingston, 1992). Other OE poems, unless otherwise attributed, are drawn from *The Anglo-Saxon Poetic Records*, ed. G.P. KRAPP and E.V.K. DOBBIE, 6 vols. (New York, 1931-1953). In all OE text I mark long vowels.

Sensory Perception in the Medieval West, ed. Simon C. THOMSON and Michael D.J. BINTLEY, *Utrecht Studies in Medieval Literacy*, 34 (Turnhout: Brepols, 2016), pp. 7-26.

BREPOLS PUBLISHERS DOI 10.1484/M.USML-EB.5.109502

ductive: the terror of sinning against God. Enabling this substitution to take place is the Seafarer's intuition of heaven, which comes about through sensory perception. Let us see how this works.

The Fearful Landlubber

Although *The Seafarer* ends like many others less nautical in the Old English canon, by enjoining the good Christian life, its method, to persuade us to replace the fear of dying with one of God, appears less common. The poet works his persuasion through sustained descriptive passages on the toil, hardship and cares of seafaring, four times breaking off for comparison with a landlubber who lives in blissful ignorance (lines 12-17, 27-30, 39-46 and 55-57). By developing this contrast the speaker slowly introduces the element of fear: not in himself, but in members of his audience. In his own case, he bewails the cold and danger of seafaring and then reveals that he plans to sail to "*elþēodigra eard*" ("a homeland of foreigners", line 37). This plan has been read as a *volte face*, even as proof that *The Seafarer* is truly a dialogue with a young sailor now taking over.[3] Not helping our prosaic confusion are the poem's six *forþon* conjunctions, of which the most recent consensus advocates "indeed" as with Latin *autem* or *vero*: a looser rendering than "and so" or "and yet".[4] By now in the poem, in any case, it is clear that there is no contradiction. The old Seafarer is so in love with the ocean that he has become an ascetic. Only by embracing the terrors of a life on the deep does he begin to feel the prospect of heaven. Indeed, in the exact middle of the poem, with a strange image of his mind as a bird, a yelling "*ānfloga*" ("lone flier", line 62), the Seafarer tells us to look for heaven over the horizon. His following sermon

[3] M. RIEGER, "Der *Seefahrer* als Dialog hergestellt", *Zeitschrift für deutsche Philologie* 1 (1869), pp. 330-339; J.C. POPE, "Dramatic voices in *The Wanderer* and *The Seafarer*", in: *Franciplegius: Medieval and Linguistic Studies in Honor of Francis Peabody Magoun, Jr.*, ed. J.B. BESSINGER and S.J. KAHRL (Hamden, CT, 1968), pp. 533-570 (speeches in lines 133a and 33b-102 and then an epilogue in lines 103-124). Pope changed his mind: J.C. POPE, "Second thoughts on the interpretation of *The Seafarer*", *Anglo-Saxon England* 3 (1974), pp. 75-86.

[4] Lines 33, 39, 58, 64, 72, 108. *Seafarer*, ed. MITCHELL and ROBINSON, p. 278 (note to line 27). B. MITCHELL, *Old English Syntax*, 2 vols., 1, *Concord, the Parts of Speech, and the Sentence*, 2, *Subordination, Independent Elements, and Element Order* (New York and Oxford, 1985), §§ 3081-3084; KLINCK, *Old English Elegies*, p. 130; S.L. HIGLEY, *Between Languages: The Uncooperative Text in Early Welsh and Old English Nature Poetry* (Philadelphia, PA, 1993), pp. 39-45.

confirms the possibility of any man's place there by urging good works against the devil, whereby the good life with men, women and wealth is converted into a better one with angels in heaven. At this point not only the human body but also the world as a whole is revealed to be in terminal decline. Bereavement is considered as but a heartbeat before the survivor's own demise, whereby his, our, flesh becomes insensate, inoperable and mindless. Beyond that, says the Seafarer, no man can buy entry into an afterlife, either for his brother or himself. It has been suggested that his quasi-heathen image of a brother depositing gold in a grave (lines 97-102), renders Psalm 48: 8-9 of the Vulgate:[5]

> 8. *Frater non redimit, redimet homo:*
> *Non dabit Deo placationem suam,*
> 9. *Et pretium redemptionis animae suae,*
> *Et laborabit in aeternum.*[6]

> 8. A brother does not pay ransom, let the man pay ransom:
> He will not give God satisfaction for himself,
> 9. Nor the price of the ransom of his soul,
> And he will toil [for this] into eternity.

Thus it is shown that gold, unless donated before death, will not help a sinner against that bigger *post mortem* dread which only God can inspire. Towards the end of *The Seafarer*, the speaker dwells on the proper fear of God, on the grace which comes with this, on His love and on the resulting stability of the old ascetic's mind as he nears his end. Fate in the long run is said to be stronger than any of the friendly or hostile ties that bind (lines 111-116). All that remains for us, says the speaker in the final exegesis of his seafaring (in lines 117-124), is to set course for our true home, thanking God for giving us the chance to live there.

In the beginning, because the Seafarer presents himself as sailing in winter "*wræccan lāstum*" ("on an exile's tracks", line 15), some readers believe that his desired voyage is *peregrinatio pro amore Dei* ('a pilgrimage for the love of God'). Whether literal or symbolic, this type of figure would refer to St Augus-

[5] K. SISAM, "*The Seafarer* lines 97-102", *Review of English Studies* 21 (1945), pp. 316-317. For the recommended giving of alms as the meaning here: J.F. VICKREY, "'The Seafarer' 97-102: 'Dives' and the burial of treasure", *Journal of English and Germanic Philology* 94 (1995), pp. 19-30, esp. p. 27.

[6] *Biblia Sacra iuxta Vulgatam Clementinam*, ed. A. COLUNGA and L. TURRADO, 9th edn. (Madrid, 1985), p. 491 (Ps 48 (49): 8-9).

tine's post-imperial doctrine of man in exile from heaven, his true home.[7] The fact that the Seafarer's imagined voyaging does not end in the promised landfall has not escaped notice, but is treated as proof that he does not advocate pilgrimage to a fixed destination in the literal sense of the word. It has even been suggested that the Seafarer is a fisherman who dislikes the sea, his poem a bricolage of earlier works.[8] As real as the voyages here appear to be, however, some idea of pilgrimage is necessary. Whether the Seafarer is like St Brendan in the Atlantic or Alcuin on a crossing to the Rhine, he has a destination in mind and this is his old home in heaven. He leaves his worldly one behind him, asking his audience to do likewise.

That the speaker interacts with audiences inside as well as outside *The Seafarer*, despite the lonely modern title, appears in the word "*sōðgied*" ("true tale", "parable") right in the first line. When the speaker says that he can "*be mē sylfum sōðgied wrecan*" ("deliver a parable about myself"), he might encourage a comparison with *Vainglory*, copied right after in the Exeter Book, in which "*wlonce wīgsmiþas winburgum in / sittaþ æt symble, sōðgied wrecað*" ("arrogant war-smiths in wine-towns, who sit at the banquet, deliver parables", or "tell true tales", lines 14-15) apparently with the aim of starting trouble.[9] There is no other instance of OE *sōðgied*. The ministry meaning 'parable' may seem at odds with the noisy hall milieu, but it is supported by the terms "*soðcuido ł giedd*" and "*soðcwide ł ged*", which are respectively Lindisfarne and Rushworth glosses for "*proverbium*" ("parable") in John 10:6.[10] The Seafarer's opening context is thus communal; with his first reference to the landlubber, he returns to this: "*Þæt se mon ne wat / þe him on foldan fægrost limpeð*" ("That man does not know, whose lot is the fairest on land", lines 12-13) with what wretched cares the Seafarer has spent his exile. The next social context is more provocative: "*Forþon him gelȳfeð lȳt, se þe āh līfes wyn / gebiden in burgum*" ("Indeed he little believes, he who has experienced life's

[7] D. WHITELOCK, "The interpretation of *The Seafarer*", in: *The Early Cultures of Northwest Europe*, ed. C. FOX and B. DICKINS (Cambridge, 1950), pp. 442-457; G.V. SMITHERS, "The meaning of *The Seafarer* and *The Wanderer*", *Medium Ævum* 26 (1957), pp. 137-153, esp. pp. 147-151. Qualified in: *Seafarer*, ed. GORDON, pp. 4-7; and KLINCK, *Old English Elegies*, p. 137.

[8] S.I. SOBIESKI, "The interpretation of *The Seafarer*: A re-examination of the pilgrimage theory", *Neophilologus* 92 (2008), pp. 127-139, esp. pp. 130, 137-138.

[9] *Longman Anthology of Old English, Old Icelandic and Anglo-Norman Literatures*, ed. and trans. R. NORTH and J. ALLARD, with P. GILLIES (Harlow, 2011), pp. 196-202, esp. p. 198.

[10] *The Four Gospels in Anglo-Saxon, Northumbrian, and Old Mercian Versions*, ed. W.W. SKEAT, 2 vols. (Cambridge, 1871-1887), 2, p. 97. *Biblia Sacra*, ed. COLUNGA and TURRADO, p. 1053.

joy in the towns", lines 27-28). So it follows from his ignorance that the landlubber, who is also "*wlonc and wīngāl*" ("arrogant and wine-flushed" or even "licentious with wine", line 29), does not believe what the Seafarer told him about weariness and seabirds as his viable alternative to communal joy and drinking. That not the generalising present, but the specific past tense is then used to tell of hail in a shore-bound winter, in the following two and a half lines (31-33a), is probably meant to give the speaker as an ancient mariner who has been rejected or even ejected by the people in the hall.

The speaker's third allusion to landlubberly proceeding deserves quoting in full. First, in riposte to the wintry sterility of the previous shore-leave situation, the Seafarer declares his desire to seek the land of foreigners. Then:

Forþon nis þæs mōdwlonc mon ofer eorþan,
ne his gifena þæs gōd, ne in geoguþe tō þæs hwæt,
ne in his dǣdum tō þæs dēor, ne him his dryhten tō þæs hold,
þæt hē ā his sǣfōre sorge næbbe,
tō hwon hine dryhten gedōn wille.
Ne biþ him tō hearpan hyge ne tō hringþege,
ne tō wīfe wyn ne tō worulde hyht,
ne ymbe ōwiht elles, nefne ymb ȳða gewealc,
ac ā hafað longunge se þe on lagu fundað. (lines 39-47)

Indeed there is no man across the earth so proud in mind,
nor so well-endowed in gifts, nor so sharp in his youth,
nor so daring in his deeds, nor his lord so loyal to him
that he may never have anxiety on his sea-journey
about what the Lord will do with him.
He has no mind for lyre nor for receiving rings,
no joy in woman either, nor use for the world
or for any other thing but the rolling of the waves,
but ever has he longing who hastens on the flood.

Despite the fact that the subject here has been treated as the Seafarer himself, there is enough descriptive detail to show that it is none but the landlubber, right until his contrast with the Seafarer at the end.[11] If this man was ever a

[11] For the Seafarer: *Seafarer*, ed. GORDON, p. 39; *Seafarer*, ed. MITCHELL and ROBINSON, p. 279; KLINCK, *Old English Elegies*, p. 134. For the landlubber: A *Choice of Anglo-Saxon Verse*, ed. and trans. R. HAMER (London, 1970), p. 189; R.F. LESLIE, "The meaning and structure of *The Seafarer*", in: *The Old English Elegies: New Essays in Criticism and Research*, ed. M. GREEN

seafarer, it was all too long ago. With "*ofer eorþan*" ("across the earth"), on the other hand, the "*mon*" ("man") is typified for three lines as the most successful landsman of his time who one day finds himself required to go to sea. The word "*sorge*" ("sorrow", line 42) appears in the poem for the first time here, despite the many trials reported earlier. The Seafarer calls these trials "*geswinc-*" ("toil", line 2), "*earfoð-*" ("hardship", line 3), "*ceare*" ("cares", lines 4, 5, 10), "*hungor*" ("hunger", line 11): sufferings on a practical level. OE *sorge*, however, runs deeper, as it does with the cuckoo's foreboding on line 54.

The terse line with "*dryhten gedōn*" halfway through this passage has likewise been regarded practically, as an expression for the Seafarer's worry about what his "earthly lord" might be willing to "do for him" in return for his services.[12] However, the *dryhten* in question is probably God. Fred Robinson translates a nearly identical line differently in *The Rewards of Piety*, where, to italicise within his translation of the larger sentence, he renders "*tō hwan þē þīn drihten gedōn wille*" (line 61) as "It is unknown to you / *at what point your Lord may wish to determine / for you* when you may no longer enjoy life".[13] Consequently it is likely that the line with *gedōn* in *The Seafarer* also refers to God and what He will "determine for" or "do with"[14] the landsman at sea. Giving every wave his full attention, the landlubber seems too much out of his element to think of entertainment, money, women and the world. The *ac*-conjunction on line 47 makes a bold contrast between the landlubber's grief about drowning, implied in "*sorge*", and the "*longunge*" ("longing") of the Seafarer when this ascetic has the wind in his sails.

In his fourth social digression, having told us of spring and how it urges a man to sail, and then of the cuckoo whose singing bodes biting sorrows, the Seafarer returns to ignorance as the hallmark of the man on land. It is worth noting that he returns to the construction on lines 12-13 with which he began his comparisons:

(Toronto, 1983), pp. 96-122, esp. pp. 103-104.

[12] *Seafarer*, ed. MITCHELL and ROBINSON, p. 279 (note to lines 41-43).

[13] F.C. ROBINSON, "'The rewards of piety': Two Old English poems in their manuscript context", in: *The Editing of Old English*, ed. F.C. ROBINSON (Oxford and Cambridge, MA, 1994), pp. 180-195, esp. p. 191. Noted in P.R. ORTON, "The form and structure of *The Seafarer*", *Studia Neophilologica* 63 (1991), pp. 37-55, esp. p. 44.

[14] KLINCK, *Old English Elegies*, p. 134.

Þæt se beorn ne wāt,
eft ēadig secg, hwæt þā sume drēogað
þe þā wræclāstas wīdost lecgað. (lines 55b-57)

That trooper does not know,
the fellow wealthy in later years, what those few men experience
who lay those tracks of exile furthest out.

The phrase "*eft ēadig*", though it has been emended to make "*ēstēadig*" ("wealthy in favour") or "*sēftēadig*" ("comfort-blessed"), has enough alliterative and semantic viability as it is.[15]Contrasted here with the wake of a ship on the world's edge, it is also found in *The Fortunes of Men*, of a man who with God's help shall on "*yldo eft ēadig weorþan*" ("become wealthy later in old age", line 60). As a formula, it shows the rich landlubber of *The Seafarer* to be old and beyond help, identifiable with the aged survivor who puts gold in his brother's grave (lines 91-99). In the short passage above, by contrast, the old sailor alludes to himself and now others as well as a privileged few, party to a mystical experience on the outer limits. And so he begins to persuade his audience. Although the experience is hardly communicable in words alone, the poet seeks to tell us of the cause of his longing by means of the "*ānfloga*" halfway through. To fathom the intuition on which his bird-image is founded, let us now look at his language of sensory perception.

Flying Aim and Mood-Sense

The Seafarer begins by relating what has happened to him. In contrast with the "*ānhaga*" ("lone dweller") who stirs the sea with (an oar under) his hands in *The Wanderer* (line 1), this able bodied seaman gives himself as the object of sufferings mostly in the passive voice. He has endured days of toil, times of hardship, biting breast-cares (lines 2-4), while many times the ship's sides have been a shelter from the care of "*atol þa gewealc*" ("the terrible rolling of waves", line 6). There the ship's nightwatch "*mec oft bigeat*" ("has often got me", line 6) as she pitches by the cliffs. Gradually he reveals his suffering body and then mind: his feet crushed with freezing shackles, the cares that "*seofedun*" ("sighed", or perhaps "whistled" from Latin *sifilare*) hot about his heart

[15] A. Bammesberger, "Old English *eft eadig secg* (*The Seafarer* line 56a)", *Notes & Queries* 61 (2014), pp. 181-182.

(lines 10-11), and the hunger from within that "*slāt / merewērges mōd*" ("tore at the mind of the sea-wearied man", lines 11-12). The word *mōd*, etymon of MnE 'mood', also shares some of the latter's meaning, although, in the mind-self duality of the OE poetic conception of mind, this word is best defined as an inner wilfulness, which sometimes controls the self and which at other times the self must control. With some 2,700 occurrences in prose as well as verse, OE *mōd* is the commonest OE term for 'mind', and in *The Seafarer* it suffers hunger, the most extreme privation.[16]

The speaker, claiming to have found nothing but ignorance on shore, defines himself as an exiled mariner without friends or family and covered with icicles in a storm. His auditory sense becomes alive: "*Þǣr ic ne gehȳrde būtan hlimman sǣ, / īscealdne wǣg*" ("There I heard nothing but sea resound, the ice-cold wave", lines 18-19). The murmuring onomatopoeia of "*hlimman*" gives us a potentially hypnotic aspect to the sea by which the speaker zones himself out. Rather as *The Wanderer*'s exiled *ānhaga*, who is said there to see "*brimfuglas*" ("ocean birds") bathing and ruffling wings on the wintry seas (line 47), he studies sea-birds. On the other hand, *The Seafarer* far exceeds the generality of *The Wanderer* through its birds' names ("*ylfete*", "*ganet*", "*huilpe*", "*mǣw*", "*stearn*", "*earn*") and their number. As Eric Lacey has shown, it "uses aurality to capture experiences of them".[17] The interaction of these birds with the Seafarer is made consistent with their properties. Respectively these are: wingbeats, honking, laughing for singing, and entertainment and laughter ("mute swan", "gannet", "curlew / whimbrel", lines 19-21); wailing in place of mead and conversation ("seagull", "little gull", lines 22-23); and the yelling of a dewy figure which presides ("white-tailed eagle", lines 24-25).[18] The question is not how much the Seafarer bemoans all this feathered wildlife as a poor substitute for hall-joys, but how soon he comes to regard it as superior.[19] His

[16] M.J. PHILLIPS, *Heart, Mind and Soul in Old English: A Semantic Study* (unpublished doctoral thesis, University of Illinois at Urbana-Champaign, 1985), p. 96; cf. pp. 172-232 and 293. M. GODDEN, "Anglo-Saxons on the mind", in: *Learning and Literature in Anglo-Saxon England: Studies Presented to Peter Clemoes on the Occasion of his Sixty-Fifth Birthday*, ed. M. LAPIDGE and H. GNEUSS (Cambridge, 1985), pp. 271-298, esp. p. 292: "an inner self or consciousness which the conscious self cannot penetrate". See also S.-A. LOW, "Pride, courage, and anger: The polysemousness of Old English *mod*", in: *Verbal Encounters: Anglo-Saxon and Old Norse Studies for Roberta Frank*, ed. A. HARBUS and R. POOLE (Toronto, 2005), pp. 81-88.

[17] E.M. LACEY, *Birds and Birdlore in the Literature of Anglo-Saxon England* (unpublished doctoral thesis, University College London, 2014), p. 84.

[18] LACEY, *Birds and Birdlore*, pp. 84-97.

[19] The birds are regarded as "pathetically inadequate substitutes" in ORTON, "Form and

Coleridgean second digression, on the incredulous wine-bibber in lines 27-30, calls these times "*bealosīþa*" ("journeys of horror", line 28), but the Seafarer also implies that if not one of his kinsmen is there to console him for all the loneliness (lines 25-26), the eagle and his party are welcome to take their place.

These birds show that the Seafarer's suffering has put him into another world, some time before the moment where some have seen a *volte face*. The man's decision to sail is revealed in a picture of interacting mental functions:[20]

Forþon cnyssað nū
heortan geþōhtas   þæt ic hēan strēamas,
sealtȳða gelāc   sylf cunnige;
monað mōdes lust   mǣla gehwylce
ferð tō fēran,   þæt ic feor heonan
elþēodigra   eard gesēce. (lines 33b-38)

Indeed now the thoughts
dash against the heart that I should try
the high currents, the salt-waves' play for myself;
fancy of the mood each moment urges
temperament to sail, that far from here
I may seek the homeland of foreigners.

Tending towards the waves, his "*geþōhtas*" become the waves; his "*heorte*", the ship's sides. Far from rejecting this world, the Seafarer has identified himself with it. His mind appears to work as follows: in response to the thoughts, his "*mōd*", the emotional will, creates a "*lust*" in order to goad the "*fer(h)ð*", his latent life force, into bringing the "*sylf*", his whole person, to the foreign land.[21] Whether this destination is meant to be heaven or northern Germany (some would see no difference), the Seafarer foregrounds his "mood" as the operative element. That the senses have not been cited is perhaps because they inspired the "*geþōhtas*".

structure of *The Seafarer*", p. 40.

[20] See A. Harbus, *The Life of the Mind in Old English Poetry* (Amsterdam, 2002), p. 187.

[21] For *fer(h)ð*, as a peripheral "non-transcendental soul-term" which takes over some functions of *feorh* ('life-force'), see: Phillips, "Heart, mind and soul", pp. 64-81 and 292-293; L. Lockett, *Anglo-Saxon Psychologies in the Vernacular and Latin Traditions* (Toronto, 2011), pp. 51-53. For the opening metaphor: A. Harbus, *Cognitive Approaches to Old English Poetry* (Cambridge, 2012), p. 44.

After the digression in which the landlubber's fear of dying is exposed (lines 39-47), the Seafarer creates a breath-taking image of spring, blossoming towns and plains, and the world hastening on (lines 48-49). This combined stimulus to a man's departure involves sensory perception on a deeper level of *mōd*:

> *Ealle þā gemoniað mōdes fūsne*
> *sefan tō sīþe þām þe swā þenceð*
> *on flōdwegas feor gewītan.* (lines 50-52)

> All these things urge the mood's keen
> feeling to a journey in him who thus thinks
> on flood-ways to move out far.

The interpretation of this passage has been vexed by the poet's apparent shift between lines, from a man implicit in "*fūsne*" to the "*sefan*" which is part of him, both objects of the verb of encouragement.[22] Technically, however, "*sefan*" goes with "*fūsne*".[23] Hereby the first line runs on in a way which links "*sefan*" with "*mōdes*" before: "the mood's keen feeling". A collocation "*mōdes sefa*" is unusual, with no more than one parallel, in a sentence from an English rubric to a Latin ritual of *c.* 1061: "*Ǣrest þinga ðū mōst þā digelnysse ðīnes mōdes sefan ðurh sōþe andetnisse geyppan and unðēawa geswicennysse behātan*" ("First business is that you must bring to light the hiddenness of your mind's feeling through true confession, and promise cessation of vices").[24] However, this collocation recalls the popular poetic compound *mōdsefa* which denotes the 'mind' some 46 times (with a similarly useful cognate in Old Saxon *môdseƀo*).[25] If the Seafarer's "*mōdes sefa*" stands for *mōdsefa*, he reanimates this compound in such a way as to spell out the inner workings of perception.

[22] *Seafarer*, ed. MITCHELL, pp. 279-280: "'urge (the one) eager of spirit, (urge) the mind to the journey by which (he [*mōdes fūs*]) (*or* it [*sefa*]) thus thinks to travel far on the ocean ways'" (notes to lines 50-51).

[23] KLINCK, *Old English Elegies*, p. 136: "Heart eager of mind".

[24] Lengths marked for text from MS Cambridge, Corpus Christi College 422, in: B. FEHR, "Altenglische Ritualtexte für Krankenbesuch, heilige Ölung und Begräbnis", in *Texte und Forschungen zur englischen Kulturgeschichte: Festgabe für Felix Liebermann,* ed. H. BOEHMER *et al.* (Halle a. S., 1921), pp. 20-67, esp. p. 50 (translation mine).

[25] R. NORTH, *Pagan Words and Christian Meanings* (Amsterdam and Atlanta, GA, 1991), pp. 72-5.

Simplex OE *sefa*, which is cognate with Latin *sapere* ('to taste, know'), is an archaic word with 93 instances in verse as against only six in prose.[26] The remaining 14 cases of *sefa* all gloss Latin *sensus* ('sense'), as in the Arundel Psalter: "*āsend on mē sefan 7 andgyt*" for "*mitte in me sensum. & intellegentiam*" ("send into me sense and intelligence"); or, with more emphasis, "*syle mē heortan sēo þē ondrǣde sefan se þē ongyte ēagan þā þē geseōn ēaran þā þē gehȳran*", for "*da mihi cor quod te timeat, sensum qui te intellegat, oculos qui te videant, aures quę te audiant*" ("give me a heart to fear you, a sense to perceive you, eyes to see you, ears to hear you").[27] OE *sefa* often plays in conjunction with the other mental terms, such as the faculties *fer(h)ð* ('temperament') and *hyge* ('inclination'), as well as the organs *heorte* and *hreðer* ('insides', 'gut') which sometimes denote the mind metonymously.[28] Less common is *myne* ('impulse', 'desire', 'love'), which, unlike *hyge*, can take an infinitive and so appears more impulsive.[29] The derivative of *myne* is *gemynd* ('memory'), for English historically the most important word of all. In short, there are so many terms that a need for variety in translation is rather obvious: repeating 'mind' will not do. Although Michael Phillips, in his discussion of most of these terms, has shown many subtle patterns of individual use, with verbal collocations giving particular roles, a strange belief persists that *hyge*, *sefa*, *mōd* and *fer(h)ð* are used nearly interchangeably and can all be translated as 'mind', and that if they have any separate functions, these do not matter.[30]

The test case arises at the heart of *The Seafarer*, in lines 58-64, where the speaker declares a present-time intuition of heaven. He has already given the "*gēac*" ("cuckoo", line 53) as a new bird in the poem (his seventh), the "*sumeres weard*" ("summer's sentinel", line 54) boding sorrow to all men who fall back on easy living. The speaker has further entered into his fourth digres-

[26] PHILLIPS, "Heart, mind and soul", p. 43; S.E. FLOWERS, "Toward an ancient Germanic psychology", *Journal of Indo-European Studies* 11 (1983), pp. 117-138, esp. p. 129: "a sentient aspect of the psychic complex".

[27] D. KUHN, *Der lateinisch-altenglische* libellus precum *in der Handschrift London, British Library, Arundel 155* (Frankfurt a. M., 2014: *Münchener Universitätsschriften: Texte und Untersuchungen zur Englischen Philologie* 41), pp. 217 (VI.2-3), 239 (XVII.11-12); cf. p. 228 (XII.38-40).

[28] PHILLIPS, "Heart, mind and soul", pp. 51-62. On the *Second Lorsch Riddle* (*c.* 800), for which *heorte* may be the solution, see LOCKETT, *Anglo-Saxon Psychologies*, pp. 275-279.

[29] PHILLIPS, "Heart, mind and soul", p. 31.

[30] GODDEN, "Anglo-Saxons on the mind", p. 289. S.-A. LOW, *The Anglo-Saxon Mind: Metaphor and Common Sense Psychology in Old English Literature* (unpublished doctoral thesis, University of Toronto, 1988), p. 20; LOCKETT, *Anglo-Saxon Psychologies*, p. 34 and n. 38; PHILLIPS, "Heart, mind and soul"; NORTH, *Pagan Words*, pp. 63-98.

sion on the landlubber's ignorance (lines 55-57): such men have no idea of what it is to be in exile on the high seas. Now at last the Seafarer tells us about himself. His perception becomes transcendental:

Forþon nū mīn hyge hweorfeð   ofer hreþerlocan,
mīn mōdsefa   mid mereflōde
ofer hwæles ēþel   hweorfeð wīde,
eorþan scēatas,   cymeð eft tō mē
gīfre ond grǣdig;   gielleð ānfloga,
hweteð on <h>wælweg   hreþer unwearnum
ofer holma gelagu.   Forþon mē hātran sind
dryhtnes drēamas   þonne þis dēade līf,
lǣne on londe;   ic gelȳfe nō
þæt him eorðwelan   ēce stondað. (lines 58-65)

So now my aim moves beyond breast-locker,
my mood-sense with the sea's flood,
over whale's domain moves widely,
over earth's surfaces, comes back to me
ravening and greedy; the lone flier yells,
incites the breast to the whale-path irresistibly,
over waters of oceans. For more hot to me
are the Lord's nirvanas than this dead life,
lent to us on land; believe will I never
that earthly riches stand eternally there.

The power of this passage lies in its suggestion. Other than Smithers' unpersuasive attempt to leave "*wælweg*" unemended in line 63, as "way to the abode of the dead", there is no proof that heaven is what the "lone flier" has seen.[31] In comparison with the technicolour lines 859-891 of *Andreas*, in which St Andrew's disciples tell him their dream vision of kingdom come, heaven in *The Seafarer* seems a long way away. But perhaps that is the point. This passage from *The Seafarer* is more powerful for being so oblique. The imagery prevails over narrative, as the comparison with *Andreas* shows, while a theological argument, such as that promoted by the Alcuinian advocates of the unitary *anima* ('soul') for *hyge* and *mōdsefa* here, is equally hard to find.[32] The

[31] G.V. SMITHERS, "The meaning of *The Seafarer* and *The Wanderer*", *Medium Ævum* 28 (1959), pp. 1-22, 99-104, esp. p. 20.

[32] P.A.M. CLEMOES, "*Mens absentia cogitans* in *The Seafarer* and *The Wanderer*", in:

two *forþon*-conjunctions may be correlative, even if the prosaic renderings "for this reason" ... "because" look unwieldy for the looser verse syntax.[33]The causal meaning is that because the Seafarer feels that a life with God is the only one worth living, his senses fly out of him to acquire it.

Guiding the Seafarer's *mōdsefa* on this journey is his *hyge*, a word which occurs 139 times and mostly in verse. *Hyge* has been taken to connote a "longing (...) which results in action" and also to be the agent of cognitive function.[34] Although there are no reliable glosses, the phrase "*beheldende mid hyge*", which renders Latin "*intendentes*" ("intending") in the *Paris Psalter* (129:2), shows that *hyge* means "purpose" or "aim".[35] Its collocation with *mōdsefa* is relatively rare: *hyge* is more often collocated with simplex *mōd* or *sefa* or *heorte*. In collocation, however, *hyge* is always put before *mōdsefa*, as *hugi* is before *môdsebo* three times in the Old Saxon *Heliand*.[36] When St Guthlac's servant is sorrowful, he carries "*hyge geomurne, / mēðne mōdsefan*" ("lamenting purpose, a weary feeling of mind", *Guthlac* (B), lines 1336b-7a). The speaker of *Homiletic Fragment II* commands "*heald hordlocan, hyge fæste bind / mid mōdsefan*" ("keep shut the hoard-locker, bind fast the purpose with presence of mind", lines 3-4a). In overweening Belshazzar, "*wearð him hȳrra hyge and on heortan geðanc / māra <on> mōdsefan þonne gemet wǣre*" ("resolve became higher and thought in heart, [in] sense of mind, bigger than would be fitting", *Daniel*, lines 490-491).

In the above *ānfloga* passage, the speaker's *hyge-mōdsefa* collocation reveals his "aim" and "mood's sense" in that order. The Seafarer's *hyge* leads and his sensory *mōdsefa* follows, but with the same verb *hweorfeð*, in lines 58 and 60, these elements blend into one entity. This is shown when the verb of

Medieval Literature and Civilization: Studies in Memory of G.N. Garmonsway, ed. D.A. Pearsall and R.A. Waldron (London, 1969), pp. 62-77, esp. pp. 69-73; F.N.M. Diekstra, "*The Seafarer* 58-66a: The flight of the exiled soul to its fatherland", *Neophilologus* 55 (1971), pp. 433-446, esp. p. 443. Modified in N. Hultin, "The external soul in 'The Seafarer' and 'The Wanderer'", *Folklore* 88 (1977), pp. 39-45, esp. p. 41.

[33] *Seafarer*, ed. Mitchell and Robinson, p. 280 (note to l. 58). Mitchell, *Old English Syntax*, § 1174.

[34] Phillips, "Heart, mind and soul", pp. 23-40, esp. p. 30. North, *Pagan Words*, pp. 84-88, esp. p. 85. Flowers, "Germanic psychology", p. 131: "functioned as the seat of the various cognitive aspects from an extremely early time".

[35] *The Paris Psalter and the Meters of Boethius*, ed. in: *Anglo-Saxon Poetic Records* 5, G.P. Krapp (New York and London, 1932), p. 125. *Biblia Sacra*, ed. Colunga and Turrado, p. 568 (Ps 129 (130)).

[36] North, *Pagan Words*, pp. 73-75. With *hugi-môdsebo*, used of mass mentality, at *Heliand*, lines 2765-2766, 2923-2924, 5241-5242.

their return, *cymeð*, is given in the singular, and here the *mōdsefa* is suddenly dominant. With this word it is the speaker's sensory perception which comes back "*gīfre ond grǣdig*" ("ravening and greedy"). His flying "mood-sense" is now like a bird of prey, and there is no better identification for the shrieking "*ānfloga*" ("lone flier", line 62) which immediately follows. Some have called this bird the cuckoo, which bodes sorrow about the passing of summer not long before in lines 53-55.[37] But the cuckoo lacks the ferocity, either of this bird or of the poem's first six.[38] The *ānfloga* defies more precise identification. Most likely it is meant to come in the high black shape of a predator. The woodland cuckoo, in comparison, is in *ubi sunt*-mourning for transience; as a changeling, he is also likely to be an expression for the human soul, in exile from heaven and born into a world where it does not belong; but he is not a bird of prey.[39]

Elsewhere I have argued that the *ānfloga* and his cries are intended to convey the message of heaven through an image of augury.[40] This cannot be the lone flier's only function, however. Although the mind's ravening cries show it to resemble a bird expecting a meal in exchange for information, they also recall the Seafarer's "*hungor*" early into the poem (line 11). By this token his physical privations have transformed into hunger of a violent spiritual kind. For this transformation no explanation seems better than that his senses transcend the body in order to feel the prospect of heaven. It follows that the material *mōdsefa*, when it returns, cannot get enough of this feeling and wants the whole person, the soul, to fly back there.

These most mystical lines of *The Seafarer* are probably based on a passage on the divine and human mind by Lactantius, which Leslie Lockett has confirmed to be their most plausible source.[41] To quote the words in *De opificio Dei* (*On the Workings of God*, *c*. 304), which the poet appears to have internalised:[42]

[37] *Die altenglische Elegie*, ed. and trans. E. SIEPER (Strasbourg, 1915), p. 277; *Seafarer*, ed. GORDON, pp. 41-42 (note to l. 62b); P.R. ORTON, "*The Seafarer* 58-64a", *Neophilologus* 66 (1983), pp. 450-459, esp. p. 451.

[38] LACEY, *Birds and Bird-Lore*, pp. 97-100.

[39] J.E. CROSS, "*Ubi sunt* passages in Old English – Sources and relationships", *Vetenskaps-Societetens i Lund Årsbok* (Lund, 1956), pp. 25-44.

[40] NORTH, *Pagan Words*, pp. 99-121. On augury, see further LACEY, *Birds and Bird-Lore*.

[41] LOCKETT, *Anglo-Saxon Psychologies*, pp. 213-227, esp. pp. 223-224, and pp. 290-298, 424-425.

[42] LOCKETT, *Anglo-Saxon Psychologies*, pp. 291-292.

> *Nec etiam aliquis potest satis admirari, quod sensus ille uiuus atque caelestis, qui mens uel animus nuncupatur, tantae mobilitatis est ut ne tum quidem, cum sopitus est, conquiescat: tantae celeritatis ut uno temporis puncto coelum collustret, et si uelit, maria peruolet, terras et urbes peragret: omnia denique, quae libuerit, quamuis longe lateque submota sint, in conspectu sibi ipse cogitando constituat.* (16.9)
>
> Nor can anyone marvel enough that the faculty of perception which is living and heavenly, which is named *mens* or *animus*, is of such great mobility that even when it sleeps, it does not lie still: of such great speed that it may survey the heavens in one point of time, and if it wishes, may fly over the seas, wander over lands and cities: in short, all the things it desires, however far and wide they may be removed, it places within its sight just by thinking of them.

The dominance of *mōdsefa* in *The Seafarer* is fully in keeping with, and probably derives from, this statement of Lactantius that "*mens*" ("mind") or "*animus*" ("spirit") are one with the "*sensus*" ("faculty of perception"). That this faculty "*coelum collustret*" ("may survey the heavens") and "*maria peruolet*" ("may fly over the seas") is circumstantial evidence that the Seafarer's *mōdsefa* also acquires a taste of heaven. The flight over earth, sea and sky is otherwise the same, while the "*urbes*" ("cities") of the Latin may be represented earlier in the poem as the "*burgum*" and "*byrig*" of lines 28 and 48 respectively. In all, there is little doubt that Lactantius' work lies at the heart of *The Seafarer*, along with his Stoicising insistence that the mind and soul are both corporeal and separate; and that the mind may wander while the soul, except at death, does not.[43] Also it seems plausible that the poet's flying "aim" and "mood-sense" is inspired by this conception of *sensus*, *mens* and *animus* in flight. What remains here is to study the poet's materialisation of *hyge* and *mōdsefa* into a bird of prey. This is his true liberty in the likely borrowing from Lactantius. Let us see how he may have built his material image of sensory perception.

Christian Doctrine, Heathen Folklore

This poet's mechanism for materialising the directing and sensory elements of mind appears to predate his society's acquisition of that Latin learning

[43] LOCKETT, *Anglo-Saxon Psychologies*, pp. 193-199.

which inspired him to his poem. This is firstly clear in the OE language itself, in which senses move out to find impressions. So, for example, when St Giles stands praying on the shore, and "*þā geseah hē ān scip ūt on þǣre sǣ*" ("then he saw a ship out on the sea"), we have *ūt*, not *ūte*: an adverb of motion, not of place.[44] The same obtains in Old Icelandic, as with a shepherd in *Eyrbyggja saga*, who "*sá inn í fjallit elda stóra ok heyrði þanga mikinn glaum ok hornaskvǫl*" ("saw great fires inside within the mountain and heard there great sounds of revelry and squealing of pipes", ch. 11).[45] Here a man sends out his seeing and hearing to acquire impressions: respectively these sensory excursions require *inn* and *þangat*, not *inni* and *þar*. The sense gathers memory in exactly the same way. In *The Wanderer*, the "Wise Man" "*feor oft gemon / wælsleahta worn*" ("often remembers from far back a number of murderous battles", lines 90-91). In *Andreas*, it is said that the heart will be lifted in any man "*þe feor oððe nēah / on mōde geman hū se maga fremede*" ("who remembers far or near in mind how the young man [Jesus] performed", lines 638-639). Here we have sense moving towards memory within the *mōd*, not receiving it from there: *feor* and *nēah*, rather than *feorran* and *nēan*.

The word *sefa* denotes perception, and in this way it may also stand for a hidden receptacle of mind: as in *Daniel*, where "*ælmihtig ēacenne gāst in sefan sende, / snyttro cræftas*" ("the Almighty sent His teeming spirit, His powers of cleverness, into [Daniel's] sense", lines 484-485a); or in *Beowulf*, where Hrothgar says "*þē þā wordcwydas wigtig drihten / on sefan sende*" ("these pronouncements the mighty Lord has sent into your sense" to Beowulf (lines 1841-1842a)). But as the faculty of perception, *sefa* may also move of its own accord. It moves into the memory, in search of things held within: in Zacharias, about to pronounce from memory in *Elene*, "*sefa dēop gewōd, / wīsdōmes gewitt*" ("sense moved deep, wisdom's intelligence", lines 1189-1190). As we have seen in the Arundel Psalter, the word *sefa* is grouped with *andgyt* ("intellect"), whose related verb is *ongietan* ('to perceive', shading into 'understand'). In *Deor*, in token of the grey area between catching and incorporating, Beadohild "*on sefan (...) gearolīce ongieten hæfde*" ("in her feeling had suddenly perceived", lines 9-10) that she was pregnant. Strictly, *ongietan* means only 'to get' or 'to acquire'.[46] This mechanism is implicit in *sefa*'s movement

[44] *The Old English Life of St Nicholas with the Old English Life of St Giles*, ed. E. TREHARNE (Leeds, 1997), p. 133.

[45] *Eyrbyggja saga*, ed. E.Ól. SVEINSSON and M. ÞÓRÐARSON (Reykjavik, 1935: *Íslenzk fornrit* 4), p. 19.

[46] Some 800 instances. Strictly used as 'perceive' in 11 or 12 out of 12 instances in *Beowulf*:

in search of things outside the body. In *The Wanderer*, for example, after the heathen exile wakes up to wintry seabirds, he appears not to search his memory, but rather to scan the horizon for signs, which include auguries:[47]

Cearo bið genīwad
þām þe sendan sceal swīþe geneahhe
ofer waþema gebind wērigne sefan. (lines 55-57)

Care is renewed
for him who must send very constantly
over the waves' binding a weary sense.

The chief difference between this scene and *The Seafarer*'s flight of mind is that the perception is sent by the self, rather than moving of its own accord.

The element of mind which directs any such mental or physical movement is intention, OE *hyge*, which we have seen guiding *mōdsefa* in *The Seafarer*. When Grendel takes fright at meeting Beowulf, "*hyge wæs him hinfūs, wolde on heolster flēon*" ("his aim was keen for out of there, would flee into darkness", *Beowulf*, line 755). At a primal level this agency is expressed by *myne*, as when the Mermedonians wish to save their lives: "*wæs him ūt myne / flēon fealone strēam*" ("Their impulse went outwards, to flee the fallow stream", *Andreas*, lines 1536-1537). Moreover, the implication of OE "*myne witan*" ("to know the desire") is that OE *myne*, like Homeric Greek *μένος* (*menos*, 'impulse') and Old Icelandic *munr* ('impulse', 'difference'), can be implanted through the psychic intervention of one mind upon another.[48]

The associated verbs, *hycgan* ('to consider') and *munan* ('to be mindful of') respectively, retain a corresponding sense of direction. In the wider spread of Germanic languages it is possible to see these activities personified. In the thirteenth-century *Gylfaginning*, when a humanoid *Hugi* outruns the fastest sprinter alive, his illusionist master says "*þat var hugr minn, ok var Þjálfa eigi vænt at þreyta skjótfæri hans*" ("that was my thought, and of Þjálfi it wasn't to

M. LAPIDGE, "*Beowulf* and perception", *Proceedings of the British Academy* 111 (2001), pp. 61-97, esp. pp. 90-91.

[47] LACEY, *Birds and Bird-Lore*, pp. 143-145; R. NORTH, "Boethius and the mercenary in *The Wanderer*", in: *Pagans and Christians: The Interplay between Christian Latin and Traditional Germanic Culture in Early Medieval Europe*, ed. T. HOFSTRA, L.A.J.R. HOUWEN and A.A. MACDONALD (Groningen, 1995), pp. 71-98, esp. pp. 88-90.

[48] J. BREMMER, *The Early Greek Concept of the Soul* (Princeton, NJ, 1983), pp. 57-58; NORTH, *Pagan Words*, pp. 34-38.

be expected he would match the speed of that", ch. 47).[49] The same type of personification is latent in *Beowulf*, when Hrothgar decides to build Heorot: "*Him on mōd bearn / þæt healreced hātan wolde*" ("it ran into his mind that he would order a hall-building", *Beowulf*, lines 67-68). OE literature, however, retains only traces of old personifications which are more widely reflected in Icelandic. In Iceland, when a dreamer sees some attackers approaching his farm, he see them as wolves, "*ok veit ek víst, at þat er manna hugir*" ("I know for sure that these are the intentions of men", *Hávarðar saga Ísfirðings*, ch. 20).[50] For pale comparison, we might note Eormanric's "*wylfenne geþōht*" in *Deor* ("wolfish intention", line 22). Critical discussions of such psychic materialisations have confused the issue by treating *hugr* here as 'soul', when it might better be defined as a '(hostile) thought-projection'.[51] The terms 'free soul', 'dream-soul', even 'transcendental soul' are acceptable, so long as we remember that these refer to 'thought': they have nothing to do with the 'unitary soul', which is a development in Plato's philosophy and in the Augustinian theology which derived from this.[52]

The third type of personification, to do with flying, is the most commonplace. As we have seen, it is implied in Lactantius' use of Latin *peruolare* ('to fly over') for mental wandering in his *De opificio Dei*. This topos underlies his rhetorical comparison between man's thought and the mind of God:

> *Et miratur aliquis si diuina mens dei per uniuersas mundi partes intenta discurrit et omnia regit, omnia moderatur, ubique praesens, ubique diffusa, cum tanta sit uis et potestas mentis humanae intra mortale corpus inclusae, ut ne saeptis quidem grauis huius ac pigri corporis, cum quo inligata est, coerceri ullo modo possit quominus sibi liberam uagandi facultatem quietis impatiens largiatur?* (16.10)[53]

[49] *Snorri Sturluson: Edda: Prologue and Gylfaginning*, ed. A. FAULKES (Oxford, 1982), p. 43, lines 10-11.

[50] *Vestfirðinga Sögur*, ed. G. JÓNSSON (Reykjavik, 1946), pp. 349-350. NORTH, *Pagan Words*, pp. 108-110.

[51] SMITHERS, "Meaning of *The Seafarer*" (1957), pp. 137-139, 152; V. SALMON, "*The Wanderer* and *The Seafarer*, and the Old English conception of the soul", *Modern Language Review* 55 (1960), pp. 1-10; ORTON, "*Seafarer* 58-64a", p. 26.

[52] E.R. DODDS, *The Greeks and the Irrational* (Berkeley, CA, and London, 1951), pp. 207-235, esp. pp. 209-211; BREMMER, *Early Greek Concept of the Soul*, pp. 10, 66-67; LOCKETT, *Anglo-Saxon Psychologies*, pp. 182-184, 316-325. Nor may 'shamanism' be used to describe this: see C. TOLLEY, *Shamanism in Norse Myth and Magic*, 2 vols. (Helsinki, 2009), 1, pp. 176-199, esp. pp. 187-188.

[53] LOCKETT, *Anglo-Saxon Psychologies*, p. 292.

> And does anyone wonder that the divine mind of God, intent through every part of the universe, runs through and rules over all things, establishing a boundary around all things, being present everywhere and poured out everywhere, when such is the strength and power of the human mind enclosed within the mortal body that it cannot be constrained in any way by the confines of this heavy and lazy body in which it is bound, from allowing itself, impatient of rest, the free power of wandering?

A simile from the *Iliad*, with *νόος* (*no-os*, 'understanding, sense, thought'), *μενοινάω* (*menoinaō*, 'I desire') and flying, renders a similar human-divine comparative topos in older (and more succinct) form:

> ὡς δ᾽ ὅτ᾽ ἂν ἀΐξῃ νόος ἀνέρος, ὅς τ᾽ ἐπὶ πολλὴν
> γαῖαν ἐληλουθὼς φρεσὶ πευκαλίμῃσι νοήσῃ
> ἔνθ‘ εἴην ἢ ἔνθα, μενοινήῃσί τε πολλά,
> ὣς κραιπνῶς μεμαυῖα διέπτατο πότνια Ἥρη (XV.80-83)[54]
>
> Just as when speeds the thought of a man who, gone
> to many a land, in his perceptive organs will think
> "Were I here, were I there", and desire many things,
> just as quick did Lady Hera, having desired this, fly over.

This archaic Greek flight of mind is no metaphor, however. By now it should be just as clear that, on the level of language, the analogous multitude of OE terms for mind, with *hyge*, *(mōd)sefa*, *myne*, *hreðer* and so forth, more resembles Homer than it does any borrowed construction of philosophy, such as Alcuin's *De ratione animae* (*On the Reason of the Soul*, *c.* 800: his pasteurising revision of Lactantius) or even that of Lactantius himself. That the Anglo-Saxons strove to acquire these constructions does not mean that their poetic language, pre-Christian as its diction is, changed itself to keep up.[55]

To conclude, *The Seafarer* is more about nautical fact than figure. Here is an 'elegy' into which the most advanced Alcuinian Neo-Platonist theology and allegorical technique have been read. Each time a scholar brings out the Augus-

[54] *Ilias*, ed. J.W. FUCHS (The Hague, 1966: *Classica Hagana* 8), O. 80-84 [no pagination]. Cf. BREMMER, *Early Greek Concept of the Soul*, pp. 40-41 (esp. 41 n.), 57.

[55] See further E.G. STANLEY, "Old English poetic diction and the interpretation of *The Wanderer*, *The Seafarer* and *The Penitent's Prayer*", *Anglia* 73 (1956), pp. 413-466, esp. p. 453: "The Anglo-Saxons treated allegory in a manner which revealed a relation of fact to figure so close that the figure was an inseparable aspect of the fact". KLINCK, *Old English Elegies*, p. 37.

tinian notion of unitary soul, this poem is dated ever later, even to the end of the reform period of the late tenth century.[56] But the seafaring is real enough, and so is the shrieking bird at the centre. The topos to which this personified perception of the Seafarer comes closest, may be seen in the heathen Norse *Grímnismál* (*Lay of Grímnir*), in which Óðinn plays on the names of his ravens:

> *Huginn oc Muninn fliúga hverian dag*
> *iǫrmungrund yfir;*
> *óumc ek of Hugin, at hann aptr né komið,*
> *þó siámc meirr um Munin.* (st. 20)[57]

> Thought and Desire fly each day
> across the colossal earth;
> I fear about Thought that he won't come back,
> yet I worry even more about Desire.

This stanza is an analogue, in that it has birds and "*aptr koma*", as with OE "*eft cuman*" in *The Seafarer*, line 61. It is most likely that the names *hug-inn* and *mun-inn*, as with the form of the adjectives *gull-inn* ('golden'), *eik-inn* ('oaken'), mean respectively 'made of *hugr*' and 'made of *munr*'.[58] This Norse materialisation of mind shows us on what pre-Christian basis the English poet personifies his elements of mind into a bird of prey. Certainly he has used Christian doctrines: his Lactantius, along with an array of other mostly biblical sources. At the same time, however, the licence with which he builds his *ānfloga* comes closer to heathen folklore. In its language of sensory perception, *The Seafarer* may be among the oldest English poems that we have.

[56] CLEMOES, "*Mens absentia cogitans*"; DIEKSTRA, "Flight of the exiled soul", p. 443: "interiorisation, by which man's celestial nature, the soul, raises itself above its baser nature, the body"; J.C. CONDE SILVESTRE, "The semiotics of allegory in early medieval hermeneutics and the interpretation of *The Seafarer*", *Atlantis* 16 (1994), pp. 71-90, esp. p. 73 (near to *c.* 1000 date) and p. 88: "It must be accepted that the first part of *The Seafarer* functions as an extended symbol which aims to exemplify the doctrines exhibited in the second part".

[57] *Edda: Die Lieder des Codex Regius nebst verwandten Denkmälern*, ed. G. NECKEL, rev. H. KUHN, 5th edn. (Heidelberg, 1983), p. 61.

[58] A change to my earlier interpretation: NORTH, *Pagan Words*, p. 106: "endowed with *hugr*, *munr*".

The Sensory Cost of Remediation; or, Sniffing in the Gutter of Anglo-Saxon Manuscripts

JONATHAN WILCOX

Digital facsimiles are revolutionising manuscript studies. The stunning images now available are enabling a new-found and newly-wide-spread appreciation of medieval manuscripts. Digitised images allow a viewer not just to examine ink and pigment in minute detail (although you can), not just to see the quill-strokes made by scribes as never before (although you can), but even to study the substrate of the book itself, to investigate blemishes on the page, to scrutinise incisions and scrapings in the surfaces of the skin. You get so close you can parse the pen strokes, see the follicles, almost feel the grain, and almost smell the parchment. But there's the rub: even as you can see incredible detail, you can't touch, you can't smell, and you can't fully control the visual point of view. Some details, particularly of the craft of production, get left behind. Viewers of digital facsimiles aren't relating to the original – and there is surely something lost in that, even as much is also gained. Centring on the example of Anglo-Saxon manuscripts and with particular reference to the Blickling Homilies, this essay considers both the benefits of the plenitude of newly accessible manuscript material and what is lost, with particular attention to the missing sensory perception.

Sensory Perception in the Medieval West, ed. Simon C. THOMSON and Michael D.J. BINTLEY, *Utrecht Studies in Medieval Literacy*, 34 (Turnhout: Brepols, 2016), pp. 27-51.

BREPOLS PUBLISHERS DOI 10.1484/M.USML-EB.5.109503

Anglo-Saxon Manuscripts in Digital Facsimiles

All three major repositories of Anglo-Saxon manuscripts (the British Library, the Bodleian Library, and the Parker Library) make at least some of their manuscripts available online, as do many other libraries containing relevant material. Digital manuscript representations come in differing formats with differing rules of access, while new projects are making more material available all the time, so that it is hard to know what manuscripts are presently available or what to expect from a particular online collection. One clear desideratum of the present digital age is for an exhaustive and updated online manuscript catalogue. Anglo-Saxon studies have been exceptionally well served in the past with bibliographical aids, including an impressive sequence of manuscript catalogues, and so the current lack is all the more striking.[1] In the course of making an argument for more material engagement within the digital world, this essay will touch on some of the key online manuscript resources now available for Anglo-Saxonists, but is far from an exhaustive treatment.

The British Library was relatively late in making manuscripts available online, but now is perhaps the leader in the field, setting a standard for free access and a pleasingly usable format. The British Library collection of *Digitised Manuscripts* provides completely free access to images of every page of a manuscript.[2] Manuscripts are provided with a useful catalogue description, including an impressive bibliography. Presentation of the images can be formatted by the page or the opening or, more oddly, by the folio, showing recto and verso beside each other. A drop-down menu of page or folio numbers allows easy navigation between pages. A user can zoom in on a page for breathtaking detail. The result is a web presentation that is easy to use and highly informative, apparently replacing the earlier, rather clunky, *Turning the Pages* format once favoured by the British Library. Some further images of illustrations are available through a separate project, the *Catalogue of Illuminated Manuscripts*, but this does not provide complete manuscripts.[3]

Perhaps the most idiosyncratic element of the British Library's *Digitised Manuscripts* has been the way it has been created and augmented with very

[1] Note, most recently, H. GNEUSS and M. LAPIDGE, *Anglo-Saxon Manuscripts: A Bibliographical Handlist of Manuscripts and Manuscript Fragments Written or Owned in England Up To 1100* (Toronto, 2014), which, although a magisterial achievement, does not include notices of online digital facsimiles.

[2] <http://www.bl.uk/manuscripts/Default.aspx>.

[3] <http://www.bl.uk/catalogues/illuminatedmanuscripts/welcome.htm>.

little fanfare, so that at times it feels like a stealth collection. Presumably, manuscripts are added as opportunity (and funding) allows. The *Digitised Manuscripts* site currently (in June 2015) has 7236 manuscripts available. The somewhat awkward search function can make it hard to track which Anglo-Saxon manuscripts are included. Manuscripts of interest to Anglo-Saxonists already there include, among others:[4]

Cotton Nero D. iv (the Lindisfarne Gospels, **343**);
Add 89000 (the St. Cuthbert Gospel, **501.2**);
Cotton Domitian A VII (the Durham Liber Vitae, **327**);
Royal 1 E vi (the Royal Bible, **448**);
Cotton Galba A XVIII (the Athelstan Psalter, **334**);
Cotton Tiberius A. II (the Athelstan Gospels, **362**);
Harley 2904 (the Ramsey Psalter, **430**);
Cotton Vespasian A. I (the Vespasian Psalter, **381**);
Cotton Vespasian A. VIII (King Edgar's New Minster Refoundation Charter, **382**);
Cotton Vitellius A. XV (the Beowulf MS, **399**);
Cotton Claudius B. IV (The Illustrated Hexateuch, **315**);
Add 49598 (the Benedictional of St Æthelwold, **301**);
Harley 76 (the Bury Gospels, **413**);
Harley 603 (the Harley Psalter, **422**);
Royal 1 D IX (the Cnut Gospels, **447**);
Cotton Tiberius C. VI (the Tiberius Psalter, **378**);
Stowe 944 (the New Minster Liber Vitae, **500**).

One useful source of further information about the project is the *Medieval Manuscripts Blog*,[5] which includes some wonderful discussion and illustration of a whole range of British Library medieval manuscripts, if only occasional details about the digitisation in progress. Even as it is therefore unclear what further manuscripts will get added and when, the British Library's *Digitised Manuscripts* site constitutes a wonderful, and expanding, resource for manuscript studies of all kinds.

More exhaustive in its coverage, but more restrictive in its access, is *Parker Library on the Web*.[6] This provides digital images of all of the medieval manuscripts assembled in Matthew Parker's collection housed at Corpus Chris-

[4] Listed by short manuscript name and, in parentheses, a commonly used informal name with the catalogue reference used by GNEUSS and LAPIDGE, *Bibliographical Handlist*.

[5] <http://britishlibrary.typepad.co.uk/digitisedmanuscripts/index.html>.

[6] <http://parkerweb.stanford.edu/>.

ti College, Cambridge. The images come with a nice intuitive presentation that allows browsing with views of a complete opening, detailed inspection of a single page, which can be heavily magnified, and easy navigation to and from a catalogue description. The quality and completeness of the images make them very useful for scholarship and teaching, but full functionality, including use of the zoom, is only available to those who subscribe to the database, which comes with a hefty enough subscription rate to make this a resource fully accessible only to academics in well-funded research institutions.

The third great repository of Anglo-Saxon manuscripts, the Bodleian Library, provides a few Anglo-Saxon manuscripts on the site *Early Manuscripts at Oxford University*.[7] This project was undertaken relatively early in the process of digitising and, as a consequence, the format now looks awkward, although it is still usable. The site provides free access to some eighty complete medieval manuscripts from collections at Oxford, but with no new manuscripts being added. Navigation is not quite as easy as with the later collections, but can be achieved through thumbnail images. Clicking on a thumbnail brings up a particularly large image that is rich in detail but not scalable, without intermediate sizes and without any guiding image, so that the pages are somewhat hard to look at. Descriptions are minimal. For all such drawbacks, the images are high quality and freely accessible, and so provide a useful, if limited resource for study and teaching. In addition to a wealth of Celtic material, Anglo-Saxon manuscripts include:

Bodleian Library, Junius 11 (the Cædmon Manuscript, **640**);
Bodleian Library, Auct. D. 2. 16 (includes Leofric's list of donations to Exeter, **530**);
Bodleian Library, Auct. F. 4. 32 (Dunstan's classbook, **538**);
Bodleian Library, Rawl. Q. e. 20 (damaged fragment of Life of St. Basil, **355**);
Corpus Christi College 197 (Rule of St. Benedict, **672**);
St. John's College 28 (Gregory's *De cura pastoralis*, **684**);
St. John's College 154 (Ælfric's Grammar, **686**).

The images here are so detailed, they allow for good inspection of the parchment. Clicking on f. 18v of MS Auct. F. 4. 32, for example,[8] brings up the final page of an anonymous homily on the Finding of the Holy Cross that occupies a single quire, ff. 10-18. This homily evidently once circulated as a separate

7 <http://image.ox.ac.uk/>.

8 <http://image.ox.ac.uk/show?collection=bodleian&manuscript=msauctf432>.

booklet since there is a vertical fold in the parchment which, along with the consequent chafing, is clearly visible in the reproduction of f. 18v.

Other digitised manuscript collections abound, including other libraries in Cambridge (Trinity College is particularly good,[9] as is Cambridge University Library[10]), other collections throughout the UK, many of the major Continental collections (including Paris[11] and Switzerland[12]), most of the major holdings in the United States (including the Pierpont Morgan library, available through the *Corsair* catalogue[13]), and many other library collections throughout the United States that contain some medieval manuscripts. The private Schøyen collection is publicly available through some low-quality digital images, along with full descriptions of provenance, and some impressive illustrations of medieval bindings.[14]

While a website gathering references to all of these collections and listing their contents would obviously be ideal, the task of keeping track looks increasingly challenging. The UCLA *Catalogue of Digitized Medieval Manuscripts*[15] once aimed for complete coverage but has since given up the attempt, with the following rather plaintive explanation:

> Please note that in 2013 active development on the CDMMSS ceased (for now). The 3129 manuscripts listed here, drawn from 139 institutions, are an increasingly partial subset of manuscripts that have been digitized in their entirety and made available on the web. Institutions large and small have continued to digitize manuscripts at an ever-quickening pace. We hope you continue to find that Catalogue useful, but the results it provides are not comprehensive.

Another, more limited, attempt at a meta-site is provided by *Manuscripts Online*,[16] a UK-based project that "enables you to search a diverse body of online primary resources relating to written and early printed culture in Britain during the period 1000 to 1500". More promising is the *Digitized Medieval Manuscripts app*,[17] a site that maps libraries that include digital medieval

9 <http://sites.trin.cam.ac.uk/james/>.
10 <http://cudl.lib.cam.ac.uk/>.
11 <http://gallica.bnf.fr/>.
12 <http://www.e-codices.unifr.ch/en>.
13 <http://corsair.morganlibrary.org/>.
14 <http://www.schoyencollection.com/>.
15 <http://manuscripts.cmrs.ucla.edu/index.php>.
16 <https://www.manuscriptsonline.org/>.
17 <http://digitizedmedievalmanuscripts.org>.

manuscripts. A label associated with each location includes a URL that allows access to the digital library website. The site currently shows 300+ digital libraries, "and is constantly updated", benefiting from crowd sourcing. This wealth of information is probably the best current source for indexing digital collections, if inevitably showing some oversights. (At the present time it indicates just three institutions in Cambridge with online collections, for example, omitting Cambridge University Library.) If the site can be maintained, it will provide a useful key to available collections, even if not the more ambitious listing of all manuscripts digitally available.

All of the digital manuscript reproductions described so far are available online on the web, which is an ample arena for present scholarly excitement. It is a predictable feature of the digital landscape, though, that there will be new opportunities for digital manuscript studies in the new platforms of the future, just as there are always risks of obsolescence as old platforms become outmoded. In terms of promise, as online manuscript images become more widely available, they will surely inform a generation of new editions that can present more information than what has become customary in traditional print editions. The *New Testament Virtual Manuscript Room*[18] provides an example from a neighbouring field, the study of the Greek New Testament, of the presentation of manuscript images that are tied to transcriptions, provided with additional bibliographical data, and add up to the materials for an edition and one that makes manifest more manuscript evidence than was ever thinkable in print. In Anglo-Saxon studies, editions that make full use of manuscript images have so far mostly circulated on CD-ROM or DVD, which risk obsolescence. Perhaps most impressive for presenting Old English poetry is an edition by Bernard Muir of *The Exeter Book*, with easy linking between edited text and manuscript image in multiple linked windows, and an abundance of additional evidence from transcripts and images neatly gathered.[19] Kevin Kiernan's *Electronic Beowulf* project has demonstrated both the potential and the pitfalls, with a pioneering manuscript-image-rich edition released in different digital forms that each became unusable with age.[20]

[18] <http://ntvmr.uni-muenster.de/>.

[19] *The Exeter Anthology of Old English Poetry*, ed. B.J. MUIR, and N. KENNEDY, software (DVD-ROM, Exeter, 2006); see also *A Digital Facsimile of Oxford, Bodleian Library, MS. Junius 11*, ed. B.J. MUIR (CD-ROM, Oxford, 2004).

[20] *Electronic Beowulf*, ed. K.S. KIERNAN, with A. PRESCOTT (2 CDs for computer, London, 1999); *Electronic Beowulf 2.0*, ed. K.S. KIERNAN, with A. PRESCOTT (2 CD-ROMS, London, 2004); *Electronic Beowulf*, third edition, ed. K.S. KIERNAN, with I.E. IACOB, programmer (CD-

In addition to the digital facsimiles provided by libraries, a few other projects make available images of manuscripts in relation to a specific digital humanities project. One example of particular value for Anglo-Saxonists is the collection of single-sheet Anglo-Saxon charters available at the *Kemble* website,[21] associated with the *Electronic Sawyer*.[22] This makes available (after registration) modern digital images of the great majority of the three hundred or so surviving single-sheet charters from Anglo-Saxon England. A slightly later period is covered by the website for the *Production and Use of Early English Manuscripts, 1060 to 1220*,[23] which includes a few images among the catalogue descriptions. Digital scholarship itself is the object of attention in the large-grant project "Digitally Enabled Scholarship with Medieval Manuscripts" undertaken since 2012 at Yale University by the Yale Digital Collections Center (YDC2),[24] although this gives little attention to early medieval examples. Some relevant digital projects in the field have apparently already succumbed to obsolescence, such as the MANCASS C11 database of eleventh-century spellings with associated images of scribal forms.[25]

The current round of digital images are particularly useful for the study of letter forms, and that potential is engaged for Anglo-Saxon manuscript studies by the web-based project, *DigiPal*.[26] Centring on the period 1000-1100, this is a web resource "designed to allow you to see samples of handwriting from the period and to compare them with each other quickly and easily". As clarified in the description of "The Project":

> The project aims to bring digital technology to bear on scholarly discussion in new and innovative ways. It combines digital photographs of medieval handwriting with detailed descriptions and characterisations of the writing, as well as the text in which it is found, and the content and structure of the manuscript or document as a whole. It incorporates different ways of exploring and manipulating the informa-

ROM, London, 2011). An online edition is now available: *Electronic Beowulf*, online fourth edition, ed. K. KIERNAN, programmed by I.E. IACOB (2015), <http://ebeowulf.uky.edu/ebeo4.0/start.html>.

21 <http://www.kemble.asnc.cam.ac.uk/>.

22 <http://www.esawyer.org.uk/about/index.html>.

23 <http://www.le.ac.uk/english/em1060to1220/>.

24 <http://ydc2.yale.edu/research-support/digitally-enabled-scholarship-medieval-manuscripts>.

25 See K. POWELL, "The MANCASS C11 database: A tool for studying script and spelling in the eleventh century", *Old English Newsletter* 38 (Fall 2004), pp. 29-34. The database is currently (June 2015) not accessible at the address given here or elsewhere on the web.

26 <http://www.digipal.eu/>.

> tion, such as annotated images, as well as more conventional text-based browse and search. It therefore allows scholars to apply new developments in palaeographical method which have been discussed in theory but which have proven difficult or impossible to implement in practice.[27]

Thus the new technologies are advancing old-fashioned palaeography, with an outcome that can be seen in a recent exciting publication drawing from this database.[28]

Newly-available digital images, then, are revolutionising what is possible in manuscript studies, providing a rich resource that is an appropriate subject for scholarly reflection. Some of the paradoxes of the power of these digital copies was brought home to me while studying MS Princeton, University Library, Scheide M. 71, the Blickling Homilies. After considerable effort to travel to the library, to be admitted as a *bona fide* manuscript scholar, and to comply with the rules of this particular Special Collections Library, I was sitting in Princeton University Library Special Collections looking at the Blickling Homilies through a magnifying glass, trying to confirm Willard's reading of the cropped quire signature on f. 8v,[29] when it occurred to me to make use of the library's WiFi set-up and the laptop on which I was taking notes to conjure up Princeton University's Digital Library[30] and look at the online digital representation of the manuscript.[31] For all the effort of going to see the original, the vetting and divesting necessary to get into the inner sanctum of the manuscript reading room, I discovered I could see the page better in the publicly-available facsimile than in the original (see the possible cropped *e* of the quire signature in the lower margin of f. 8v (Fig. 3.1),[32] alongside the clearer example of a quire signature, the *.p.* on f. 73v, available at (Fig. 3.2).[33] This raised forcefully for me the question of the status of the original in an age of electronic repro-

[27] <http://www.digipal.eu/about/the-project/>.

[28] P.A. STOKES, *Vernacular Minuscule from Æthelred to Cnut, circa 990-circa 1035* (Cambridge, 2014).

[29] *The Blickling Homilies: The John H. Scheide Library, Titusville Pennsylvania*, ed. R. WILLARD (Copenhagen, 1960), p. 39. My description of the manuscript is published in *Homilies by Ælfric and Other Homilies* (Tempe, AZ, 2008), pp. 129-142.

[30] <http://pudl.princeton.edu/>.

[31] Available at <http://pudl.princeton.edu/objects/x346d4176>.

[32] <http://pudl.princeton.edu/viewer.php?obj=x346d4176#page/40/mode/2up>.

[33] Available at <http://pudl.princeton.edu/viewer.php?obj=x346d4176#page/170/mode/2up>.

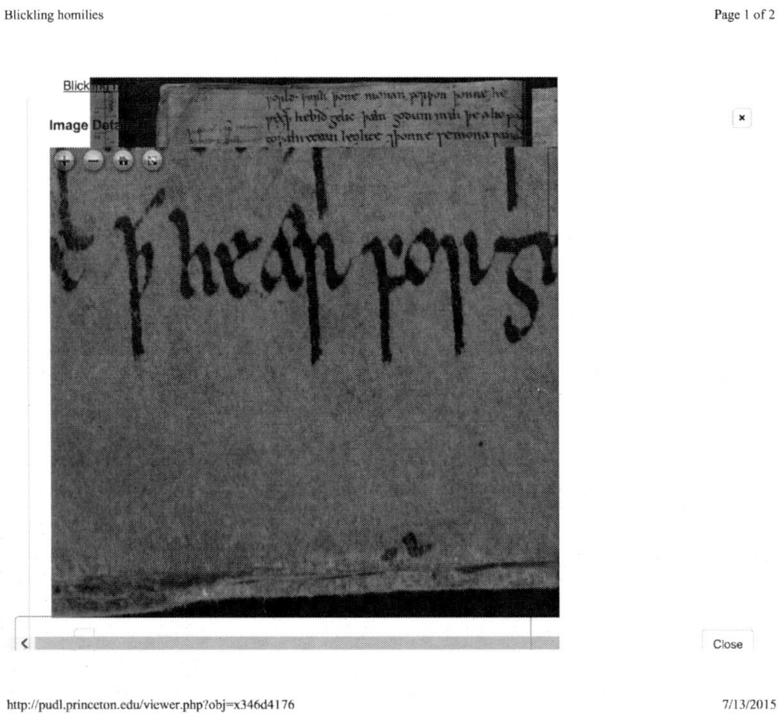

Fig. 3.1 Screenshot of MS Princeton University Library, Scheide M. 71 (the Blickling Homilies) f. 8v (detail) (<http://pudl.princeton.edu/>), courtesy of Scheide Library, Princeton University Library.

duction. For visual purposes, the copy can provide better access than the original, and yet, surely, the original gave me something not available in the representation.

Theorising the Digital Turn

The turn to new media has been the subject of considerable scholarly scrutiny. Walter Benjamin provides the most famous theory of the copy in his essay "The work of art in the age of mechanical reproduction", written in 1936, just

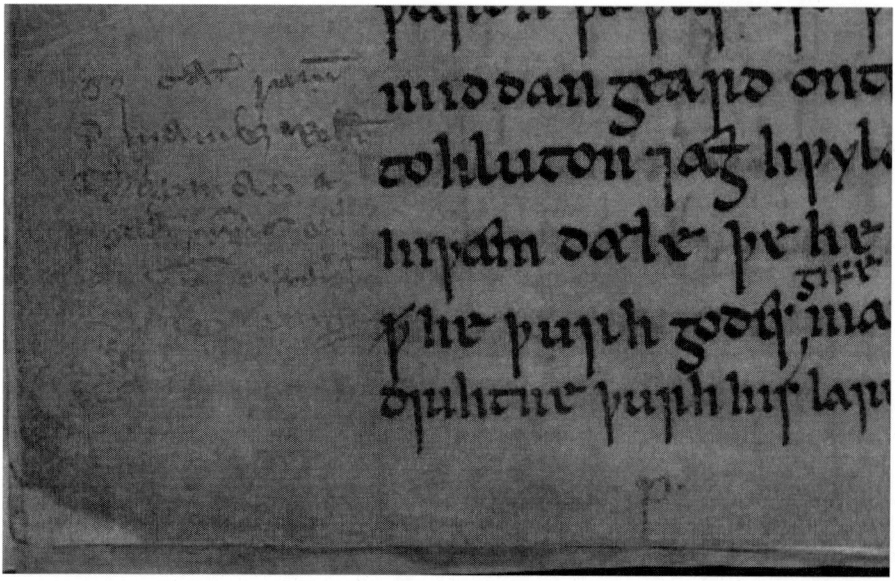

Fig. 3.2 MS Princeton University Library, Scheide M. 71 (the Blickling Homilies) f. 73v (detail) taken from the screenshot of Princeton University's Digital Library (<http://pudl.princeton.edu/>), courtesy of Scheide Library, Princeton University Library.

as the technology of photography and film was reaching its maturity.[34] Benjamin helps pinpoint the underlying issues by describing how an original work of art carries with it an aura, in part a reflection of its accumulated history, in part a result of the veneration or ritual power that an audience is willing to give it. Surely the rituals of access to Special Collections help maintain the aura of manuscript originals. Usefully, though, Benjamin argues in favour of the new technology of his day, which he sees as a political force for good. "The progressive reaction", which he considers enabled by mechanical reproduction, "is characterized by the direct, intimate fusion of visual and emotional enjoyment with the orientation of the expert" (section 12), suggesting a democratising both of pleasure and of access. Benjamin hints at how such copies may actually

[34] Translated H. ZOHN (1968) and available freely online: <https://www.marxists.org/reference/subject/philosophy/works/ge/benjamin.htm> [accessed 23 July 2015].

increase the aura of the original even as his analysis celebrates mass reproduction. Theorists of the internet draw heavily on Benjamin as they show how the internet is a medium of the copy par excellence. This transfers value from the unique to the multiple and facilitates the kind of poaching and appropriation described by the likes of de Certeau and Berger.[35] One consequence of the digital turn, then, is a democratisation of access that is surely salutary for manuscript studies. This erstwhile restricted field is thriving now that images of medieval manuscripts are so widely available and every user of *Wikipedia* who types in "Old English poetry" or "Beowulf" gets to see at least one manuscript page displayed. The gatekeepers who had to work to preserve the material originals are now bypassed with ease, even as the role of the expert interpreter remains crucial. Indeed, since most *Wikipedia*-viewers presumably can't read the insular minuscule of the *Beowulf*-manuscript, and presumably couldn't understand the language even if they could read the script, the image is there above all as some kind of infinitely-reproducible totem of pastness and of materiality. Widespread reproduction may serve to bolster the aura afforded to the original and suggest a kind of aura of the copy.

The aura of the high-quality digital image comes in part from the apparent access it provides to the original and in part from its display of the latest technology. I for one find myself wowed every time I zoom in on any of the scalable images described above. The very fact of a zoom that allows me to control entry into the manuscript and that gets me so close to the texture of the page pulls me into the object in some emotional as well as visual way. Magnification is hardly the only trick available to the new technology, even if it is the one that most commonly satisfies me as viewer. Bill Endres, of the University of Kentucky, demonstrates the creation of digital flyovers on the pages of the St Chad Gospels in "The St Chad Gospels: Potentials for 3D in the study of manuscripts" (2012).[36] By swooping in on a manuscript page constructed with various textures, the viewer is presented with a thrilling sense of closeness to an almost three-dimensional page, presented in a video precisely revelling in the technique even as it shows the outcome of that technique. Such closeness not only pays homage to the original, although it does do that; it also parades the effectiveness of the new medium, showing reverence both to medieval object and to modern cleverness that can create such a copy.

[35] See M. DE CERTEAU, *The Practice of Everyday Life*, trans. S. RENDALL (Berkeley, 1984); and J. BERGER, *Ways of Seeing* (Harmondsworth, 1972).

[36] On YouTube: <https://www.youtube.com/watch?v=ebr0HNnNNrs&feature=share>.

The paradoxical relation of copy to original is described well by the double-logic of remediation as explored by Bolter and Grusin.[37] They demonstrate how new media often fulfill two apparently contradictory impulses simultaneously. One is the logic of hypermediacy, a displaying of all the multiple levels of accumulated technology lying behind the latest media. Frames, pages, and bookmarks are some of the obvious ways in which internet formats draw on and insistently parade many of the forms of earlier media, both appropriating the language of earlier technologies and building their display into the new medium.[38] The other logic driving new media is that of immediacy: the desire to provide intimate, apparently unmediated, access to an underlying object or experience. In the world of online gaming, viewers often report a kind of complete immersion that blocks out the everyday world and the passage of time, a kind of immediacy despite all the intervening frames. In most of the digital manuscript reproductions, the viewer gets to see the frames and the multiple markers of the media gathered around or superimposed upon the manuscript page. Thus the viewer is presented with all the reassuring icons for controlling and framing the object under scrutiny, hinting at the fragmentary and accumulative logic of hypermediacy. And yet, for all that parading of the mechanism of the technology, whenever I zoom in on a manuscript page, I think at some level that I am getting close to the parchment itself, fulfilling the logic of immediacy as I imaginatively screen out the framing processes to be drawn to the thing itself. The zoom function and the digital flyover have me imagining that I am able to interact intimately with the manuscript (immediacy), even as the multiple layers of approach, the surrounding commentary, access to embedded video or different kinds of pictures, have me revelling in the accretive and deeply-mediated presentation of the object (hypermediacy).

Both logics are well served by the current technology, and yet not quite well enough. I appreciate the bibliography provided by the *British Library Digitised Manuscripts* site, but I would like live links to access all those commentaries more easily. If the script is hard for me to read, I would appreciate a transcription tied to the manuscript. And if a transcription, why not also an edition, so that I could read the text with the help of editorial conventions? And if the text is in a language I can't understand, why not also have it tied to a

[37] J.D. BOLTER and R. GRUSIN, *Remediation: Understanding New Media* (Cambridge, MA, 2000; first published in 1999).

[38] Such language and practices are critiqued by Johanna Drucker in multiple essays, including "The virtual codex: From page space to e-space", in: *A Companion to Digital Literary Studies*, ed. R. SIEMENS, S. SCHREIBMAN, and A. LIU (Malden, MA, 2007), pp. 216-232.

translation? As explored above, the time is surely close for effective digital editions that will exploit the logic of hypermediacy. Meanwhile, the zoom function of the *British Library Digitised Manuscripts* or of *Parker on the Web* stops with a magnification that captures individual letters with great clarity, but I would like to go further still. I want more immediacy to get more fully under the skin that appears to be in front of me. In another paradox of the digital age, there is never enough hypermediacy nor enough immediacy.

But I want more immediacy in another way, too. The digital representations described here are all tied to just one of the senses. In the state of current technology, it is certainly possible to embed audio files to augment an exclusively visual representation, as Kiss *et al.* show in their persuasive analysis of the latest digital editions.[39] But even with the addition of sound, the reproduction is still going to be lacking much of the embodied nature of the original. The art historian Michael Camille is eloquent on how medieval manuscripts appeal to all the senses, not just sight and sound.[40] All those flowers in the borders of Books of Hours suggest the olfactory as, with less sweetness, do those farting grotesques Camille so intriguingly uncovered.[41] Parchment itself gives off a distinct odour. Fruits and harvest scenes in the margins suggest the gustatory, picking up on the famous biblical images of eating the wisdom of books (Ezekiel 3:1-3, Apoc. 10:9-11). And the tactile is everywhere in the operation of a real book, but absent from the digital simulacrum. Parchment alerts an attentive hand to the difference between flesh side and hair side, while the book asserts values of weight and heft, portability and haptic involvement to those who hold it.

The thing itself carries epistemological weight as object, as a current critical turn towards thing theory would remind us.[42] Attentiveness to things as objects has blossomed, perhaps not coincidentally, at the same time as the digital revolution represents the apparent triumph of the disembodied. Object Oriented Ontology provides an extreme instantiation, suggesting a perspective

[39] F.G. KISS, E. POLEG, L. DOLEŽALOVÁ, and R. WÓJCIK, "Old light on new media: Medieval practices in the digital age", *Digital Philology* 2 (2013), pp. 16-34.

[40] M. CAMILLE, "Sensations of the page: Imaging technologies and medieval illuminated manuscripts", in: *The Iconic Page in Manuscript, Print, and Digital Culture*, ed. G. BORNSTEIN and T. TINKLE (Ann Arbor, 1998), pp. 33-53.

[41] See M. CAMILLE, *Image on the Edge: The Margins in Medieval Art* (Cambridge, MA, 1992).

[42] See *Things*, ed. B. BROWN (Chicago, 2004).

that in this instance might ponder the point of view and the ethical rights of the book itself.[43]

One other aspect of engagement with materiality may be particularly relevant here. Consciousness of materiality should involve acknowledgement of the craft that went into producing an object. Such craft involves a kind of embodied cognition that has long been practised and that may acquire renewed intellectual respect when described by a philosopher like Richard Sennet.[44] Digital representation removes an object from the craftiness of its material construction, even as a complementary interpretive move has involved some analysts engaging with the materiality and craft of the digital representation.[45] I would like to suggest that the current crop of digital manuscript reproductions could be more sensitive to the underlying craft they can help uncover.

How can a material turn be well served by the current digital revolution and a medium that is apparently so immaterial? Can what is missing in the digital be brought back through scholarship in other ways? I would like to briefly consider the issue in relation to a particular conundrum of my own research, evidence for the binding of the Blickling Homilies, before suggesting some conclusions that play up the craft of these objects of study and the many senses that a book works to engage.

A Case Study of Manuscript Materiality

One of the issues I was considering in looking at the Blickling Homilies was how this particular book circulated in the Anglo-Saxon period. Mary Jane Toswell, building on the work of Donald Scragg and P.R. Robinson, suggested that the quires may have circulated unbound.[46] That kind of circulation would

[43] B. HOLSINGER, "Of pigs and parchment: Medieval studies and the coming of the animal", *Proceedings of the Modern Language Association of America* 124 (2009), pp. 616-623, ponders some of the issues and posits the Old English book / Bible riddle as a self-conscious engagement from the period.

[44] R. SENNET, *The Craftsman* (New Haven, 2008).

[45] See, for example, J. DRUCKER, "Humanistic theory and digital scholarship", in: *Debates in the Digital Humanities*, ed. M.K. GOLD (Minneapolis, 2012), pp. 85-95.

[46] M.J. TOSWELL, "The codicology of Anglo-Saxon homiletic manuscripts, especially the Blickling Homilies", in: *The Old English Homily: Precedent, Practice, and Appropriation*, ed. A.J. KLEIST (Turnhout, 2007), pp. 209-226, building on P.R. ROBINSON, "Self-contained units in composite manuscripts of the Anglo-Saxon period", *Anglo-Saxon England* 7 (1978), pp. 231-238; D.G. SCRAGG, "The homilies of the Blickling manuscript", in: *Learning and Literature in*

make it more likely that these homilies were preached in the field rather than being preserved in a copy more intended for study than for performance.[47] The Blickling Homilies provide an interesting case study for approaching this question, since there is extensive evidence for the later medieval use of this book in Lincoln, although little for its early circulation. By 1304, the manuscript was in the possession of Lincoln city corporation, where it was used as an oath book and a book of record, with the noting of names and some city affairs in the margins and blank spaces. Early in this re-use the manuscript was likely rebound in view of the addition to the front of the book of a fourteenth-century quire providing the gospel sequentiae that make it particularly suitable for an oath book. The book was presumably rebound again with the addition of a further quire at the front containing a fifteenth-century calendar. Other rebindings during this period of use are possible. In the modern period, the book was further rebound at least three times: by the shop of Charles Lewis in the 1840s or 1850s, by Marguerite Duprez-Lahey at the Pierpont Morgan Library in 1956-1957, and by Scott Husby at Princeton in 2007.[48] Is there evidence in the surviving manuscript, I wondered, of how the collection was bound in the early medieval period before all those rebindings?

The sewing of a permanent binding involves creating holes in the parchment at the fold of the bifolios once they are gathered into a quire. The parchment is most straightforwardly cut by a knife at the necessary sewing stations, leaving slit-shaped holes in the parchment known as kerfs, although the hole could be made by the sewing needle, leaving a more circular hole. In permanent bindings from early medieval Europe, the quires are generally stitched onto sewing supports, which are then attached to the covers in various ingenious ways.[49] If the quires circulated without a cover or permanent binding, they might have been held in place with minimal sewing or tacketing. This would most likely involve making just two stabs through the parchment to sew

Anglo-Saxon England: Studies Presented to Peter Clemoes, ed. M. LAPIDGE and H. GNEUSS (Cambridge, 1981), pp. 299-316.

[47] See my "The use of Ælfric's homilies: MSS Oxford, Bodleian Library, Junius 85 and 86 in the field", in: *A Companion to Ælfric*, ed. H. MAGENNIS and M. SWAN (Leiden, 2009), pp. 345-368, for a discussion of the phenomenon and the example of a homily by Ælfric.

[48] For details, see the introduction to the Willard facsimile and my description, both cited in n. 29 above.

[49] For a brief general account of the binding process, see R. CLEMENS and T. GRAHAM, *Introduction to Manuscript Studies* (Ithaca, NY, 2007), chapter 4; for full details see J.A. SZIRMAI, *The Archaeology of Medieval Bookbinding* (Aldershot, 1999).

thread that would hold the quires loosely together.[50] One way of understanding the prior circulation of the Blickling Homilies would be to see if there is any evidence of sewing stations from before the addition of the fourteenth-century gospel sequentiae or the fifteenth-century calendar. This involves looking in the gutter of the manuscript to see the kerfs and holes that accommodate the sewing and looking at the sewing support. There is no theoretical reason that such evidence of craft should not be as visible in a digital facsimile as the sequence of pen strokes on the page, particularly if the manuscript was photographed disbound, but the digital representation of the Blickling Homilies presents images of the page that have been trimmed as if to avoid any indecorous gaze falling into the gutter. Not only is there no picture of the open book from above or below, but even when the images are displayed as a full verso-to-recto opening, they in fact present two separate, neatly-cropped single-page images placed side by side rather than a picture of an opening spread.

Such occlusion of evidence for craft proves to be normal in many of the digital facsimiles described in this essay. Even when a manuscript is displayed as an opening on the *British Library Digital Manuscripts* website, two cropped images of pages appear side by side, with the consequent loss of some evidence for the craft of production. In the case of British Library, the single page image generally does seem to include a sliver of the other page of the opening, thus allowing some view of the gutter. *Early Manuscripts at Oxford University* does not make available images of an opening, although the single page cropping generally includes a good view of the gutter. *The Parker Library on the Web*, on the other hand, does present a picture of a complete opening in one of its views, although the zoom function only operates on an image of separate individual pages. Choices about the formation and presentation of the digital image which may seem minor or inevitable, such as the choice to neatly crop the view of the page, exert inevitable control on the viewing experience and have considerable consequences for the kind of study possible through the digital medium. Even as digital images can be stunning for showing details of the surface, choices made in the way they are formed are not necessarily conducive to presenting full evidence for the craft of the book's creation.

Of course, it is not always possible to uncover a book's past, even when viewing it in the flesh. Mending and re-use obscures earlier evidence. The kerfs served for each of the three rebindings of the modern period and the same holes

[50] See SZIRMAI, *Bookbinding*, chap. 10, on limp bindings.

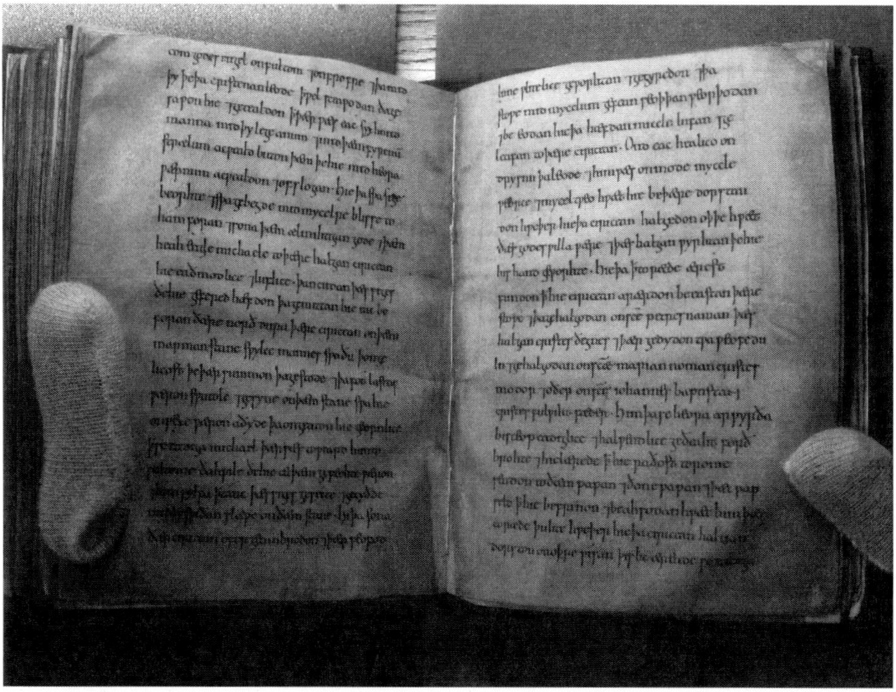

Fig. 3.3 MS Princeton University Library, Scheide M. 71 (the Blickling Homilies) f. 123v/124r, courtesy of Scheide Library, Princeton University Library.

may have served previous bindings, too.[51] A pair of holes visible on some pages towards the top of the book (about 35 mm and 58 mm down from the top edge) and somewhat off the centre of the bifolios may possibly have served a tacketed binding. These punctures are generally visible on ff. 109 to 135 (part-way through Quire XV to the end of Quire XVIII), with a possible second at places (such as f. 135). These possible tacket holes can now be seen particularly well at the f. 123v/124r opening (see Fig. 3.3, full 123v/124r spread, and Fig. 3.4, close up). However, in a telling paradox, they are not visible in the online image, here and in many other places (see Fig. 3.5, f. 124r, top part, in digital image).

The reason for this is that the digital photographs were taken at a time when the book was unbound but the pages still carried the repairs of Margue-

[51] Scott Husby reported that he used the sewing locations used by Marguerite Duprez-Lahey and by the shop of Charles Lewis; personal communication, e-mail of 8/15/2008.

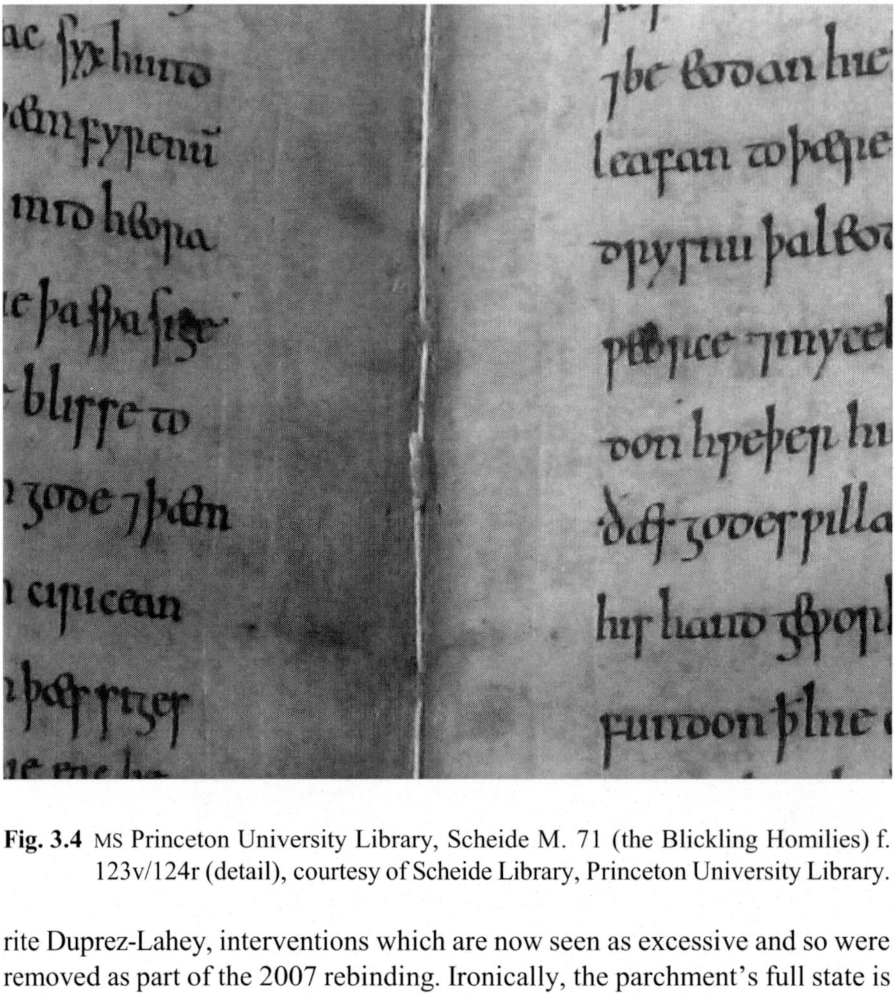

Fig. 3.4 MS Princeton University Library, Scheide M. 71 (the Blickling Homilies) f. 123v/124r (detail), courtesy of Scheide Library, Princeton University Library.

rite Duprez-Lahey, interventions which are now seen as excessive and so were removed as part of the 2007 rebinding. Ironically, the parchment's full state is better captured in the black and white print facsimile of 1960, the photography for which was undertaken before the mending associated with the 1950s binding (Figure 3.6, full 123v/124r spread in 1960 print facsimile). My point here is not just that conservation practises change, but rather that the apparent quality of the digital reproduction can give it a definitive air that it doesn't deserve. The digital image looks so good, it is seductively convincing as a stand-in for reality, even though that reality is contingent on constraints that are not always obvious and is no more the thing itself than any other reproduction.

The stabbed punctures are probably evidence of holding folios together with a tacket binding, even though the date or duration of such binding is hard

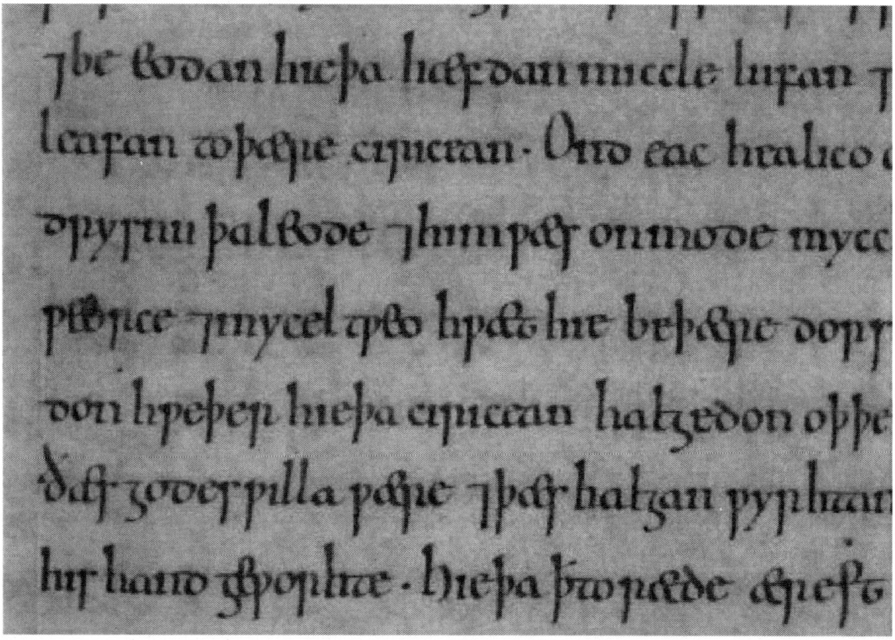

Fig. 3.5 MS Princeton University Library, Scheide M. 71 (the Blickling Homilies) f. 124r (detail), taken from a screenshot of Princeton University's Digital Library (<http://pudl. princeton.edu/>), courtesy of Scheide Library, Princeton University Library.

The stabbed punctures are probably evidence of holding folios together with a tacket binding, even though the date or duration of such binding is hard to establish. More evidence for Anglo-Saxon practice is provided by the alphabetical quire signatures in the centre of the bottom margin of the last folio of a quire (a second sequence comes from a later medieval date). Many have been lost to cropping, which clearly occurred in the course of the multiple rebindings, with the loss of some text; others may have been erased in campaigns to clear the margins when the manuscript was prepared for sale. Still surviving quire signatures are clear on ff. 73v (see Fig. 3.2), 110v (see Fig. 3.7), and 119v, and these are probably Anglo-Saxon.[52] Quire signatures suggest that the

[52] Willard thinks they are written by Hand A, the scribe of most of the Anglo-Saxon manuscript.

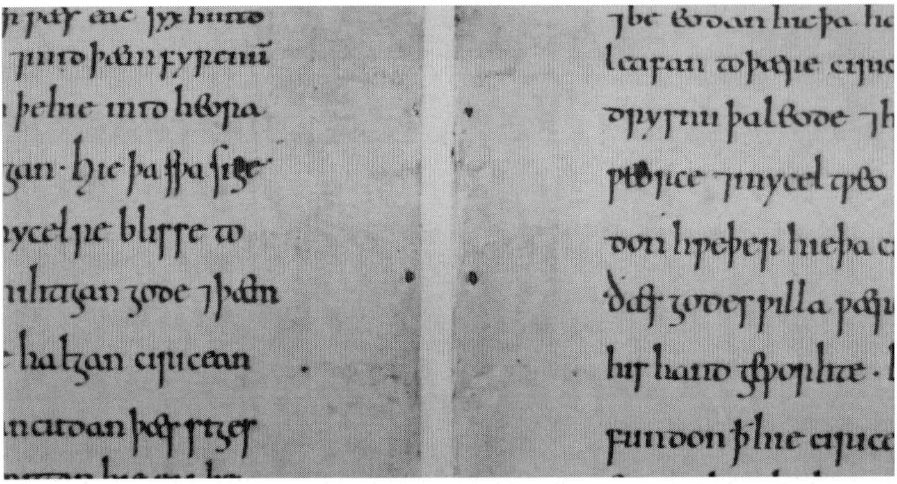

Fig. 3.6 MS Princeton University Library, Scheide Collection M. 71 (the Blickling Homilies): ff. 123v/124r (detail), in 1960 print facsimile.

gatherings needed sequencing, but was this because they had circulated separately, or was this a normal part of Anglo-Saxon binding practice? Ker lists twenty-seven Anglo-Saxon manuscripts which contain possibly original quire signatures.[53] This is an aspect of Anglo-Saxon manuscript practice that would benefit from further study.

One further clue also hints at tactile engagement of this book: the outer leaves of a quire are often soiled, perhaps suggesting circulation unprotected by a binding. Again, the evidence is obscured by the later use of the book, when the book presumably experienced much handling as an oath book. This may have been the time of the loss of four quires from the beginning of the Anglo-Saxon material (as can be inferred from the quire signatures) as well as material from the end. Heavy soiling, discolouration, or rubbing is evident at some quire ends, such as ff. 1r, 31v/32r, 39v/40r, 49v/50r, 64v/65r, 73v/74r, 79v/80r, 86v/87r, 110v/111r (see Fig. 3.7), 120v/121r, 135v/136r, although a similar degree of soiling is evident on a number of openings from within a quire, too, in a book which evidently experienced some rough handling.

Evidence for production and early circulation, then, proves tantalisingly inconclusive in the case of the Blickling Homilies manuscript. Even so, this

[53] N.R. KER, *Catalogue of Manuscripts Containing Anglo-Saxon* (Oxford, 1957; repr. 1990), p. XL, out of the 402 manuscripts that he examines.

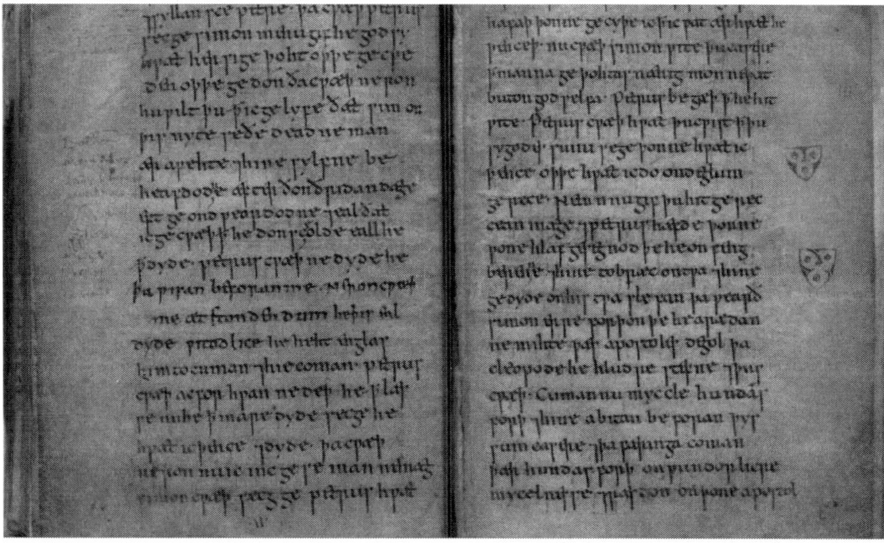

Fig. 3.7 MS Princeton University Libary, Scheide M. 71 (the Blickling Homilies) ff.110v/111r, taken from a screenshot of Princeton University's Digital Library (<http://pudl. princeton.edu/>), courtesy of Scheide Library, Princeton University Library.

case study illustrates how the evidence of craft easily gets lost in a digital presentation. Binding evidence is ill-served by most digital facsimiles. The *British Library Digital Manuscripts* website pleasingly includes images of the cover and of the full sequence of end leaves, even if these are blank. It does not, however, include pictures of the open book seen from above or below, which would facilitate a visual sense of the book's opening action. Just as scale is often ill served by current digital reproductions,[54] so too is point of view. Even if digital images will never provide the same experience as engaging with the book itself, some relatively easy supplements to the current record would allow better engagement with the craft of the book.

[54] As explored by E. TREHARNE, "Fleshing out the text: The transcendent manuscript in the digital age", *postmedieval* 4 (2013), pp. 465-478.

Animating the Disembodied: A New Philology of Touch and Smell

An emphasis on the aura of the original, on embodiment, and on the craft processes involved in creation seems to play up those facets least served by the current digital revolution, but perhaps this does not have to be so. It is almost possible to imagine a future age of virtual manuscript reproduction in which touch and smell and hearing will be served as well as sight. For now, though, the sense of sight predominates, and while some aspects of sight are not yet adequately accounted for, at their best the current crop of digital facsimiles draw viewers into the book and into the page with an intimacy that I want to suggest establishes some kind of aura of the copy. While the digital copy lacks the accumulated history of the original and the veneration that we are willing to accord that, it makes up for it in using the wow factor of new technology to convey through sight an intimacy with an absent object venerated through a kind of digital cleverness.

The paradoxically disengaged engagement of the double logic of remediation works well to spark interest in medieval manuscripts today. It may also spark interest in what is missing – the tactile and olfactory, the sound of the pages and the taste of the words chewed over – and that lack may best be made good through a different contemporary turn, a wealth of craft-centred workshops on book arts. A recent survey of the field shows how book arts and crafts are thriving at precisely this moment of the apogee of the disembodied digital copy, and it charts the array of short-course and institutional opportunities.[55] Creation of books and a revival of book arts may be an effective antidote to what the new technology risks leaving behind.

In yet another paradox, the most important source fuelling this renewed engagement with hands-on book arts is probably the explosion of digital representation. This essay has suggested that the repositories of digital manuscripts provide ready access to images with an aura, if only through the power of magnification and widespread dissemination. Online courses potentially bring the study of the craft of medieval manuscripts to larger audiences. The Institute for Historical Research at the University of London, for example, offers *InScribe: Palaeography Learning Materials* as an online opportunity,[56] while Stanford

[55] E. VASDALL ELLIS, "The east-west, then-now binding nexus", in: *Scraped, Stroked, and Bound: Materially Engaged Readings of Medieval Manuscripts*, ed. J. WILCOX (Turnhout, 2013: *Utrecht Studies in Medieval Literacy* 23), pp. 135-157.

[56] <http://www.history.ac.uk/research-training/courses/online-palaeography>.

University has offered a MOOC on medieval manuscripts: *Digging Deeper: Making Manuscripts*.[57] These disembodied delivery systems can exploit the wide distribution of digital resources to give a taste of hands-on manuscript engagement, albeit mediated by the disembodied new media.

Indeed, web-based presentations on the creation of medieval manuscripts abound. A search for "Making Medieval Manuscripts" on YouTube will currently return about 1,880 relevant returns, incorporating many useful how-to videos on aspects of craft. Some of these make good use of the medium for conveying the craft of manuscript production. A particularly appealing example is *Making Art: Medieval Manuscripts*, provided as part of the *Pharos* website by the Fitzwilliam Museum,[58] which centres on a wonderful animation of the making of the Metz Pontifical (an incomplete fourteenth-century French manuscript), and incorporates embedded short videos of craft technique, including footage of the Macclesfield Psalter being rebound. Another excellent craft video is *Making Manuscripts* released by the Getty Museum,[59] including footage on parchment creating and binding (partly featuring the legendary binder Bill Anthony, who died in 1989), in addition to writing and illustration. A modern example of the creation of an illuminated manuscript, namely the St John Bible created for the contemporary monastic community in Minnesota,[60] also enables handy digital documentation of the craft of manuscript creation.[61]

Digital resources, then, can go some way to telling the story of book craft in a paradoxically hands-on way, even as the best complement to the current digital turn probably lies in a return to the tactile, olfactory, embodied experience of the old-fashioned in-person craft classroom. Jerome McGann suggests in a recent polemical essay that one of the most valuable elements for the continued life of philology has been the Rare Book School at the University of Virginia.[62] The University of Iowa Center for the Book provides professional training in book arts and crafts in an academic context, which makes it part of a growing institutional category recognised through the creation in 2008 of a new professional organisation, the College Book Art Association.

[57] <https://lagunita.stanford.edu/courses/English/DiggingDeeper1/Winter2015/about>.

[58] <http://www.fitzmuseum.cam.ac.uk/pharos/sections/making_art/manuscript.html>.

[59] <https://www.youtube.com/watch?v=nuNfdHNTv9o>.

[60] <http://www.saintjohnsbible.org/>.

[61] <http://www.kbtc.org/page.php?id=330>.

[62] J. McGann, "Philology in a new key", *Critical Inquiry* 39 (2013), pp. 327-346. See also <https://rarebookschool.org/>.

Tactile book studies for medievalists are particularly well served by short courses over the summer. The University of London is a leader in the field, with the Institute of English Studies offering a London International Palaeography Summer School and short courses from the London Rare Books School.[63] In the United States, Timothy Graham has been leading a biannual summer seminar, "Paleography and Codicology: A Seminar on Medieval Manuscript Studies", at the University of New Mexico since 2006.[64] Such hands-on engagement can use the tools that are a traditional strength of the humanities – small group, in-person teaching – augmented by a respect for craft instruction to complement an area of inquiry opened up through the new opportunities of the digital humanities.

This is a trend that has been recognised by the National Endowment for the Humanities, who supported a summer seminar for College and University teachers in the "Materiality of Medieval Manuscripts: Interpretation through Production" that I directed in Summer 2015.[65] This kind of seminar allows scholars drawn by the newly-ubiquitous digital facsimiles to complement the visual acuity provided by the digital image with a taste of embodied craft knowledge of the book that comes from scraping, stretching, and smoothing skin soaked in lime to make parchment; from cutting a quill and then using oak-gall ink to write on the prepared parchment surface; from ruling and designing the layout of a manuscript page; and from stitching and sewing gatherings and preparing and attaching oak boards. Craft practitioners have traditionally handed on such skills through apprenticeships, whereby the new practitioner internalises through repetition the bodily realities of a craft.[66] While a seminar can never imbue expertise in such areas, even brief engagement with the activity encourages a different kind of embodied knowledge of the books that medievalists study. A workshop in such craft skills for academics creates a context for bringing together embodied knowledge with an object of deep academic study. It enables both a critique of what is lacking in the current world of digital humanities and an appreciation of what the digital world is

[63] <http://www.ies.sas.ac.uk/studytraining/research-training-courses>.

[64] <http://www.unm.edu/~medinst/academics/paleography-2014/index.html> [accessed 23 July 2015]. See R.L. McDaniel, "Palaeography and Codicology: A Seminar on Medieval Manuscript Studies, University of New Mexico, Institute for Medieval Studies, June 9-July 3, 2008", *Old English Newsletter* 41.3, <http://www.oenewsletter.org/OEN/print.php/reports/mcdaniel41_3/Array> [accessed 23 July 2015].

[65] See <http://www.uiowa.edu/manuscript-materiality/>.

[66] As described well by Sennet, *The Craftsman*.

making possible. An appreciation of the digital tools combined with a sensory engagement with manuscript craft allows a medievalist scholar to imagine a study of the whole book as perceived through all the body's senses, or what might be considered a philology of touch and smell.[67]

Conclusion

In conclusion, I certainly don't want to downplay the positive value of the digital revolution, which is proving so useful for manuscript study. The present turn from print to digital media gives renewed interest to what can be learned from the earlier medium of the parchment manuscript. Digital reproductions provide unparalleled tools for the study of medieval manuscripts, but the seductiveness of the apparent immediacy should raise cautions over what is missing. A volume centring on sensory perception is a good place to attempt the articulation of a Philology of Smell that takes seriously the complete bodily engagement with the materiality of manuscripts. In a final paradox, the digital revolution and a new-found respect for the academic study of craft may be the perfect combination for an engagement with medieval manuscript studies that draws on all the senses.

[67] See *Scraped, Stroked, and Bound*, which contains the essays of a group of scholars who went through a seminar based on a similar premise in 2008.

The *York Mystery Plays*: Exploring Sound and Hearing in Medieval Vernacular Drama

MARIANA LOPEZ

The *York Mystery Plays* are a series of forty-eight plays in Middle English that narrate events of relevance to the Christian faith and were linked to the Corpus Christi feast. They originated late in the fourteenth century and were performed regularly in York until 1569.[1] The plays had three main aims: to honour and reverence Jesus, to manifest the wealth of the city, and to elicit the devotion of the audiences while eliminating vices.[2] The City Council would issue billets authorising the craft guilds to prepare for the performance,[3] which was outdoors and used wagons specifically constructed for the occasion. The wagons were manhandled through the streets following a predetermined route through the city (the pageant route) and stopping at different street spaces (stations) to perform for an audience.

1 *REED: York*, ed. A. JOHNSTON and M. DORRELL (Toronto, 1979).

2 *REED: York*.

3 E. WHITE, *People and Places: The Social and Topographical Context of Drama in York 1554-1609* (unpublished doctoral thesis, University of Leeds, 1984).

Sensory Perception in the Medieval West, ed. Simon C. THOMSON and Michael D.J. BINTLEY, *Utrecht Studies in Medieval Literacy*, 34 (Turnhout: Brepols, 2016), pp. 53-73.

BREPOLS PUBLISHERS DOI 10.1484/M.USML-EB.5.109504

The importance of the sense of hearing for religious purposes in medieval times, coupled with the significance of hearing in the *York Mystery Plays*, which is noted in the predominance of words over actions as well as the reference of the stations as places to 'hear' the plays,[4] highlights the importance of including discussions on sound in the study of medieval drama. The importance of acoustics has been argued for in connection to Elizabethan theatre but has only received limited attention in the field of medieval drama. Smith has pointed out that actors and directors in the Elizabethan period considered the wooden frames of the theatres as an essential part of a company's tools that could be transported and that influenced the production and propagation of sound.[5] This essay argues that an acoustical analysis of the *York Mystery Plays* may help elucidate whether the importance of acoustical considerations can be extended to medieval York. The findings presented in this article invite scholars to reconsider the importance of the different senses in the medieval period, by suggesting that hearing may have been the primary sense for experiencing dramatic performances.

Performing the York Mystery Plays*: Acting and Singing*

Although extant records of the *York Mystery Plays* provide little information on the actors involved, their training or performance style, there are references to the importance of voice projection in a proclamation from 1415 and an ordinance from 1476.[6] The importance of audibility in the plays can also be linked to the preponderance of words over actions observed in the plays. King has analysed three situations in which this can be observed: voices off, the direction of the audience's attention, and the constraint of actions.[7] She believes that some plays may have included lines that were delivered by a character that was out of the audience's sight ('voice off'), generating suspense by delaying the action and making the actor invisible to the audience. Spoken lines were also used to manipulate the audience's attention. Calls for attention

[4] P. KING, "Seeing and hearing: Looking and listening", *Early Theatre* 3 (2000), pp. 155-166; *REED: York*.

[5] B. SMITH, *The Acoustic World of Early Modern England: Attending to the O-Factor* (Chicago, 1999).

[6] *REED: York*; M. ROGERSON, "Devotional acting: Sydney 2008 and medieval York", in: *The York Mystery Plays: Performance in the City*, ed. M. ROGERSON (York, 2011), pp. 205-225.

[7] KING, "Seeing and hearing".

can be found at the openings of several of the plays and in many cases they are requests to the audience to listen instead of requests for silence.[8] Words can also provide restrictions to the actions; for example, it is Mary's *planctus* at the cross that expresses her grief, not the action of weeping.[9]

'How' the lines were delivered is also of relevance.[10] Questions of volume and pitch may have been essential to the performance; the inclusion of tyrannical characters would have resulted in exceptionally loud voices used to convey a sense of bullying.[11] Voice projection can also be related to the plays. Training in such skill was common to many occupations, including preachers, therefore the fact that twenty-two plays have openings that resemble preaching may be an indication of the mode of delivery.[12]

Music was an important part of life in the Middle Ages, and York was no exception. Music was performed within religious institutions such as parish churches, monasteries and the Minster, as well as in secular contexts where it was performed by minstrels.[13] Religious music could be monophonic (only one melodic line) or polyphonic (two or more melodic lines), and it was monophonic plainchant that was most commonly used for worship.[14] Singers were trained in cathedrals and monastic schools and their training would have included learning the Psalter and the plainchant repertory by heart, as well as reading Latin and plainchant notation; a select group of singers was also trained in polyphonic singing.[15] The majority of the members of the clergy would have been able to perform plainchant items as part of the daily worship.[16]

References to singing in the *York Mystery Plays* are associated with two types of figure: angels and good human characters.[17] Angelic singing is used in the plays to benefit worthy listeners, such as the Virgin Mary, and to provide

[8] KING, "Seeing and hearing"; P. KING, "Poetics and beyond: Noisy bodies and aural variations in medieval English outdoor performance", *14th Triennial Colloquium of the Société Internationale pour l'étude du Théâtre Médiéval*, Poznań, Poland, 22-27 July 2013, available at <http://www.staff.amu.edu.pl/%7Epber/Pamela%20King.pdf> [last accessed 02/11/15].

[9] KING, "Seeing and hearing".

[10] KING, "Poetics and beyond".

[11] KING, "Poetics and beyond".

[12] KING, "Poetics and beyond".

[13] C. DAVIDSON, *Corpus Christi Plays at York: A Context for Religious Drama* (New York, 2013).

[14] R. RASTALL, *The Heaven Singing: Music in Early English Religious Drama*, 1 (Cambridge, 1996).

[15] RASTALL, *The Heaven Singing.*

[16] RASTALL, *The Heaven Singing.*

[17] RASTALL, *The Heaven Singing.*

a glimpse of Heaven.[18] Human characters that do God's will can also sing to praise God.[19] The identification of musical items in the plays is not due to the inclusion of notated music in the manuscript but to the analysis of different elements, including dramatic directions, text references and the use of Latin.[20] Dramatic directions provide references to the inclusion of vocal music, and in some cases the piece to be performed is specified by the inclusion of an *incipit*.[21] Textual references to music within the plays can also further the understanding of musical performances; for example, in *The Shepherds*, the title characters comment on the *Gloria* sung by the angel, their own imitation of this piece, and the song they sing on their way to Bethlehem.[22] The use of Latin passages sourced from the liturgy can also be an indication of a sung piece.[23]

The sparseness of notated music is related to the fact that medieval music tradition was mainly aural; music was often sourced from the liturgy and such items were often memorised. If singers needed to consult the pieces they could use their own service books by referring to the verbal *incipits* included in the text.[24] Therefore, the inclusion of *incipits* in the play texts indicates that they were sung in their customary musical setting.[25] The lack of notated music could indicate that the pieces were sung monophonically, to improvised polyphony or that there was a polyphonic version of the piece that was known to the performers; while the addition of a musical *incipit* may indicate that a particular version of a piece was used.[26] Furthermore, the non-inclusion of notated music could indicate that the music was pre-existent while its inclusion would indicate that it was a newly composed piece.[27]

The only surviving notated music from the plays is found in *The Assumption of the Virgin*. The composition dates from 1430-1440 and consists of three polyphonic pieces: *Surge, proxima mea*; *Veni de Libano, sponsa*; and *Veni,*

[18] R. RASTALL, *Minstrels Playing: Music in Early English Religious Drama*, 2 (Cambridge, 2001).

[19] RASTALL, *Minstrels Playing*.

[20] RASTALL, *The Heaven Singing*; RASTALL, *Minstrels Playing*.

[21] RASTALL, *Minstrels Playing*.

[22] RASTALL, *The Heaven Singing*; RASTALL, *Minstrels Playing*.

[23] RASTALL, *The Heaven Singing*.

[24] RASTALL, *The Heaven Singing*.

[25] RASTALL, *The Heaven Singing*.

[26] RASTALL, *The Heaven Singing*.

[27] RASTALL, *The Heaven Singing*.

electa mea.[28] The manuscript includes two polyphonic versions of each text and all pieces were composed in the same period, in two parts and in the mezzo-soprano range. The "A versions" are included in the body of the text at the appropriate points of the play. Musically, they are homorhythmic (the different voices share similar rhythmic characteristics), they present short and clear music phrases as well as simultaneous cadences.[29] The "B versions", on the other hand, are copied at the end of the play; they present free counterpoint (a more complex and less strict form of interconnection among the voices) and include overlaps at cadences.[30]

Trained singers from the York Minster and parish churches may have performed the most complex vocal pieces and may have even participated in more than one play.[31] It is also possible that the actors themselves performed the simpler, congregational chants, since they would have been familiar with the musical items from their use in liturgical services.[32]

The following sections will explore how audiences interacted with the performances as well as different theories on the staging of the plays and their impact on acting and singing.

Audiences

The performance of the *York Mystery Plays* would have included three main audience positions. The first one is the group of eminent individuals such as the Lord Mayor, the Lady Mayoress and the aldermen who would have been feasting while watching the performance from the windows of buildings along the pageant route.

A different audience position may have been the result of people hiring a place at a scaffold set up at a playing station. Evidence for the use of scaffolds dates from 1417 and is recorded in the *A/Y Memorandum Book* where it is stated that the people who receive money from the scaffolds set up before their doors in public property should pay a third of their earnings to the chamber-

[28] *Six Songs from the York Mystery Play 'The Assumption of the Virgin'*, ed. R. RASTALL (North Harton, 1984).

[29] *Six Songs*, ed. RASTALL; RASTALL, *The Heaven Singing*.

[30] *Six Songs*, ed. RASTALL; RASTALL, *The Heaven Singing*.

[31] RASTALL, *The Heaven Singing*.

[32] RASTALL, *The Heaven Singing*.

lains.[33] This reference is the only extant record of the use of scaffolds; there is no documentation indicating how they were constructed or if they were used after this year.[34] Furthermore, the record suggests that scaffolds may have been used only in 1417 and only ever in Micklegate and, possibly, in the Pavement, which were the widest sections of the pageant route.[35]

Although no information has survived regarding the characteristics of the scaffolds, it is possible to gain an insight through the analysis of Fouquet's miniature *The Martyrdom of St. Apollonia*.[36] Fouquet's depiction shows a kneeling and standing audience at ground level, quite close to the action, while the different scaffolds have floors raised by supporting posts.[37] An upper storey in each structure is formed by the inclusion of frames or rods that support the curtains, which enclose the structure at the top, sides and back.[38]

Audiences of the *York Mystery Plays* could also have watched the performance free of charge by standing at the playing stations. Meredith argues that the standing audience would have been essentially mobile, reorganising the narrative by viewing the plays, either by chance or by choice, in a different order, some pageants more than once and others not at all.[39] Rastall explains that standing audiences, due to their proximity to the actors, would have had a greater involvement in the actions portrayed.[40] Audience members could have participated by responding 'Amen' to blessings and by singing the plainchant items.[41]

[33] *REED: York*.

[34] P. MEREDITH, "The fifteenth-century audience of the York *Corpus Christi* play: Records and speculation", in: *'Divers toyes mengled': Essays on Medieval and Renaissance Culture in Honour of Andre Lascombes*, ed. M. BITOT, R. MULLINI and P. HAPPÉ (Tours, 1996), pp. 101-111.

[35] MEREDITH, "Fifteenth-century audience".

[36] D. CROUCH, "Paying to see the play: The stationholders on the route of the York *Corpus Christi* play in the fifteenth century", *Medieval English Theatre* 13 (1991), pp. 64-111.

[37] R. SOUTHERN, *The Medieval Theatre in the Round: A Study of the Staging of The Castle of Perseverance and Related Matters* (London, 1975).

[38] SOUTHERN, *Medieval Theatre in the Round.*

[39] MEREDITH, "Fifteenth-century audience".

[40] RASTALL, *The Heaven Singing.*

[41] RASTALL, *The Heaven Singing.*

Staging the York Mystery Plays

One of the most challenging aspects of research into the *York Mystery Plays* is the lack of information regarding the wagons used. The only surviving documentation on how the York wagons were constructed refers to the Mercers' guild and the play of *The Last Judgement*. The most relevant document is a 1433 indenture,[42] which indicates a complex structure, consisting of a pageant with wheels that has four iron poles, a heaven of iron, clouds, a rainbow made of timber, cloths for the back and the sides of the wagon, a seat of iron that would allow God to ascend to Heaven, and twenty artificial angels.[43]

In 1501 the Mercers commissioned the construction of a new wagon to Thomas Drawswerd, and since he was a carver it was likely to have been a wooden structure with details carved on it.[44] The roof might have been gabled and there is a mention of windows, which may indicate that the wagon was closed on three sides and they were a means to provide lighting.[45]

The information drawn from the Mercers' documentation provides an incomplete picture of what the wagons looked like. It does not represent a detailed description of how the elements in the inventories are positioned in the overall structure nor does it make reference to dimensions. As a consequence, it is important to resort to other sources. With this aim in mind scholars have studied religious processional events in continental Europe that were contemporary to the *York Mystery Plays*.

Twycross studied the Flemish *ommegangen*, which were religious processions on pageant cars that followed a predetermined route through a town, carrying relics or revered images.[46] The examination of written records as well as paintings, such as van Alsloot's *The Triumph of Archduchess Isabella* (1615), revealed their existence from the fourteenth century, when floats with religious *tableaux* started being included, but the processions existed before this date and included costumed figures representing religious characters.[47] The merchants of York who travelled to the Netherlands in the Middle Ages would

[42] *REED: York*.

[43] A. JOHNSTON and M. DORRELL, "The York mercers and their Pageant of Doomsday, 1433-1526", *Leeds Studies in English*, n.s. 6 (1973), pp. 10-35.

[44] *REED: York*; JOHNSTON and DORRELL, "The York mercers".

[45] *REED: York*; JOHNSTON and DORRELL, "The York mercers".

[46] M. TWYCROSS, "The Flemish *Ommegang* and its pageant cars", *Medieval English Theatre* 2 (1980), pp. 15-41 and pp. 80-92.

[47] TWYCROSS, "Flemish *Ommegang*".

have seen the *ommegangen* and could have returned to England with a description of the wagons, which in turn could have influenced the structures built by the craft guilds in York.[48] The wagons analysed by Twycross have a base shaped as a cube, columns holding a roof and are open on all sides, with the exception of some that include walls or balustrades built up to approximately knee height; roof structures are shown as flat or pitched.[49]

Nelson studied the processions of Good Friday in Valladolid and Holy Thursday in Medina del Campo.[50] The Valladolid procession dates from the sixteenth century and consists of twenty-four wagons that carry sculpted figures representing scenes from the Passion; the wagons used are four-wheeled, steerable, present mechanisms to raise the platform and to provide more floor space, and have curtains covering the wheels.[51] The procession in Medina del Campo includes eight scenes that are represented with sculpted figures on top of platforms and carried through the streets on the shoulders of guildsmen.[52] None of the wagons in either of these processions have roofs or canopies, which Nelson believes would obscure visibility for audiences.[53]

The study of the streets of York can give an indication of the dimensions of the wagons. Multi-level wagons would have had to be lower than the overhanging jetties of the timber-framed buildings or narrow enough to be able to go through the space between them.[54] Since the pageant route was within the city walls, the city gates did not present limitations to the wagon height, which has been suggested as approximately seven metres for a multi-level wagon.[55]

Scholars have considered two main alternatives for the orientation of the wagons during the performances: the side-on and the front-on orientations. Side-on orientation refers to the use of the longer side of the wagon as the front of the performance space, with the actors performing towards the side of the street (the left- or right-hand side of the pageant route). Front-on orientation indicates the use of the front of the wagon as the front of the stage, and in this case the performers would have been playing towards one end of the street.

[48] TWYCROSS, "Flemish *Ommegang*".

[49] TWYCROSS, "Flemish *Ommegang*".

[50] A. NELSON, "Easter Week pageants in Valladolid and Medina del Campo", *Medieval English Theatre* 1 (1979), pp. 62-70.

[51] NELSON, "Easter Week pageants".

[52] NELSON, "Easter Week pageants".

[53] NELSON, "Easter Week pageants".

[54] J. MCKINNELL, "The medieval pageant wagons at York: Their orientation and height", *Early Theatre* 3 (2000), pp. 79-104.

[55] MCKINNELL, "Medieval pageant wagons".

Although arguments for each of the orientations are often polarised, it is worth bearing in mind that staging techniques may have differed among the guilds and the same play may even have varied in its performance according to the station.[56]

In 1992, Twycross suggested that the wagons were used with a front-on orientation, which would have made the wagons more visually impactful as they made their way through the streets, stating that her previous support to the side-on theory had been influenced by the consideration of the wagon as a proscenium stage.[57]

McKinnell also argues for the front-on orientation, stating the visual impact it produces when approaching down the street, the lifting gear not overbalancing the wagon, and less manoeuvring required than with a side-on orientation, as turning to face the corresponding side of the street would not be an issue.[58] Moreover, he considers that side-on wagons would have been too wide for the streets, and in some stations the audience would have been too close to see properly. A front-on wagon, on the other hand, can use as much of the length of the street as necessary.[59] As a downside of the front-on orientation McKinnell mentions the difficulty of using the front of the wagons as an entrance for actors because of the space taken by the steering circle and undercarriage.[60]

It is also necessary to consider how the wagon orientation would have affected audience experience. On this matter, White points out that if scaffolds were placed on the sides of the street for paying audiences then the use of front-on wagons would have resulted in a restricted view that would have been the same or worse than that of the standing audience that was watching the play without charge.[61] Twycross suggests that if enclosed wagons were used, then they are less likely to have had a front-on orientation since an enclosed front-on wagon would have resulted in the view being most likely completely block-

[56] M. ROGERSON, "Raging in the streets of medieval York", *Early Theatre* 3 (2000), pp. 105-125.

[57] M. TWYCROSS, "The left-hand-side theory: A retraction", *Medieval English Theatre* 14 (1992), pp. 77-94; M. TWYCROSS, "'Places to hear the play': Pageant stations at York, 1398-1572", *REED Newsletter* 2 (1978), pp. 10-13.

[58] J. MCKINNELL, "Producing the York *Mary* plays", *Medieval English Theatre* 12 (1990), pp. 101-123.

[59] MCKINNELL, "Producing the York *Mary* plays".

[60] MCKINNELL,, "Producing the York *Mary* plays".

[61] E. WHITE, "Places for hearing the Corpus Christi play in York", *Medieval English Theatre* 9 (1987), pp. 23-63.

ed for those members of the audience (prominent individuals such as the Lord Mayor) watching the plays from windows.[62]

A further drawback of the front-on orientation is that the actors would have strained their voices in order to reach a greater number of people and ensure their involvement in the plays.[63] Moreover, differences in wagon orientation would have resulted in different actor-audience dynamics. Side-on performances in the narrow streets of York would have been more intimate, whereas performing longitudinally would have enabled a greater number of people to see the play.[64]

Questions on the use of the street space by the actors have also been key to discussions on the *York Mystery Plays*. Beadle and King consider that the wagon space would have been insufficient to perform the longer plays, and the street space would have been used.[65] Blasting,[66] on the other hand, argues that the use of street space was not related to space limitations, but to the representation of the journeys taken by the characters. Additionally, the limited space would have forced the performers to be positioned standing next to each other, making the staging technique analogous to representations in the medieval visual arts.[67]

Walsh argues that the relationship between street space and wagon space was particularly important in those plays that included travelling scenes and high places; the street space was utilised to represent the journey of the characters and the wagon represented high places that could also have symbolic significance.[68] Walsh considers the problems of visibility derived from playing at street level only relevant when considering non-paying audiences, since paying audiences would have watched from scaffolds or the windows of nearby buildings.[69] In relation to this, McKinnell suggests that the street-level may have been reserved for those scenes that were loud enough for the audiences not to

[62] TWYCROSS, "Retraction".

[63] WHITE, "Places for hearing"; E. WHITE, "Places to hear the play in York", *Early Theatre* 3 (2000), pp. 49-78.

[64] WHITE, "Places to hear the play in York".

[65] *York Mystery Plays: A Selection in Modern Spelling*, ed. R. BEADLE and P. KING (Oxford, 1995).

[66] R. BLASTING, "The pageant wagon as iconic site in the *York Cycle*", *Early Theatre* 3 (2000), pp. 127-136.

[67] BLASTING, "The pageant wagon".

[68] M. WALSH, "High places and travelling scenes: Some observations on the staging of the York Cycle", *Early Theatre* 3 (2000), pp. 137-154.

[69] WALSH, "High places and travelling scenes".

mind whether the action could be seen.[70] Walsh also points out that the audience at street level may have been accustomed to being in close proximity to the actors, and acquainted enough with the theatre codes of the time to make space for the actors in the travelling scenes.[71]

Rogerson defends the theory of on-wagon performances stating that the stage directions implicit in the dialogues are often interpreted through a modern conception of theatre in which words that refer to an action or movement will be accompanied by the corresponding action, but limited movements on the wagon could have been just as effective in creating the illusion of travelling.[72]

Acoustics, Sound and Hearing

The exploration of the importance of sound and hearing in medieval times evidences the relevance of considering acoustics in relation to the plays, by studying both speech and music, two elements that were considered integral to medieval religious practice. Central to the *York Mystery Plays* was the desire to reverence Christ. Forms of art in the Middle Ages had a didactic purpose and there was no differentiation between beauty and utility.[73] Tydeman explains that medieval drama was able to express the Christian faith in a captivating way for those who were not able to read.[74] The importance of the reverence of Christ combined with the desire to communicate religious doctrine to the audience indicates that the lines delivered and the music performed would have needed to be as intelligible and engaging as possible, so that the Christian message could be transmitted to the audience. Therefore it is difficult to imagine staging and performance decisions that did not consider aural aspects to be crucial to the performance.

Reflecting on York's 'soundscape' during the performances is key to the analysis of the experiences of actors and audiences. The term 'soundscape' refers to the perception of all sounds modified by the environment in a particu-

[70] McKinnell, "Medieval pageant wagons".

[71] Walsh, "High places and travelling scenes".

[72] Rogerson, "Raging in the streets".

[73] U. Eco, *Art and Beauty in the Middle Ages*, trans. H. Bredin (New Haven, 1986).

[74] W. Tydeman, "An introduction to medieval English theatre", in: *The Cambridge Companion to Medieval English Theatre*, ed. R. Beadle (Cambridge, 1994), pp. 1-36.

lar context. Such modifications can include the effect of meteorological conditions as well as the effects of sound reflection, absorption and diffraction.[75]

During the performances of the *York Mystery Plays* the soundscape would have included different types of sounds: those that were intentionally produced during the performance, those that were a result of the performance but were not part of the narrative, and those sounds that were independent from the performance.

The first category of sounds, those that were included intentionally as part of the performance, would include the actors' voices, music, and sound effects, such as the use of a thunder machine to represent hell.[76] An essential characteristic for the actors was the ability to project their voices and make themselves audible.[77] Furthermore, the preponderance of the word over the action described by King seems to indicate that it must have been necessary for most of the audience to be able to hear the words as clearly as possible.[78] Although voice projection and volume would have been essential in achieving audibility it is also necessary to consider the role of the acoustics of the performance spaces (playing stations and wagons) in enhancing or compromising intelligibility. Acoustic considerations in relation to the music of the plays are also essential. It is of relevance to study how the performance of plainchant items was affected by their rendition and reception in outdoor spaces, considering that these items were composed to suit the very different acoustic characteristics of religious spaces, and it was in such spaces that they would have been regularly heard.[79]

The second type of sounds populating the soundscape were a result of the performance but not part of the narrative. They included the sound of the mechanisms used to move God between Heaven and Earth in the Mercers' pageant, the sound of the wagon wheels as they were moved along the pageant route, and the conversations among men pushing the wagons from station to station.[80] Audiences would also have contributed to the soundscape by chatter-

[75] ISO 12913-1, *Acoustics – Soundscape – Part 1: Definition and conceptual framework*, International Organization for Standardization.

[76] DAVIDSON, *Corpus Christi Plays at York*; KING, "Poetics and beyond".

[77] *REED: York*; KING, "Poetics and beyond"; ROGERSON, "Devotional acting".

[78] KING, "Seeing and hearing".

[79] M. BARRON, *Auditorium Acoustics and Architectural Design* (London, 1993).

[80] DAVIDSON, *Corpus Christi Plays at York*; KING, "Poetics and beyond".

ing between plays and, in the case of those watching the plays from within buildings, there was the sound coming from their feasts.[81]

The last type of sounds includes those independent of the performance. The church bells would have rung to mark the canonical hours, and the sound from the liturgical services emanating from the religious institutions would have been audible from the city streets.[82] Sounds resulting from the presence of animals as well as sounds associated with weather conditions would have completed the soundscape.[83]

The three types of sounds listed above are interconnected, and the consideration of speech and vocal music in relation to the acoustics of the performance spaces needs to include an awareness of the possible impact other sounds had on them. It is very likely that sounds such as the church bell or the chatter of audiences affected intelligibility and the audience's involvement. Furthermore, there might have been instances in which the convergence of different types of sounds aided the overall reception of the plays. For example, music could have been used while God moved between Heaven and Earth to mask the sound produced by the lifting mechanism.[84]

The following section focuses on the study of the impact of the acoustic features of the performances spaces on speech and vocal music.

The Acoustics of the York Mystery Plays

As was observed above, researchers studying the performance of the *York Mystery Plays* face the challenge of working with information that is often scarce and open to several interpretations. Such a challenge can benefit from combining knowledge and methodologies from the humanities and sciences. Furthermore, the application of digital technologies to medieval studies can allow us to revisit research questions and analyse them in previously unthought-of ways.

My research acknowledges the importance of such interdisciplinary approaches as well as the relevance of digital technologies by applying acoustical analyses to the study of the *York Mystery Plays*. I have used a combination of

[81] DAVIDSON, *Corpus Christi Plays at York*.
[82] DAVIDSON, *Corpus Christi Plays at York*; KING, "Poetics and beyond".
[83] DAVIDSON, *Corpus Christi Plays at York*; KING, "Poetics and beyond".
[84] KING, "Poetics and beyond".

acoustic measurement techniques and computer models to further our understanding of the impact of the street spaces and wagon structures on performance and reception.[85] The use of computer models allows for numerous changes to be made to the geometry of the performance spaces, the acoustic properties of the surface materials, and the positions of actors / singers and listeners, which facilitates experimentation.

My focus has been on Stonegate, the better preserved of the playing stations, in the sixteenth century. I designed eight different computer models to reflect the unknowns linked to the space in the period of interest; the versions differed from one another in relation to the height of the buildings, the windows being open or closed, and the type of window used (in-line with the wall or projecting). I also incorporated wagons to the street simulations to explore their impact on the acoustics, as well as the repercussions of wagon orientation (side-on or front-on) and the positions of performers and audience members.

I simulated two contrasting examples of wagon structures. The first type of wagon is a multi-level design based on the 1433 Mercers' wagon of *The Last Judgement* with its lower section representing Earth closed on three sides with curtains and with a wooden deck. The upper deck, which represents Heaven, has a wooden base, and a wooden surface is also included at the back.

The second type of wagon is based on *The Nativity*-wagon in van Alsloot's painting *The Triumph of Archduchess Isabella* (1615). It consists of a wooden deck and a wooden pitched roof supported by four wooden columns. Both wagons have a depth of 1.83 metres, a length of 3.66 metres and include curtains covering the wheels. The first wagon is 6.7 metres high and the second 6.17 metres.

Below I present a short introduction to room acoustics to help with the interpretation of my research results.

[85] M. Lopez, S. Pauletto and G. Kearney, "The application of impulse response measurement techniques to the study of the acoustics of *Stonegate*, a performance space used in medieval English drama", *Acta Acustica united with Acustica* 99 (2013), pp. 98-109; M. Lopez, "Objective evaluation of a simulation of the acoustics of a medieval urban space used for dramatic performances", *Applied Acoustics* 88 (2015), pp. 38-43; Ead., "Using multiple computer models to study the acoustics of a sixteenth-century performance space", *Applied Acoustics* 94 (2015), pp. 14-19; Ead., "Acoustics, performers and audiences in medieval English drama", *Auditorium Acoustics 2015*, Paris, France, 29-31 October 2015; Ead., "An acoustical approach to the study of the wagons of the *York Mystery Plays*: Structure and orientation", *Early Theatre Journal* 18.2 (2015), pp. 11-36.

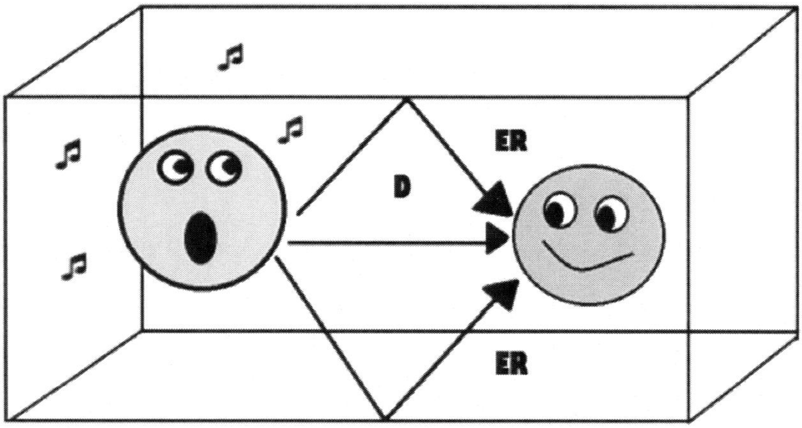

Fig. 4.1 Representation of *direct sound* (D) and the *early reflections* (ER) arriving at the listener.

Acoustical Concepts

Research into room acoustics considers the components of the sound arriving at the listener, which are the 'direct sound', the 'early reflections' and the 'reverberant sound'. 'Direct sound' is the sound that travels in a straight line, which is the shortest path between sound source and listener. It is heard first and provides information about the location of the sound source; it is essential to intelligibility. 'Early reflections' are the discrete sounds that arrive at the listener after the 'direct sound', and which have reflected off one or more surfaces (see Fig. 4.1). 'Early reflections' are highly dependent on the position of the source and listener as well as on the shape of the space. They increase the sense of loudness, augment the sense of spaciousness (if arriving at the side of the listener), increase intelligibility and provide a sense of intimacy.[86] The 'reverberant sound' arrives after the 'early reflections', having travelled through numerous paths. Reflections arrive at the listener very close one from the other and from all directions. 'Reverberant sound' remains constant regardless of changes in source and listener positions; it is diffuse, that is, there is equal probability of it visiting any of the parts of the space. The drop in levels of both 'early reflections' and 'reverberant sound' is affected by sound absorp-

[86] BARRON, *Auditorium Acoustics*.

tion, which is the removal of acoustic energy from a space due to the presence of different surface materials.

The acoustical analysis presented in this article applies the components described above through four objective parameters: reverberation time (T30), clarity (C50, C80) and spatial impression (IACC_{E3}/Interaural Cross-Correlation Coefficient-Early). Reverberation time is the time in seconds that it takes for sound to decay by 60dB after the sound source has stopped emitting sound. It is a result of the dimensions of the space as well as the absorption properties of the surface materials. The optimum reverberation time for a space depends on its function. If a space is used mainly for the spoken word then speech intelligibility is of the utmost importance; therefore, short reverberation times will be preferred. If a space is used for music performances, the optimum reverberation time depends on the type of music performed. Music that is characterised by short notes and complex rhythmic patterns will benefit from short reverberation times that will enable the listener to distinguish every note, while music that is slow and rhythmically simple would benefit from longer reverberation times.[87]

Clarity is an early-to-late arriving energy ratio expressed in decibels (dB), which can be calculated using C50 or C80. C50 considers the division between early and late energy as 50 milliseconds and gives an indication of speech intelligibility and definition in a space, whereas C80 is more suitable for the analysis of music and uses 80 milliseconds to divide early from late energy. Both direct sound and early reflections are considered within the early energy, whereas reverberant sound constitutes the late arriving energy. A predominance of early energy will result in higher clarity values, since early reflections fuse with the direct sound and provide higher definition,[88] which results in better speech intelligibility and the perception of musical detail. Furthermore, clarity is higher when the listener is nearer to the source due to the prominence of the direct sound. In the case of rhythmically complex musical items high levels of clarity will be preferable since each sound will be more distinct, whereas in the case of performances of, for instance, plainchant items, which present slow melodic lines, lower values of C80 would be beneficial.

The IACC_{E3} parameter is used to study Apparent Source Width (ASW), which is associated with the perceptual broadening of the sound source and is

[87] L. BERANEK, *Music, Acoustics & Architecture* (New York and London, 1962).

[88] G. SOULODRE and J. BRADLEY, "Subjective evaluation of new room acoustic measures", *Journal of the Acoustical Society of America* 98.1 (1995), pp. 294-301.

determined by the presence of early lateral reflections. The connection between an increase in the ASW and early lateral reflections is a result of the fusion of direct sound and early reflections, which increases the perceived level of the direct sound.[89] Reflections arriving at the sides of the listener (90 degrees) result in the most prominent effects.[90] The $IACC_{E3}$ parameter measures the dissimilarity of signals arriving at both ears considering the first 80 milliseconds of the energy averaged across 500Hz-2kHz. Music audiences prefer lower values, which correspond to a greater dissimilarity between the signals and indicate a larger ASW.[91]

Acoustical Analysis of the York Mystery Plays

Although most acoustical analyses focus on absolute numerical values, my research has instead centred on the differences that result from analysing possible characteristics of the street space as well as a variety of staging configurations. Furthermore, objective parameters cannot tell us how the plays were perceived and experienced in past cultures; they can only indicate possible changes connected to alterations in the performance space. Caution should be exercised when arriving at conclusions, as modern forms of listening should not be assigned to past cultures.[92]

The analysis of the eight different computer models of sixteenth-century Stonegate indicated that the alternation between buildings with open and closed windows resulted in changes in reverberation time and clarity, with the models that had no windows resulting in shorter reverberation times and higher clarity values. This simulated the effect produced if all windows had been opened for people to watch the performances from inside. Differences in the height of the street facades also produced variations in the reverberation time

[89] SOULODRE and BRADLEY, "Subjective evaluation".

[90] M. BARRON and H. MARSHALL, "Spatial impression due to early lateral reflections in concert halls: The derivation of a physical measure", *Journal of Sound and Vibration* 77.2 (1981), pp. 211-232.

[91] Y. ANDO, *Concert Hall Acoustics* (Berlin, 1985); M.R. SCHROEDER, D. GOTTLOB and K.F. SIEBRASSE, "Comparative study of European concert halls: Correlation of subjective preference with geometric and acoustic parameters", *Journal of the Acoustical Society of America* 56.4 (1974), pp. 1195-1201.

[92] The present essay does not include the numerical analysis of the results linked to the different acoustical parameters; instead it focuses on the main findings. For full acoustical analyses, see the articles listed in n. 85.

and clarity, higher buildings resulting in longer reverberation time and lower clarity. Changes in the window type did not produce any significant differences, and $IACC_{E3}$ presented negligible variations as a result of the changes across the virtual models. These findings show that buildings with higher facades and closed windows would have resulted in a better acoustic experience for both performers and audiences. However, details on every building on Stonegate and their use in the period of interest remain unknown, so all possible alternatives need to be considered.

Research also demonstrated that reverberation time and clarity were affected by the incorporation of wagon structures, with the former presenting, in general, a drop in values, and the latter evidencing an increase. The inclusion of wagon structures also affected $IACC_{E3}$ values by indicating a general tendency towards an improvement in the ASW.

The results showed there were differences in all acoustical parameters as a result of the change of wagon orientation, and these were particularly evident when the wagon closed on three sides was used. The side-on orientation resulted in a longer reverberation time than the front-on wagon, whereas the front-on wagon resulted in higher clarity and a larger ASW. It is important to bear in mind that, although values for clarity and ASW are lower for the side-on orientation, they are still within the range considered appropriate for speech and music. Furthermore, the increase in clarity in the front-on wagon is detrimental to the performance of plainchant items, and it is at the expense of the reverberation time. As a result, it is the side-on orientation that provided the most suitable acoustic setting.

Another point for analysis was focussed on the effects of changes in the performers' location. The comparison of performers positioned on the Heaven deck to those at street level and on the lower deck (representing the Earth) demonstrated that the use of sound sources on the upper deck resulted in longer reverberation times, lower clarity and an increase in ASW, particularly emphasised when using a front-on orientation. These acoustical characteristics are fitting to the use of the Heaven deck for musical performances representing angelic singing, bringing visual and aural aspects together during the performance.

The effect of audiences was analysed through the addition of two standing audience areas at the sides of the wagons and scaffolds placed against the right-hand side of the pageant route. Scaffolds were modelled consisting of three

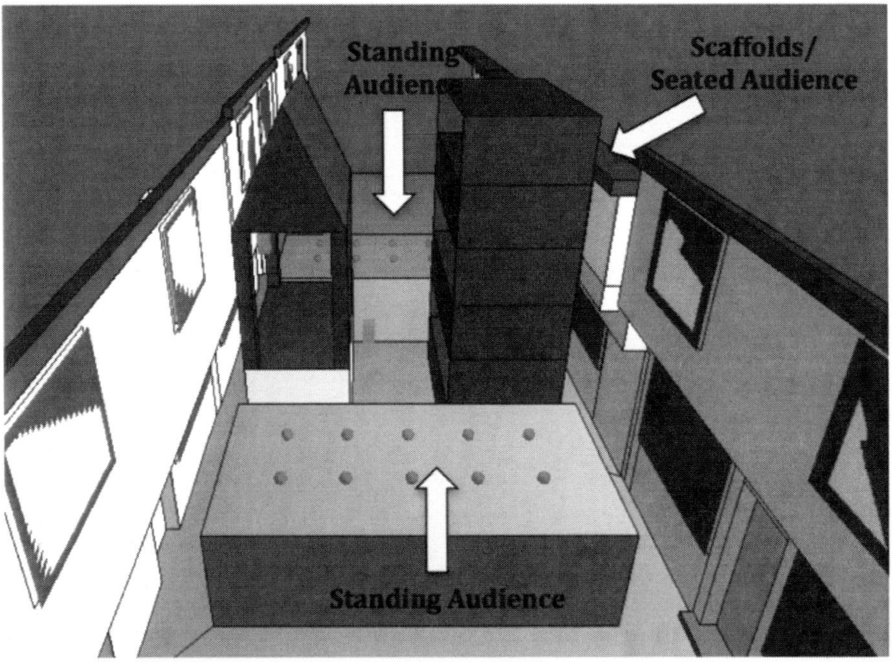

Fig. 4.2 Simulation of medieval Stonegate with a wagon, a three-levelled scaffold for paying audiences and two areas for standing audiences. The surfaces in different purple shades indicate sound absorption and scattering associated with the presence of an audience whereas the green surfaces indicate a wooden structure. The red spheres represent the listeners.

different levels and simulated as wooden structures 6 metres high, 2 metres deep and 3.66 metres long. It should be noted that, due to the very sparse evidence on the appearance and use of scaffolds for the *York Mystery Plays*, the manner in which this was modelled represents only one out of many possible interpretations of their design and implementation. The idea of having audiences at different levels was drawn from Fouquet's painting *The Martyrdom of St. Apollonia*. Southern's analysis of Fouquet's painting only identifies audiences at two levels and suggests that the scaffolds were built using supporting frames and that they were covered by curtains on the sides, top and back. The virtual models I used were only partially based on Southern's analysis, as the intention was to determine the effect on the acoustics of Stonegate resulting from a structure that consisted of surfaces with low absorption coefficients. The objective of this decision was to arrive at an understanding of what may have been the longest reverberation times achievable through a modification of the audience area, whilst still using a plausible design.

When studying the acoustics of theatres or concert halls, acousticians often warn venue designers of the impact of the presence of audiences on the acoustics, since they introduce additional absorption and scattering. However, the introduction of audience areas to Stonegate had a positive acoustical effect: the reverberation time increased, in particular in relation to the second and third levels of the scaffolds, making the space more suitable for vocal performances. Moreover, it is interesting to explore how different acoustical characteristics can be associated with different audience areas. Seated audiences, who would have paid for their seats, seem to have been at positions where the reverberation time is longer while still retaining high levels of clarity. These characteristics seem to indicate that paying audiences had better seats for both the spoken and sung extracts from the plays. However, when considering the ASW, it is standing audiences that would have enjoyed better positions. These differences prompt questions on the aural preferences of audiences at the time of the performances, which may be relevant to the period studied but may not be the same characteristics preferred by modern audiences. Equations used in modern acoustics for the calculation of parameters attempt to reproduce auditory perception by assuming that it is identical in all individuals across cultures, but that is not necessarily the case.[93] Studies have shown that even changes in whether listeners are musicians or non-musicians, or whether they own a recorded version of a piece they are listening to or not, may have effects on the perception of room acoustics.[94] If such changes within the same culture produce variations in perception it can be safely assumed that the acoustic preferences of audiences in medieval times were different from ours. Research into other medieval spaces used for both speech and music can start to shed light on what those preferences were and how they might be used to reinterpret our findings.

[93] B. BLESSER and L.-R. SALTER, *Spaces Speak, Are you Listening?* (Cambridge, MA, 2007).

[94] T. COX and B. SHIELD, "Audience questionnaire survey of the acoustics of the Royal Festival Hall, London, England", *Acustica* 85.4 (1999), pp. 547-559.

Conclusions

The differences in acoustics due to changes in the staging of the plays makes it possible to argue that the organisers could have used the street spaces and their wagons to make the most of the acoustic characteristics. Although the physical reasons behind these differences in acoustics may not have been understood, they may have been explored through a process of trial-and-error. The wagons themselves might have been built in different manners to accommodate the need for better-suited acoustics.

When discussing Elizabethan drama above, it was mentioned that companies of actors considered the wooden frames of their theatres as an essential part of their equipment and that they could transport them if necessary. It may be possible to apply a similar notion to the guilds and their wagons. These wagons were also an essential tool for the performances; guilds were willing to maintain them throughout the years, preserve them from damages, rebuild or adapt them, and pay for special places for their storage. Therefore, they may have been to the guilds as precious as the wooden frames used for Elizabethan theatres to their actors, and they may have also been aware of how their use modified sound during performances.

The evidence of the relevance of acoustics in the *York Mystery Plays* explored in this article highlights the importance of sound in the period and paves the way for further studies on the sense of hearing in relation to other forms of medieval drama across Europe. It also urges scholars to reconsider the primacy of the different senses and to analyse how performance and staging decisions might have followed an 'aural approach' instead of a visual one.

Birds and Words: Aurality, Semantics, and Species in Anglo-Saxon England

ERIC LACEY

The hearing ear, and the seeing eye, the Lord hath made even both of them – Proverbs 20:12

The King James Bible's rendition of Proverbs 20:12 can be read variously, depending on whether 'even' is read adjectivally (i.e. they are made equal) or adverbially (i.e. the Lord made them indeed). Whichever is the case is more or less irrelevant here, as these two senses – hearing and seeing – are repeatedly invoked in the Bible as those which grant or allow access to knowledge.[1] This would have been as true for the majority of Anglo-Saxons, too: even literacy, the privilege of the religious and a select few among the

[1] E.g. Genesis 24:30; Exodus 3:7; Numbers 24:4; Deuteronomy 4:12, 18:16 and 29:4; 1 Samuel 3:11; 1 Kings 3:28 and 10:7; 2 Kings 6:30, 19:16 and 20:5; Nehemiah 9:9; Job 29:11; Isaiah 5:7; Ezekiel 1:28; Luke 23:8; Acts 7:31 and 8:6; Revelation 22:8.

Sensory Perception in the Medieval West, ed. Simon C. THOMSON and Michael D.J. BINTLEY, *Utrecht Studies in Medieval Literacy*, 34 (Turnhout: Brepols, 2016), pp. 75-98.

BREPOLS PUBLISHERS DOI 10.1484/M.USML-EB.5.109505

laity, depended on these two senses for its acquisition and practice.[2] Sight and sound would have been the principal faculties used for quotidian tasks, and would have frequently prefaced any other kind of stimulation: objects are seen before they are touched, people and animals are (often) heard before they are seen, food is seen (or smelled) before it is tasted, and so on. There is a bias towards the visual in scholarship: historically, scientific enquiry privileged the observable, and observable data (whether written or illustrative) was well-suited to being textually transmitted.[3] This is a bias which we must confront when embarking on recovery of sensory perception in the medieval world, in which the unseen was at least as influential as the seen.[4] Blindness and partial-sightedness might be considered some of the more significant barriers to functional independence today, but that is because priority is placed on interacting with the visual: reading, writing, navigating and so on. However, in the Middle Ages, deafness was a greater impediment to the wellbeing of individuals because it precluded them from hearing – and therefore understanding – the word of God.[5] In the chiefly oral society of the Anglo-Saxons, wherein speaking and hearing were the main means of exchange between individuals, aurality would have been the primary means of receiving and imparting knowledge.

[2] On literacy see H. MAGENNIS, "Audience(s), reception, literacy", in: *A Companion to Anglo-Saxon Literature*, ed. P. PULSIANO and E. TREHARNE (Oxford, 2008), pp. 84-101; G.H. BROWN, "The dynamics of literacy in Anglo-Saxon England", in: *Textual and Material Culture in Anglo-Saxon England: Thomas Northcote Toller and The Toller Memorial Lectures*, ed. D. SCRAGG (Cambridge, 2003), pp. 183-212, and D.H. GREEN, *Medieval Listening and Reading: The Primary Reception of German Literature, 800-1300* (Cambridge, 2005).

[3] This tendency is implicit, but nonetheless clear, in the histories of science, biology and ornithology. For general histories of science see D.C. LINDBERG, *The Beginnings of Western Science* (Chicago, 1992); E. GRANT, *The Foundations of Modern Science in the Middle Ages: Their Religious, Institutional and Cultural Contexts* (Cambridge, 1996); E. GRANT, *Science and Religion, 400 B.C. to A.D. 1550* (Baltimore, 2004); E. GRANT, *A History of Natural Philosophy: From the Ancient World to the Nineteenth Century* (Cambridge, 2007). A history specifically on biology is E. MAYR, *The Growth of Biological Thought: Diversity, Evolution and Inheritance* (London, 1982); histories specifically concerning ornithology are E. STRESEMAN, *Ornithology: From Aristotle to the Present* (London, 1975); M. WALTERS, *A Concise History of Ornithology* (London, 2003); and P. BIRCHAM, *A History of Ornithology* (London, 2007).

[4] This is arguably more true for the perceived workings of the Christian God than it is for those superstitious elements in traditional culture; see A. HALL, *Elves in Anglo-Saxon England: Matters of Health, Gender, and Identity* (Woodbridge, 2007), esp. pp. 67-68.

[5] I. METZLER, *A Social History of Disability in the Middle Ages: Cultural Considerations of Physical Impairment* (Abingdon, 2013), esp. pp. 200-201.

The importance of aurality (and orality) in Anglo-Saxon culture has been well considered in some respects, but not in others.[6] The Anglo-Saxon perception of birds falls into the latter. While the importance of bird calls has frequently been noted as underlying (at least) some Old English bird names,[7] discussions of these have almost always been predicated on equating these bird names with the visually-oriented identifications given pride of place today. Essentially, they fall into the fallacy of supposing that "the Anglo-Saxons' way of looking at the world is essentially the same as the modern one, except that the words are different".[8] Underlying this mentality, too, is the assumption that there is some kind of objectivity inherent in the categorisation – i.e. the speciation – we have of birds today. There is not. This mentality, which we may term an essentialist approach, derives ultimately from the Aristotelian tradition of essences, and it asserts that there is some objective essential basis by which species are differentiated.[9]

Semantics, Species and Taxonomies

Speciation is categorisation.[10] These acts of vernacular quotidian speciation are commonly known as 'folk-taxonomies', and they are closely bound up with

[6] See, for example, the essays in *Orality and Textuality in the Middle Ages*, ed. A.N. DOANE and C. BRAUN PASTERNACK (London, 1991); A. JORGENSEN, "The trumpet and the wolf: Noises of battle in Old English poetry", *Oral Tradition* 24.2 (2009), pp. 319-326; R. DANCE, "*Þær wearð hream ahafen*: A note on Old English spelling and the sound of *The Battle of Maldon*", in: *The Power of Words: Anglo-Saxon Studies Presented to Donald G. Scragg on his Seventieth Birthday*, ed. J. WILCOX and H. MAGENNIS (Morgantown, 2006), pp. 278-317. In relation to birds see K. POOLE and E. LACEY, "Avian aurality in Anglo-Saxon England", *World Archaeology* 46.3 (2014), pp. 400-415; E. LACEY, "When is a *hroc* not a *hroc*? When it is a *crawe* or a *hrefn*!: A case-study in recovering Old English folk taxonomies", in: *The Art, Literature and Material Culture of the Medieval World*, ed. M. BOULTON, J. HAWKES, and M. HERMAN (Dublin, 2015), pp. 138-152.

[7] W.B. LOCKWOOD, *Oxford Book of British Bird Names* (Oxford, 1984), *passim*; LACEY, "When is a *hroc* not a *hroc*?", pp. 142-148.

[8] This point is made by E.A. ANDERSON, *Folk-Taxonomies in Early English* (Madison, WI, 2003), p. 19; see also LACEY, "When is a *hroc* not a *hroc*?", pp. 138-140.

[9] J. HAFFER, "The history of the biological species concept", *Acta Zoologica Sinica* 52 (2006), pp. 415-420; W. KUNZ, *Do Species Exist? Principles of Taxonomic Classification* (Weinheim, 2012).

[10] Walter Bock differentiates 'species concept', 'species categories', and 'species taxa': the 'species concept' comprises such evolutionary biological concerns as genetic and reproductive isolation (and applies only to sexually reproducing organisms), whereas the category and taxa

how users of a language perceive and organise the world around them.[11] These folk-taxonomies underpin present-day scientific systematics,[12] and for many people there is no difference between folk taxonomies and scientific taxonomies:[13] they are both heterogeneous hierarchies which can be formed in multiple ways and according to varying criteria.[14] We cannot, therefore, labour under the impression that there is some fundamental and essential quality that distinguishes species, nor can we assert that folk-taxonomies are somehow inferior or less true.[15] We must also remember that the fixedness of present-day speciation is arbitrary, and that species are liable to recategorisation, separation, and merging in light of new evidence.[16] While present-day species con-

pertain to the relatively arbitrary compartmentalisation and arrangement of these organisms within hierarchies. This hierarchical organisation is the same thing as folk taxonomies. See W. BOCK, "Species: the concept, category, taxon", *Journal of Zoological Systematics and Evolutionary Research* 42 (2004), pp. 178-190; W. BOCK, "Species concepts versus species category versus species taxa", *Acta Zoologica Sinica* 52 (2006), pp. 421-424; see also ANDERSON, *Folk Taxonomies*, pp. 21-54; LACEY, "When is a *hroc* a *hroc*?", pp. 138-139; MAYR, *The Growth of Biological Thought*, pp. 147-300.

[11] The concept is known variously as 'ethnobiological classification', 'folk biological nomenclature' and 'biological kind classification' too. The most fulsome study of this kind is ANDERSON, *Folk-Taxonomies*; see further LACEY, "When is a *hroc* not a *hroc*?", pp. 138-142; S. ATRAN, "The nature of folk-biological life forms", *American Anthropologist* 87.2 (1985), pp. 298-315; B. BERLIN *et al.*, "General principles of classification and nomenclature in folk biology", *American Anthropologist* 75.1 (1973), pp. 214-242; C.H. BROWN *et al.*, "Some general principles of biological and non-biological folk classification", *American Ethnologist* 3.1 (1976), pp. 73-85. For categorisation and thinking see G. LAKOFF, *Women, Fire, and Dangerous Things: What Categories Reveal about the Mind* (Chicago, 1987), especially pp. 5-156 and 269-303; S. HARNAD, 'To cognize is to categorize: Cognition is categorization", in: *Handbook of Categorization in Cognitive Science*, ed. H. COHEN and C. LEFEBVRE (Oxford, 2005), pp. 20-45; J. BOSTER, "Categories and cognitive anthropology", in: *Handbook of Categorization*, pp. 92-118.

[12] MAYR, *The Growth of Biological Thought*, pp. 147-208; K. DE QUIEROZ, "Branches in the line of descent: Charles Darwin and the evolution of the species concept", *Biological Journal of the Linnaean Society* 103 (2011), pp. 19-35; P.H. RAVEN *et al.*, "The origins of taxonomy", *Science* 174.4015 (1971), pp. 1210-1213.

[13] LACEY, "When is a *hroc* not a *hroc*?", pp. 139-142.

[14] LACEY, "When is a *hroc* not a *hroc*?", pp. 141-142 (and nn. 19-26); see also KUNZ, *Do Species Exist?*, the essays in *Species Concepts and Phylogenetic Theory: A Debate*, ed. Q.D. WHEELER and R. MEIER (New York, 2000) and K. DE QUIEROZ, "Species concepts and species delimitations", *Systematic Biology* 56.6 (2007), pp. 879-886, especially p. 880.

[15] See also BOCK, "Species", p. 179.

[16] For example, the gannet (*Sula bassanus*) was recategorised from the genus *Morus*; hooded crows (*Corvus cornix*) and carrion crows (*Corvus corone*) used to be considered the same species (see KUNZ, *Do Species Exist*, pp. 99-100); see also P. AGAPOW, "Species: Demarcation and diversity", in: *Phylogeny and Conservation*, ed. A. PURVIS *et al.* (Cambridge, 2005), pp. 57-75 (at pp. 61-63).

cepts are concerned more with phylogeny and branches of evolution, historical species concepts were predicated, like folk-taxonomies, on features which were arbitrarily deemed significant: reproductivity, ecological niches, and even – in the case of phenetic species concepts – morphologically.[17] It is important to remember that these criteria reflect contemporary notions of accurate observation (e.g. genetics, ecology, ethnology), and so, when considering how and why speakers of Old English made the distinctions they did with regards to animals, we must think of the Anglo-Saxons' notions of accurate observation.

Bede, in his *De natura rerum* (*On the Nature of Things*), was, like the earliest students of the natural world, concerned with natural order.[18] Aristotle sought groupings of animals in order to distinguish common features that may elucidate a natural architecture and a deeper understanding of the universe (i.e. a cosmic teleology);[19] Isidore of Seville sought the essence and nature of things in the origins of their words;[20] and even the dizzyingly fulsome catalogue in Pliny's *Natural History* has natural order at the heart of it: the content of the different books is generally governed by what present-day semanticists would call 'basic level categories', and the movement across subjects within the books is governed by associations across the natural world.[21] After the Anglo-Saxons, the pioneering systematists were concerned with grouping things according to 'kind', though precisely what these 'kinds' comprised was varied and arbitrary. They could be motivated by utility, as was the case for Frederick II of Hohenstaufen's division of hunted birds into waterfowl, land birds and 'neutral birds' (I.2), and also a duality of raptorial / non-raptorial birds (I.3), or they could be motivated by "totally artificial" ordering principles like the hardness of beaks, the perceived harmoniousness of their singing or whether they bathe in dust or water.[22] Where we have ordered lists of birds in Old English,

[17] DE QUIEROZ, "Species concepts", pp. 880-882; DE QUIEROZ, "Branches in the line of descent".

[18] Bede, *De natura rerum*, ed. and trans. C. KENDALL and F. WALLIS (Liverpool, 2010), pp. 1-12.

[19] LINDBERG, *The Beginnings of Western Science*, p. 63; Aristotle, *On the Parts of Animals* I.5, trans. J.G. LENNOX, *Aristotle: On the Parts of Animals I-IV* (Oxford, 2001), pp. 13-15; see further A. FALCON, *Aristotle and the Science of Nature: Unity without Uniformity* (Cambridge, 2008).

[20] *The Etymologies of Isidore of Seville*, trans. S.A. BARNEY, W.J. LEWIS, J.A. BEACH and O. BERGANHOF (Cambridge, 2006) , pp. 18-24.

[21] T. MURPHY, *Pliny the Elder's Natural History: The Empire in Encyclopedia* (Oxford, 2004), pp. 29-48. For "basic level categories" see E. ROSCH, "Principles of categorization", in: *Cognition and Categorization,* ed. E. ROSCH and B. LLOYD (Hillsdale, 1978), pp. 27-48.

[22] Frederick II of Hohenstaufen, *The Art of Falconry, Being the* De arte venandi cum avibus

they are arranged alphabetically in the glossaries and are therefore of no use for inferring the underlying systems of categorisation. Some insight, however, may be gleaned from close analysis of the bird names themselves.

Bird Identification in Old English

Bird names in Old English can be broadly arranged into four groups: names motivated by appearance, names motivated by behaviour, names motivated by sound, and those which do not clearly (or we do not currently know enough about to) fit into one of the other categories. In the following table I translate the Old English literally without specifying which birds were the referents: as we shall see below, the relationship between lexeme and referent does not match up easily with our present-day categories.[23]

	Name	Name elements	Literal meaning
Behaviour	*Dopened*	*Dop* < OE **dopian* ('to dip', cf.ON *deypa*, OHG *toufen*, OS *dopian*)[24] + *ened*	Dip-duck
	Duce	*Duce* < OE **ducan* ('to dive', cf. German *tauchen*, Dutch *duiken*)[25]	Diver
	Dufedoppe	*Dufe* < OE *dufan* 'to dive'	Dive-dipper
	Feolofor	*Feolu* 'much' + *for* < *faran* 'travel'[26]	Much-travelled
	Frecmase	*Frec* = 'greedy' + *mase*	Greedy-*mase*

of Frederick II of Hohenstaufen, ed. C. Wood and F. Fyfe (London, 1943), pp. 7-15; Mayr, *Growth of Biological Thought*, p. 168.

[23] The names in this table comprise only those which are attested in Old English – those which are reconstructed on the basis of later evidence, like many of those in Kitson, "Old English bird-names (I)" and id., "Old English bird-names (II)", are not included here. There is no space to discuss every name analysis fully here, though in some cases a discussion or supporting evidence is referenced.

[24] G. Kroonen, *Etymological Dictionary of Proto-Germanic* (Leiden, 2013), s.v. "*daupjan"; V. Orel, *Handbook of Germanic Etymology* (Leiden, 2003), s.v. "*daupjanan".

[25] Kroonen, *Etymological Dictionary*, s.v. "*dūkan".

[26] Kitson, "Old English bird-names (I)", p. 487.

	Giw	< Proto-Germanic **giwo*, related to ON *gjá* 'gap'[27]	Gaper
	Glida	< OE *glidan* 'to glide'	Glider
	Hafoc	Related to OE *hebban* 'to lift' and Latin *capere* 'to seize' + *-oc* (hypocoristic suffix)[28]	Seizer
	Hleapewinc	*Hleap* < OE *hleapan* 'to leap' + **winc* < Proto-Germanic **wenkjanan* 'to move sideways'[29]	Sideways leaper
	Putta / puttoc	< Proto-Germanic **putjan*, cognate with Present-day 'put'[30] + *-oc* suffix	Putter[31]
	Rindeclifer	*Rind* 'bark' + *clifer* 'cleaver'	Bark-cleaver
	Yrðling	*Yrð* = *eorð* 'earth' + *-ling* diminutive	Little earth thing
Appearance	*Amer*	*Amer* 'coat'	Coated
	Colmase	*Col* 'coal' + *mase*	Coal-coloured *mase*
	Ganot	Ultimately from the same root as *gander* 'goose'	Long-necked squat-bodied bird[32]

[27] KROONEN, *Etymological Dictionary*, s.v. "*giwōjan"; KITSON, "Old English bird-names (II)", p. 8.

[28] LOCKWOOD, *Oxford Book of British Bird Names*, s.v. "(-ock".

[29] OREL, *Handbook*, s.v. "*wenkjanan".

[30] KROONEN, *Etymological Dictionary*, s.v. "*put(t)ōn".

[31] See KITSON, "Old English bird-names (II)", p. 9.

[32] M.E.R. LACEY, *Birds and Bird-Lore in the Literature of Anglo-Saxon England* (unpublished doctoral thesis, University College London, 2014), pp. 72-82.

	Geoluwearte	*Gealwe* 'yellow' + *earte* (of Proto-Indo-European antiquity, meaning some kind of small water-bird)[33]	Yellow water-bird
	Goldfinc	*Gold* 'gold' + *finc*	Golden *finc*
	Isern	*Is* 'ice' + *earn* 'eagle'	Ice-eagle
	Rædda / ruddoc	< *Ræd* 'red' + *-oc* suffix	Red thing
	Reodmuða	*Reod* 'red' + *muða* 'mouth'	Red-mouth
	Sweartling	*Sweart* 'black' + *-ling* diminutive	Little black thing
	Ylfete	< Proto-Indo-European *h_2elb^h-*o*- 'white'[34]	White thing
Habitat	*Ceaffinc*	*Ceaf* 'chaff' + *finc*	*Finc* which lives among chaff
	Clodamer	*Clod* 'clod' + *amer*	*Amer* which lives among clod
	Edischen	*Edisc* 'park' + *hen*	*Hen* which lives in the park
	Erschen	*Ersc* 'park' + *hen*	*Hen* which lives in the park
	Feldfara	*Feld* 'field' + *fara* 'to go'	Field-journeyer
	Stæðswealwe	*Stæð* 'bank' + *swealwe*	*Swealwe* which lives at the bank
	Wuduculfre	*Wudu* 'wood' + *culfre* 'dove'	Dove which lives in the woods
	Wudusnite	*Wudu* 'wood' + *snite*	*Snite* which lives in the woods

[33] KROONEN, *Etymological Dictionary*, s.v. "*artō(n)-".
[34] KROONEN, *Etymological Dictionary*, s.v. "*albut-".

Sound	*Agu*	Onomatopoeic root (**ag*)[35]	[ag]-sounding thing
	Ceo	Onomatopoeic	[tʃeu]-sounding thing
	Cicen	Onomatopoeic + *-en* suffix	[tʃik]-sounding thing
	Cocc	Onomatopoeic	[kok]-sounding thing
	Cran	Onomatopoeic root (**gr*)[36]	[gɹ]-sounding thing
	Crawe	Onomatopoeic	[kɹa]-sounding thing
	Cyta	Onomatopoeic	[kiːtə]-sounding thing
	Đisteltwige	*Đistel* 'thistle' + onomatopoeic [twi], folk-etymologised under influence of *twig* 'branch'	[twi]-sounding thing found on thistles
	Finc / pinca	Onomatopoeic	[pɪŋk] / [spɪŋk]-sounding thing[37]
	Geac	Onomatopoeic origin < **gaukaz*	[gauːkə]-sounding thing
	Hen / hana	Root meaning 'singer'[38]	Singer
	Hæferblæte	*Hæfer* 'goat' + *blætan* 'to bleat'	Goat-bleater
	(Hege)-sucga	*Hege* 'hedge' + *sucga* < *sucgan* 'to suck'	Sucking-noise-making hedge-dweller

[35] Kroonen, *Etymological Dictionary*, s.v. "*ag/kkōn". Compare W. Lehmann, *A Gothic Etymological Dictionary* (Leiden, 1986), s.v. "ahaks".

[36] Kroonen, *Etymological Dictionary*, s.v. "*krana/ōn-".

[37] Forms with and without initial /s/ are common in words of Indo-European antiquity.

[38] Orel, *Handbook*, s.v. "*xanōn"; Kroonen, *Etymological Dictionary*, s.v. "*hanan-".

	Higera	Onomatopoeic root	[χiχ]-sounding thing
	Hraga	Onomatopoeic root	[χɹai]-sounding thing[39]
	Hrefn	Onomatopoeic	[χɹaß]-sounding thing
	Hroc	Onomatopoeic	[χɹok]-sounding thing[40]
	Hulfestre	*Hulf* = onomatopoeic [hʊlf] + *-estre* agentive suffix[41]	[hulf]-sounder
	Hwilpe	Onomatopoeic	[hwilp]-sounding thing
	Linetwige > *linet*	*Lin* 'flax' + onomatopoeic [twi], folk-etymologised under influence of *twig* 'branch'	[twi]-sounding thing found on flax
	Mæw	Onomatopoeic	[mæːu]-sounding thing
	Mase	Onomatopoeic	[mas]-sounding thing
	Nihtegale	*Niht* 'night' + *gale* < *galan* 'to chant'	Night-chanter
	Pea / pawa	Onomatopoeic / Onomatopoeic borroing from Latin *pava*	[piːə]-sounding thing
	Pipere	*Pipere* 'piper'	Piper
	Pur	Onomatopoeic	[pur]-sounding thing

[39] For *higera* and *hraga* see LACEY, *Birds and Bird-Lore*, pp. 69-72.

[40] For *crawe*, *hrefn* and *hroc* in detail, see LACEY, "When is a *hroc* not a *hroc*?".

[41] R. HOGG and R. FULK, *A Grammar of Old English*, 2, *Morphology* (Chichester, 2011), p. 51.

	Rardumle	*Rarian* 'to roar' + *dumle* of uncertain meaning. Possibly onomatopoeic[42]	? [dum]-roarer
	Scric	Onomatopoeic	[skriːtʃ]-sounding thing
	Secgscara	*Secg* 'sedge'+ *scara* 'shearer'	Shearing-sounding thing in the sedge[43]
	Stangella	*Stan* 'stone' + *giellan* 'to yell'	Stone-yeller
	Swan	< Proto-Indo-European **suonh*$_2$*-o-*[44]	The sound
	Swealwe	Related to *swelgan* 'to swallow'; compare *sucga*	Swallowing / sucking-sounding bird
	Þrostle / strostle	Onomatopoeic	See discussion below
	Þrysce	Onomatopoeic	See discussion below
	Ufe	Onomatopoeic	[uːf]-sounding thing
	Ule	Onomatopoeic	[uːl]-sounding thing
	Worhana	Onomatopoeic [wɔ:r] + *hana*	[wɔːr]-sounding *hana*
Appearance and sound	*Spicmase*	*Spic* 'blubber' + *mase* Possible that *spic* [spik] analysed onomatopoeically	Fat-*mase* [spik]-sounding *mase*

[42] See H. SUOLAHTI, *Die Deutschen Vogelnamen* (Strasbourg, 1909), p. 385.

[43] Compare KITSON, "Old English bird-names (I)", p. 497.

[44] KROONEN, *Etymological Dictionary*, s.v. "*swana-".

Unclear	*Culfre*	Borrowing of Latin *columba*[45]	-
	Cuscote	*Cu* 'cow'+ *sceotan* 'to shoot'	? Cow-shot
	Earn	Indo-European antiquity	Eagle
	Earngeot / earngeap	*Earn* + *geot* 'pour' / *geap* 'gape'	?
	Ened	Indo-European antiquity	Duck
	Fina	?	?
	Frysca / Frisca	?	?
	Gos	Indo-European antiquity	Goose
	Herefong	*Here* 'army' + *feng* 'to take'	'Army-seizer'
	Lawerce	Non-Indo-European word of Proto-Germanic antiquity[46]	Lark
	Osle	Indo-European antiquity	Small or medium bird
	Salthaga	?*Saltna* 'dance'[47] + *haga* 'hedge'	'Dance-hedge'
	Scealfor	?*Sceal* 'shoal' + *fara* 'to go'	?'shoal-traveller'
	Scræf	? related to 'scrape'(e.g. ON *skrapa*, OE *scearfian*	?scraper ?scrape-sounding thing
	Snite	?	?
	Spearwa	Common Germanic root (**sparwaz*)	Small bird

[45] LACEY, *Birds and Bird-Lore*, pp. 197-200; LOCKWOOD, *Oxford Book of British Bird Names*, s.v. "culver".

[46] P. SCHRIJVER, "Animal, vegetable and mineral: Some Western European substratum words", in: *Sound Law and Analogy: Papers in Honour of R.S. Beekes*, ed. A. LUBOTSKY (Amsterdam, 1997), pp. 293-316.

[47] KITSON, "Old English bird-names (I)", p. 486.

Stær / stærling	Indo-European antiquity[48]	Bird
Stearn	Common Germanic[49]	Some small sea-bird
Turtle	Borrowing from Latin[50]	Dove
Wrenna (also metathisised *wærna*)	Possibly Common Germanic[51]	Small bird
Wroc	Unclear	-

The 'unclear' category, as might be expected, is heterogeneous. Some of these are unclear to us (or at least to me): thus both the motivation for, and meaning of, *tysca* and *frysca* (if they are not, indeed, the same word) are buried beneath confused glossary entries and obscure morphology. Whether or not these were clear (or unclear) to speakers of Old English is unknowable. Some of the other names, like *scealfor* and *scræf*, were probably transparent to speakers of Old English, but are morphologically (and etymologically) uncertain. Others still are generally unclear, both in terms of etymology and referent, like *earngeap / earngeot* and *wroc*. The names of Indo-European and Common Germanic antiquity were probably not analysable to Old English speakers, and so the motivation for their naming is deemed unclear.

For the most part, however, bird names in Old English were transparently descriptive. This is presumably because named identification – and therefore transmission of this sort of knowledge – would have been *in situ*. In the absence of popular ornithological literature, ornithological organisations, or any other kind of regulating body, the name itself was the principle authority for its applicability to a bird. In this sense, we might term these names endogenic: the expression meaning of the word (i.e. the full range of applicable meanings) was relatively abstract, and this abstract meaning may have determined the range of possible referents.[52]

[48] KROONEN, *Etymological Dictionary*, s.v. "*star(r)a(n)"; OREL, *Handbook*, s.v. "*staraz ~ starōn".

[49] OREL, *Handbook*, s.v. "*sternaz".

[50] LACEY, *Birds and Bird-Lore*, p. 197.

[51] KROONEN, *Etymological Dictionary*, s.v. "*wrandan-(?)".

[52] Prototype semantics is useful here: each of these terms had a prototypical referent (albeit

Of particular interest here is the fact that so many names are motivated by the sound of birds. This is perhaps no surprise, given that birds are usually heard before they are seen.[53] Some birds, such as bitterns, nightingales, and cuckoos, are seldom seen but frequently heard; in some sense, they exist only as aural experiences within a landscape.[54] Even those birds which are frequently seen, however, may be marked out by their vocalisations (like the *crawe*, etymon of present-day 'crow'). The names alone demonstrate that aurality was important as a way of perceiving. However, this does not adequately stress its importance: in and amongst these aurally-motivated names are visually similar birds which are distinguished by their calls, suggesting the primacy of aural experience in these cases. In what follows, the importance of sound at rather precise levels of specification is shown, and taxonomic rank is noted by levels. Level I is the 'basic level' category, and is to some extent arbitrary (it may be 'animal' or 'bird', depending on the subject discussed), and additional levels denote specificity. The addition of A denotes a cultural and thematic criterion, e.g. 'domesticated animals' is Level IA of Level I 'animals'.[55]

Ule *and* Ufe

Here is a bird for which we have only one onomatopoeic word in modern English, but two in Old English: the owl. In modern English it is a Level II bird-name which lexicalises a range of largely, but not strictly, nocturnal birds with round heads and seemingly flat faces. The semantic range of the Old English terms is not immediately clear, as the two Old English words, *(h)ufe* and *ule*, are attested almost exclusively in the glossaries.[56] Outside of the glossaries

one that varied according to region, background and the like), and similarity to the prototype would have been grounds for inclusion. See L.E.C. De Oliveira *et al.*, "Prototypes and folk taxonomy: Artisanal fishers and snappers on the Brazilian coast", *Current Anthropology* 53.6 (2012), pp. 789-798.

[53] J. Mynott, *Birdscapes: Birds in our Imagination and Experience* (Princeton, 2009), pp. 116-119.

[54] See also Poole and Lacey, "Avian aurality", pp. 400-405.

[55] See further Anderson, *Folk Taxonomies*.

[56] *Ule*: Ælfric, *Ælfric's Glossary*, l.10, ed. J. Zupitza, *Ælfrics Grammatik und Glossar* (Berlin, 1880), p. 307; glosses to Aldhelm's prose *De laude virginitatis*, lines 533-538, ed. A. Napier, *Old English Glosses* (Oxford, 1900); Second Antwerp glossary line 986, ed. L. Kindschi, *The Latin-Old English Glossaries in Plantin-Moretus MS.32 and British Museum MS.*

we find *ule* once in Leviticus and in possibly four place-names,[57] though the *ule* is not described at all in Leviticus, and the place-names bearing *ule* are not species-specific environments. Kitson draws attention to Suffolk place-names possibly employing *(h)ufe*, though again these environments are not species-specific.[58] This means that if we are to have any chance of recovering the semantics of *(h)ufe* and *ule*, then the lexical and ornithological evidence provides us with the best means of doing so.

While *ule*, the etymon of modern English 'owl', is the more common word in Old English, the presence of cognates of *(h)ufe* in Old High German suggests the latter is not a bookish neologism, though we cannot remark on its prevalence in Old English with any certainty.[59] Although *ule* glosses a wide

Additional 32,246 (unpublished doctoral thesis, Stanford University, 1955); Brussels glossary l. 35, ed. T. WRIGHT and R. WÜLKNER, *Anglo-Saxon and Old English Vocabularies*, 2 vols. (London, 1884), 1, IX.3; Second Corpus glossary, C.119, N.138 and U.238, ed. J. HESSELS, *An Eighth-Century Glossary, Preserved in the Library of Corpus Christi College, Cambridge* (Cambridge, 1890); First Cleopatra glossary, ll. 1275 and 4281, ed. W. STRYKER, *The Latin-Old English Glossary in MS. Cotton Cleopatra A.III* (unpublished doctoral thesis, Stanford University, 1951), Second Cleopatra glossary, ll. 41 and 42, ed. J. QUINN, *The Minor Latin-Old English Glossaries in MS. Cotton Cleopatra A. III* (unpublished doctoral thesis, Stanford University, 1951), Third Cleopatra glossary, l. 1361, ed. QUINN, *The Minor Latin-Old English Glossaries*; an Old English glossary in MS London, British Library, Harley 107, l.55, ed. J. ZUPITZA, "Altenglische Glossen", *Zeitschrift für deutsches Altertum und deutsche Literatur* 33 (1989), pp. 237-242; Harley 3376 glossary, C.579, ed. R. OLIPHANT, *Harley Latin-Old English Glossary Edited from British Museum MS Harley 3376* (The Hague, 1966: *Janua linguarum, series practica* 20); MS Stowe 57 glossary, l.30, ed. R. GARRETT, "Middle English and French glosses from MS Stowe 57", *Archiv für das Studium der neueren Sprachen und Literaturen*, n.s. 21 (1908), pp. 411-412. *(H)ufe*: Brussels glossary, l.67; Second Antwerp, l.1027; Second Corpus, B.206; Épinal-Erfurt lines 142 and 161, ed. J. PHEIFER, *Old English Glosses in the Épinal-Erfurt Glossary* (Oxford, 1974); First Cleopatra l.700, among some glosses to Isidore's *Etymologiae*, l.4, ed. W. RIEHLE, "Ueber einige neuentdeckte altenglische Glossen", *Anglia* 84 (1966), pp. 150-155; and in two other glossaries edited by H.D. Meritt (Nos. 36 and 70, both on line 14 (H. MERITT, *Old English Glosses: A Collection* (New York, 1945: *MLA General Series* 16)).

[57] Leviticus 11:13, ed. S. CRAWFORD, *The Old English Version of the Heptateuch* (London, 1922). The place-names are in S 79 (*ulan wylle*, 'owls' well'), S 377 (*ulan del*, 'owls' dale'), S 1307 (*ulan bearhe*, 'owls' wood'), and S 803 (*ulan hyrste*, 'owl's copse'), where the charters are numbered as in P. SAWYER, *Anglo-Saxon Charters: An Annotated List and Bibliography* (London, 1968). The topography of South Stoke indicates that *hyrste* means 'copse' in S 803. See G. B. GRUNDY, "The Saxon land charters of Hampshire with notes on place and field names: 4th series", *Archaeological Journal* 34 (1927), pp. 160-340, at pp. 216-217.

[58] KITSON, "Old English bird-names (II)", p. 6.

[59] There are several variant forms in Old High German. J. BOSWORTH and T. TOLLER, *An Anglo-Saxon Dictionary* (London, 1898), note that the OHG *(h)uvo* can occur both "with and without initial *h*" (s.v. "huf"), and SUOLAHTI, *Die Deutschen Vogelnamen*, p. 309, gives *ûro*,

variety of Latin 'owl' words, namely *strix*, *ulula*, *noctua* and forms of *cavannus* (most often in the form *cavannarum*), (*h*)*ufe* only ever glosses *bubo* and *bufo*.[60] Later on, in the eleventh century, there are also instances where (*h*)*ufe* glosses Latin *vultur*.[61] This suggests that *ule* had a wider semantic range than (*h*)*ufe*. As *ule* never glosses *bubo* or *bufo*, Latin words which refer to the large Eagle Owl (*Bubo bubo*), the implication of the glossary evidence is as follows: firstly, that (*h*)*ufe* is a Level III term which refers exclusively to the large Eagle Owl (and then, if we can trust its glossing *vultur,* as a Level IA term for large birds of prey generally, where Level I is all birds), and secondly, that *ule* is a Level II term which lexicalises all smaller owls. The former point is supported by Suolahti's analysis of the Old High German cognates of (*h*)*ufe*, all of which, he argues, also refer to the Eagle Owl.

There is a potential problem here, however, and that is the disputed status of the Eagle Owl in Anglo-Saxon England. Derek Yalden and Umberto Albarella note that "Eagle Owls are not represented in Medieval British archaeology", and that this is "a strong argument that they had become extinct well before then",[62] though it is worth bearing in mind that the Eagle Owl's preferred habitat in the more remote portions of mountains and forests means that they are not likely to be well represented in the archaeological record.[63] The Eagle Owl is still an accidental visitor to Britain today, and it is similarly an accidental visitor to other areas where historically there were populations.[64] Because of the dearth of evidence for an Eagle Owl population in Anglo-Saxon

hû(*w*)*o*, and in n.1, *uuof* and *uuo*.

60 According to J. ANDRÉ, *Les Noms d'oiseaux en Latin* (Paris, 1967), both *bubo* and *bufo* refer to the Eagle Owl (s.v.v. "bubo, -onis" and "bufo, -onis"), whereas *noctua* (s.v.) is a vertically polysemous term which lexicalises both the Level I A meaning covering all nocturnal creatures (where Level I is 'all creatures'), and the Level III meaning of the Little Owl (*Athene noctua*). *Ulula* (s.v.) refers to the Tawny Owl (*strix aluco*), *strix* (s.v. "strix, strigis") refers to the Barn Owl (*Tyto alba*), and André identifies *cavannus* (s.v. "cauannus") as a Gaulish name for the Tawny Owl. The probable source for this lemma is given by André.

61 KITSON, "Old English bird-names (II)", p. 7, notes that two eleventh-century manuscripts of Ælfric's Grammar add *(h)ufe* to gloss *vultur*.

62 D.W. YALDEN and U. ALBARELLA, *The History of British Birds* (Oxford, 2009), p. 138.

63 For the bird's history in the British Isles, see YALDEN and ALBARELLA, *History of British Birds*, pp. 58-60, and J. FISHER, *The Shell Bird Book* (London, 1963), p. 24. Because of issues with the semantic fields of *bubo* and *ufe* we cannot unquestioningly accept Fisher's comments, on p. 324, that identify the Eagle Owl as "recorded" or "possibly native" between the eighth and eleventh centuries.

64 S. CRAMP *et al., Handbook of the Birds of Europe, the Middle East and North Africa: Birds of the Western Palearctic*, 4, *Terns to Woodpeckers* (Oxford,1985), p. 467; H. MIKKOLA, *Owls of Europe* (Calton, 1983), pp. 88-89.

England, Kitson suggests that OE (*h*)*ufe* referred to the Long-eared Owl (*Asio otis*), "as the native species most similar to the eagle owl and most different from the tawny"; he takes *ule* to refer "mainly" to the Tawny Owl.[65] This raises the stakes for an accurate identification of the (*h*)*ufe*, as it may or may not supply documentary evidence for the Eagle Owl's presence in Anglo-Saxon England.[66]

The onomatopoeic nature of *ule* and (*h*)*ufe* is beyond reasonable doubt, and they match quite well to transcriptions of owl vocalisations. Specifically, *ule* is closest to the hooting of the vocal (and nocturnal) Tawny Owl (*Strix aluco*),[67] whereas (*h*)*ufe* captures the forcefully expulsive, almost cough-like, qualities of the calls of crepuscular and nocturnal Long-eared Owl,[68] the often diurnal Short-eared Owl (*Asio flammeus*),[69] and, though the evidence for its residency in Anglo-Saxon England is basically non-existent, the nocturnal and crepuscular Eagle Owl.[70] If we combine this with the glossary evidence, then the following taxonomies are suggested.

Ule

Ule is an onomatopoeic name redolent of the Tawny Owl's hoot, but as the Tawny Owl is nocturnal and rarely seen (or, at least, rarely observed in the act of its eponymous vocalisation), *ule* could plausibly lend itself to a range of nocturnal birds. This would explain the rationale underlying the varied Latin 'owl'-terms it glosses. Moreover, the fact that it never glosses *bubo* or *bufo* suggests that it was firmly differentiated from the (*h*)*ufe*. Thus, *ule* is a verti-

[65] KITSON, "Old English bird-names (II)", p. 6.

[66] See, for example, FISHER, *The Shell Bird Book*, p. 324.

[67] The Tawny Owl's hoot is the sound most people tend to think of when imagining an owl-call. See MIKKOLA, *Owls of Europe*, pp. 140-142; CRAMP *et al.*, *Handbook*, pp. 540-542.

[68] Often transliterated as 'oh' but described as a 'deep hooting'. See L. SVENSSON *et al.*, *Collins Bird Guide: The Most Complete Guide to the Birds of Britain and Ireland and Europe* (London, 2009), p. 228; MIKKOLA, *Owls of Europe*, pp. 215-217; CRAMP *et al.*, *Handbook*, pp. 582-584.

[69] The most relevant vocalisations are the alarm-call often transliterated as 'chef', the female's 'cheh-ef', and the deep hooting flight-call often transliterated as 'uh'. See SVENSSON *et al.*, *Collins Bird Guide*, p. 228; MIKKOLA, *Owls of Europe*, pp. 235-236; CRAMP *et al.*, *Handbook*, pp. 597-598.

[70] See SVENSSON *et al.*, *Collins Bird Guide*, p. 222; MIKKOLA, *Owls of Europe*, pp. 73-79; CRAMP *et al.*, *Handbook*, pp. 470-478.

cally polysemous term which lexicalises both Level IA 'birds of the night' (where Level I is 'birds'), Level II 'non-(*h*)*ufe* owls' and possibly even Level III 'Tawny Owl'. The status of the now-resident Little Owl (*Athene noctua*) is not clear in Anglo-Saxon England. It is generally thought to have been introduced to the British Isles in the nineteenth century,[71] though Fisher notes that we have fossil evidence for their presence in Britain in the Late Ice Age.[72] It seems probable that the Little Owl, as well as the other occasional visitors such as the Scops Owl (*Otus scops*), came under *ule* too, even if only in its Level II meaning.

Ufe

(*H*)*ufe* is an onomatopoeic name that evokes the cries of not just one, but three species: the Long-eared Owl, the Short-eared Owl and the Eagle Owl. It is uncertain whether the last of these was resident in Anglo-Saxon England, though it seems to have been the primary referent of (*h*)*ufe*'s OHG cognates. Unlike the Tawny Owl, these three owls are likely to have been seen calling during the day, at dawn, or at dusk, and, moreover, are visually quite similar. The main differences are that the Eagle Owl is substantially larger (59-73 cm long, 138-170 cm wingspan) than the Long-eared or Short-eared owls (L 31-37 cm, WS 86-98 cm, and L 33-40 cm, WS 95-105 cm respectively), and only the Eagle Owl and Long-eared Owl have particularly prominent 'ear-tufts'; these are much more difficult to see on a Short-eared Owl.[73] The general colouration is nearly identical: all three are largely yellowish-brown with dark streaks, and in flight expose lighter under-wings. Therefore, I suggest that the semantic range of (*h*)*ufe* encompassed these three diurnal and crepuscular owls (to the exclusion of largely nocturnal owls, hence (*h*)*ufe* never glosses Latin *noctua*), and that identification was made on both aural and visual grounds. The taxonomic level is less clear; it seems safe to say that (*h*)*ufe* is at least Level II, though the consistency with which it glosses only *bubo* and *bufo* means that it could possibly be a Level III term too. Further support for this lexicalisation may be found in French, where our Level II 'owl' corresponds to two French

[71] KITSON, "Old English bird-names (II)", p. 6, and D.T. PARKIN and A.G. KNOX, *The Status of Birds in Britain and Ireland* (London, 2010), p. 223.

[72] FISHER, *Shell Bird Book*, p. 324.

[73] SVENSSON *et al.*, *Collins Bird Guide*, pp. 222, 228; MIKKOLA, *Owls of Europe*, pp. 69-73, 213-215, 233-235; CRAMP *et al.*, *Handbook*, pp. 466-467, 472-473, 488-489.

terms: *chouette* and *hibou*. This French evidence is particularly useful as *hibou* is a borrowing of cognates of *(h)ufe*.[74] While *chouette* is the Level II term for 'owl' generally, the onomatopoeic *hibou* is a Level III term which refers specifically to *chouette à oreilles*, ('owls with ears'; the ears are also known as *aigrettes*),[75] i.e. the Long-eared, Short-eared and Eagle Owls.

Þrysce *and* Þrostle

Another set of similar-looking species with different names in Old English are the thrushes (genus *Turdus*); in particular, the strikingly similar Song Thrush (*Turdus philomelos*) and Mistle Thrush (*Turdus viscivorus*). Both birds are medium sized Passerines (though the Mistle Thrush is slightly larger than the Song Thrush),[76] brown hued along their heads and backs, with light breasts speckled with dark spots. Their Old English names are *þrysce* and *þrostle*, which, as Kitson notes, "are closely related, Germanic variants on a root whose meaning 'thrush' is of Indo-European antiquity".[77] As there is little to disagree with in Kitson's analysis of these names and their semantic ranges,[78] I limit myself to supplementing this with a discussion on how onomatopoeia lies behind these names and their semantic fields, and what we can say about their taxonomic levels.

As Kitson has noted, *þrysce* and *þrostle*[79] were likely identified as different birds in Old English, though his strongest evidence is that they sometimes gloss different lemmata.[80] However, Kitson does not draw attention to Lockwood's

[74] M. DESFAYES, *Origine des noms des oiseaux et des mammifères d'Europe y compris l'espèce humaine* (Paris, 2000), p. 77.

[75] DESFAYES, *Origine des noms des oiseaux*, p. 139.

[76] SVENSSON *et al.*, *Collins Bird Guide*, p. 294; P. CLEMENT and R. HATHWAY, *Thrushes* (London, 2000). The Mistle Thrush averages 26-29 cm in length, whereas the Song Thrush averages 20-22 cm.

[77] KITSON, "Old English bird-names (I)", p. 484. For the Proto-Indo-European etymon **trosdos*, see J.P. MALLORY and D.Q. ADAMS, *The Oxford Introduction to Proto-Indo-European and the Proto-Indo-European World* (Oxford, 2006), p. 145. See also LOCKWOOD, *Oxford Book of British Bird Names*, s.v.v. "Throstle" and "Thrush".

[78] I.e. that they overlap with each other and also with the Starling (*Sturnus vulgaris*) and Blackbird (*Turdus merula*). See KITSON, "Old English bird-names (I)", pp. 484-485.

[79] The variation of forms with and without initial 's-' is "of Indo-European antiquity" and is noted by KITSON, "Old English bird-names (I)", p. 485, and so I have silently included OE *strosle* with *þrostle* in my analysis.

[80] KITSON, "Old English bird-names (I)", p. 484.

rather crucial observation that *þrostle* reflects the same Germanic root as *þrysce* with a diminutive ending.[81] Later usage of 'Throstle', referring to the smaller Song Thrush, is suggestive, though it is worth noting that the Song Thrush is both smaller and quieter than the Mistle Thrush, and that therefore the diminutive suffix could possibly reference either, or both, of these aspects.[82] The use of OE *þrostle* to gloss Latin *turdella* (properly *turdela,* a diminutive of *turdus*) may indicate that glossators were aware of *þrostle*'s diminutive status, and thereby provide evidence that this term was used of the Song Thrush from an early date.[83] However, this hypothesis is problematised by the fact that Latin *turdela* referred primarily to the larger Mistle Thrush,[84] and by the interpretamenta we find for *turdus*, which are never *þrysce*. When we do find *turdus* in the glossaries, its preferred interpretamentum is *scric*,[85] though it is also glossed by *stær* ('starling').[86] Indeed, *þrysce* is attested very rarely in Old English at all: *þrysce* glosses *sturtius*,[87] þrisce glosses *trutius*,[88] and *ðrae-*

[81] LOCKWOOD, *Oxford Book of British Bird Names*, s.v. "Throstle".

[82] KITSON, "Old English bird-names (I)", p. 484, makes the observation that the Mistle Thrush is both louder and larger. Compare also the sonographs in S. CRAMP *et al.*, *Handbook of the Birds of Europe, the Middle East and North Africa: The Birds of the Western Palearctic*, 5, *Tyrant Flycatchers to Thrushes* (Oxford, 1988).

[83] *Turdella* is glossed by variants of *þrostle* in Second Corpus, T. 323; Second Cleopatra, l. 51; Harley 107, l. 52; Épinal-Erfurt, l. 1011. The *Dictionary of Old English Corpus* <tapor.library.utoronto.ca/doecorpus/> [accessed 30 June 2015] transcribes a further attestation from an unedited glossary in MS Oxford, Bodleian Library, Bodley 730, with the short title "CollGl 25", where it is line 84. The unusual entries in the Second Antwerp and Brussels glossaries (line 1023: "*Turdella se mare stær*", "the starling of the sea", and line 63: "*Turdella scealfor*") are less easy to explain. The most probable explanation is that the common source for Brussels and Cleopatra drew on Isidore's *Etymologiae* XII.7.71 ("*Turdela quasi maior turdus*", "*Turdela* is the larger *turdus*"), and either understood the text and had **se mara stær* ("the greater *stær*"), or misread the *maior* as meaning 'famous' and had **se mær stær*. In either case, the adjective was subsequently misread as a genitive singular variant of *mere* / *mære* ('the sea'), which, in spite of generally declining as a masculine noun is attested with the feminine genitive singular form *mere* (see BOSWORTH and TOLLER, *An Anglo-Saxon Dictionary*, s.v. "mere"). See also ANDRÉ, *Les noms d'oiseaux en latin*, s.v. "turdela, -ae".

[84] *Ibid.* See also Isidore, *Etymologiae*, XII.7.71.

[85] Second Antwerp, l. 1011, Brussels l. 47, Second Corpus T. 324, Second Cleopatra l. 55, Leiden glossary § 47, l. 63, ed. J. HESSELS, *A Late Eighth-Century Latin-Anglo-Saxon Glossary Preserved in the Library of the Leiden University* (Cambridge, 1906), and Épinal-Erfurt, l. 1013. It is tempting to read *srheich*, which glosses *turdus* in MS Bodley 730, l.88, and *stint*, in Harley 107, l. 55, as corruptions of the *scric* interpretamentum, though see the remarks I make below.

[86] *Ælfric's Glossary*, 307.7 and Second Antwerp, l. 1022.

[87] Harley 107, l. 53.

[88] Second Cleopatra, l. 56.

sce glosses *truitius*.[89] Kitson would see these lemmata as "corruptions of *turdus*", though in each of these cases *turdus* occurs as a separate lemma.[90] Kitson may well be correct in identifying these garbled lemmata as such, but what is important for my purposes here is why the glossators kept such incomprehensible lemmata. While copying glosses out into lists must have been a slavish task, this does not deprive the scribes of having reasons for matching the lemmata and interpretamenta as they do.

Understanding both the importance of the aural perception of birds as well as the suggested taxonomic levels can go some way to explaining some of these difficulties, namely: 1) the absence of glosses where *þrysce* is the interpretamentum for *turdus* despite the pairing of the diminutives of both of these words, 2) the use of *þrysce* only for forms so garbled that they are barely recognisable as corruptions of *turdus*, and 3) the potential for *scric* and *stær* to be considered plausible glosses for *turdus*. First, the existence of a diminutive form does not necessarily indicate a diminutive meaning. The diminutive form is also used hypocoristically, for example, and many bird names are attested with hypocoristic variants which do not substantially alter the word's meaning. To take another Old English example: we find hypocoristic forms of *putta* ('kite', 'buzzard'), in *pyttel*, found only in place-names and personal names,[91] and in *puttoc*, found only as a personal name in Old English. Later attestations of both *pyttel* and *puttoc*, and their reflexes, evidence that these were names for kites and buzzards, and that their meanings were no different to that of *putta*.[92] Although we do not have Germanic cognates to help corroborate which of these is the original form, it is probable, *a priori*, that *putta* (literally 'that which puts', a reference to the bird's swooping strike)[93] represents the stem from which *pyttel* and *puttoc* derive. Despite Lockwood's reticence, we may be sure, on the basis of a wealth of available parallels, that both *–el* and *– ock* suffixes are common diminutives in Old English.[94] The implication of this

[89] Second Corpus, T. 314.

[90] KITSON, "Old English bird-names (I)", p. 484. *Turdus* occurs as a separate lemma, with different interpretamenta, to the garbled lemmata for *þrysce* in Harley 107, l. 53, Second Cleopatra, l. 55 and Second Corpus, T. 324.

[91] KITSON, "Old English bird-names (II)", p. 9.

[92] KITSON, "Old English bird-names (II)", p. 9, and LOCKWOOD, *Oxford Book of British Bird Names*, s.v. "puttock".

[93] KITSON, "Old English bird-names (II)", p. 9.

[94] See the *Oxford English Dictionary* <www.oed.com>, s.v.v. "el, suffix1", and "-ock, suffix", and LOCKWOOD, *Oxford Book of British Bird names*, s.v.v. "(-le" and "(-ock".

parallel is that *turdella* and *þrostle* may have been recognised as hypocoristic bird names, rather than as diminutives with augmentative counterparts.

The second reason that *þrostle* may gloss *turdella* at the expense of *þrysce* glossing *turdus* is that the first pair are closely onomatopoeic, evoking a similar sound in a way that the second pair does not. Both *turdella* and *þrostle* are commonly acknowledged to be onomatopoeic in origin, though some commentators remark on this quality only with respect to its Indo-European onomatopoeic roots.[95] It seems that both terms were still perceived as onomatopoeic in the Anglo-Saxon period: *þrostle* suggests a /θrostəla/, *turdella* suggests the very similar /tɜrdəla/. The sound evoked by both *þrostle* and *turdella* seems a good match for the trisyllabic beginning of the Mistle Thrush's most characteristic cry.[96]

Similarly, both *turdus* and *þrysce* were understood to be onomatopoeic too.[97] However, in this case, the sounds suggested by the names are much less alike: *turdus* evokes the part of the Song Thrush's song often transliterated as 'trrü-trrü-trrü',[98] whereas *þrysce* suggests a screechier sound like /θruːʃ)/ or /θriːskə/.[99] The sound suggested by /θruːʃə/ might explain why it only glosses garbled derivatives of *turdus*: *sturtius*,[100] trutius,[101] and *truitius*,[102]which all possess an initial dental, medial back vowel and final lingual consonant possibly redolent of the sound of *þrysce*. A combination of poor transmission and an

[95] ANDRÉ, *Les noms d'oiseaux en latin*, s.v.v. "turela, -ae" and "turdus", endorses the possibility that these names are onomatopoeic in origin, though it is not clear how far back he thinks these origins are, or if they were understood to be onomatopoeic; his explanation, s.v. "turdus", suggests the latter. MALORY and ADAMS, *The Oxford Introduction to Proto-Indo-European,* p. 145, like LOCKWOOD, *Oxford Book of British Bird Names*, s.v.v. "throstle" and "thrush", and SUOLAHTI, *Die Deutschen Vogelnamen*, p. 53, consider the Indo-European onomatopoeic origins without remarking on the possibility of contemporary speakers recognising the names as such.

[96] SVENSSON *et al.*, *Collins Bird Guide*, p. 294 ; CLEMENT and HATHWAY, *Thrushes*, pp. 397-400 ; see also the copious notes on the differing thrush calls in CRAMP *et al.*, *Handbook of the Birds of Europe, the Middle East and North Africa :The Birds of the Western Palearctic*, 5, *Tyrant Flycatches to Thrushes*.

[97] ANDRÉ, *Les noms d'oiseaux en latin*, s.v. "turdus". For the onomatopoeia of *þrysce*, see below.

[98] SVENSSON *et al.*, *Collins Bird Guide*, p. 294; CLEMENT and HATHWAY, *Thrushes*, pp. 397-400.

[99] I am grateful to Alaric Hall for bringing this phonetic change to my attention. On /ʃ/ to /sk/ see R. HOGG, *A Grammar of Old English*, 1, *Phonology* (Chichester, 2011), pp. 269-270.

[100] Harley 107, l. 53.

[101] Second Cleopatra, l. 56.

[102] Second Corpus Glossary, T. 314.

expectation of onomatopoeia may lie behind the entry *Strutio þryssce* (1.48) in the Brussels glossary, and also the gloss *Structio scric* if the Latin were understood to be onomatopoeic (i.e. on the basis of /stru:tɪjəʊ/ and /θru:ʃə/, and /stru:ktɪjəʊ/ and /skri:tʃ/).[103] Presumably a gloss such as *turdus. þrysce* is at the root of all these corrupted forms, and such a gloss could well have been based on parallelism between *þrysce* / *þrostle*, and *turdus* / *turdella*. The corruption of the lemma, however, could suggest that such linguistically oriented understanding was not widespread.

The glossing of *turdus* by *scric* and *stær*, as Kitson has remarked, could imply a regional variation in the identification of these birds.[104] I take issue, however, with his subsequent remark that Ælfric, in particular, "did not care very much about the names of small birds", and that this contributed to the use of *scric* and *stær* to gloss *turdus*.[105] Kitson adduces an entry from Ælfric's glossary (307.7) to support this, which reads "*passer spearwa oððe lytel fugel*" ("*passer*: sparrow or little bird"). There are many reasons to assume that Ælfric's statement here is indicative of a more general perception of small birds, held more pervasively than by just a few clergymen. The popularity of Ælfric's glossary and the lack of alteration to this entry in the various manuscripts suggests it was generally accepted by its audience, and we must also bear in mind the difficulty of differentiating small birds of sparrow-size. Furthermore, we must contend with the fact that *passeres* ('sparrows') is rendered *staras* (lit. 'starlings') in Matthew 10:29 and Luke 12:6,[106] and that we find reflexes of *spearwa* used of other birds in Middle English and in the realm of folk-nomen-

[103] Harley 107, l. 65. The description of the *struthio* ('ostrich') in Isidore's *Etymologiae* XII.7.20 reads: "*Struthio Graeco nomine dicitur, quod animal in similitudine avis pinnas habere videtur; tamen de terra altius non elevatur. Ova sua fovere neglegit; sed proiecta tantummodo fotu pulveris animantur*" ("The ostrich is named from the Greek, which is seen to have feathers like a bird, but it does not rise above the ground. It neglects the incubation of its eggs, and the abandoned eggs are brought to life by only by the warm dust" (*Isidori Hispalensis Episcopi Etymologiarum sive Originum*, ed. W.M. LINDSAY, 2 vols (Oxford, 1911)). This could conceivably have been understood to apply to either the blackbird or the thrushes, which tend to nest low in thick underbrush and are often seen flying close to the ground, and this may have influenced the glossator's understanding of a garbled form of *turdus*. Although KITSON, "Old English bird-names (II)", p. 22, suggests that an Old English word for the ostrich, *stryce*, goes back to Common Germanic, both the OE *stryce* and the variety of differing Old High German forms (noted in SUOLAHTI, *Die Deutschen Vogelnamen*, p. 223: *struz*, *struua*, *struth*, *stral*, *strud*, *strux* etc.) suggests that in these instances, too, the motivation for the gloss was onomatopoeia.

[104] KITSON, "Old English bird-names (I)", p. 485, and n. 1.

[105] KITSON, "Old English bird-names (I)", p. 485, and n. 1.

[106] KITSON, "Old English bird-names (I)", p. 485, and n. 1.

clature.[107] Together, this suggests that there were degrees of overlap among the small birds, and that *spearwa* could function as a Level II term (where Level I is *fugelas* ('birds')) denoting all small birds, and that Ælfric is as reliable a source as any for the birds and bird names of Anglo-Saxon England.

Aurality and Categorisation

These two case-studies (*ule* / *ufe* and *þrysce* / *þrostle*) illustrate the differing ways in which aurality was important in bird categorisation. In the former, aurality provides the means for differentiating birds which are grouped together today. In the latter, a perceived expectation of aurality underlies unusual glossarial interpretations, and that a diminutive could be applied with regards to sound rather than size. Taking this together with the general preponderance of aurally motivated names among birds, it suggests that sound was not just an important faculty for perceiving birds, but one of the most important senses for knowing about them. An *ufe* could be perceived and categorised separately from an *ule* on this basis, as could a *þrysce* and a *þrostle*. This combination of perceived difference and categorical difference amounts to an act of folk-taxonomical speciation. Birds, therefore, were perceived, categorised, and understood via both visual and aural means. While those bird names motivated by behaviour are clearly visually motivated and those based on sounds are aurally motivated, those based on habitat might be motivated by both, as birds would have both been seen and heard in those environs. As in Proverbs 20:12 (and other places in the Bible), seeing and hearing are complementary senses, where hearing can both supplement the visual and supersede it, granting knowledge where the visual cannot.

[107] *Middle English Dictionary* <ets.umdl.umich.edu/m/med/>, s.v. "sparwe (n.)", and LOCKWOOD, *Oxford Book of British Bird Names*, s.v. "Sparrow".

"Whistle While You Work": Scribal Engagement with Old English Poetic Texts

SIMON C. THOMSON

It is well known that Anglo-Saxon textual reception was mostly not a silent or individual experience, but a communal and auditory one. There is considerable evidence that scribes understood this reception context, and that some manuscripts were "deliberately designed to assist the delivery of acoustic texts".[1] It is also clearly understood that some texts were designed to be seen as well as to be heard: appearance could shape meaning.[2] Hearing and sight often worked together; in Katherine O'Brien O'Keeffe's terms, "interpretative information appears in graphic directions determined and mediated by the

[1] J. Crick, "English vernacular script", in: *The Cambridge History of the Book in Britain*, 1, *c. 400 – 1100*, ed. R. Gameson (Cambridge, 2012), pp. 174-186, at p. 182.

[2] M.P. Brown, "Mercian manuscripts: The implications of the Staffordshire Hoard, other recent discoveries, and the 'new materiality'", in: *Writing in Context: Insular Manuscript Culture 500-1200*, ed. E. Kwakkel (Leiden, 2013), pp. 23-64, at pp. 44-45; E. Treharne, "The form and function of the Vercelli Book", in: *Text, Image, Interpretation: Studies in Anglo-Saxon Literature and its Insular Context in Honour of Éamonn Ó Carragáin*, ed. A. Minnis and J. Roberts (Turnhout, 2007), pp. 253-266, at pp. 265-266; T. Graham, "Cambridge, Corpus Christi College 57 and its Anglo-Saxon users", in: *Anglo-Saxon Manuscripts and Their Heritage*, ed. P. Pulsiano and E.M. Treharne (Aldershot, 1998), pp. 21-69, at pp. 34-37.

Sensory Perception in the Medieval West, ed. Simon C. Thomson and Michael D.J. Bintley, *Utrecht Studies in Medieval Literacy*, 34 (Turnhout: Brepols, 2016), pp. 99-122.

BREPOLS PUBLISHERS DOI 10.1484/M.USML-EB.5.109506

subjectivity characteristic of oral performance".[3] In the following discussion, I consider not the sensory experience of receiving and performing texts, but the sensory experience of producing them. It is my contention that Anglo-Saxon scribes could and did engage with Old English poetic texts. This in turn implies a scriptorium where scribes did not have silently to process the individual graphemes of the texts they reproduced, but where they could hear and, to some degree, represent metrical rhythms in their writing.[4]

There are four major codices of Old English poetry, all produced within a relatively short period of time from the mid tenth to the early eleventh century. They are the Vercelli Book, the Exeter Book, Junius 11, and the Nowell Codex.[5] All four contain only Old English, though they have few other similarities. As some examples of their differences, out of the four the Vercelli Book and the Nowell Codex include prose alongside poetry; the Nowell Codex and the Exeter Book include both religious and secular pieces; the Exeter Book and the Vercelli Book have just one scribe; Junius 11 and the Nowell Codex are partially illustrated. Comparing scribal practice in each, then, is not straightforward; the challenges becomes more marked given variance between texts within individual manuscripts. As a very general rule "scribal practice has to be considered poem by poem".[6]

[3] K. O'BRIEN O'KEEFFE, *Visible Song: Transitional Literacy in Old English Verse* (Cambridge, 1990: *Cambridge Studies in Anglo-Saxon England* 4), p. 187.

[4] Cf. M.B. PARKES, *Their Hands Before Our Eyes: A Closer Look at Scribes: The Lyell Lectures Delivered in the University of Oxford 1999* (Aldershot, 2008), p. 66.

[5] The Vercelli Book is MS Vercelli, Biblioteca Capitolare, CXVII; the most recent facsimile is The Visionary Cross Project's *The Digital Vercelli Book*, <http://vbd.humnet.unipi.it/beta/104v>. The Exeter Book is MS Exeter, Cathedral Library, 3501; the most recent facsimile is *The Exeter DVD: The Exeter Anthology of Old English Poetry*, ed. B.J. MUIR, programming N. KENNEDY (Exeter, 2006). Junius 11 is MS Oxford, Bodleian Library, Junius 11; the most recent facsimile is *A Digital Facsimile of Oxford, Bodleian Library, MS Junius 11*, ed. B.J. MUIR (Oxford, 2005); images online in the Bodleian Library's *Early Manuscripts at Oxford University*, <http://image.ox.ac.uk/show-allopenings?collection=bodleian&manuscript=msjunius11>. The Nowell Codex is the second half of MS London, British Library, Cotton Vitellius A. XV; the most recent facsimile is *The Electronic 'Beowulf' 3.0*, ed. K. KIERNAN (London, 2011); images are online in The British Library's *Digitised Manuscripts Online*, <http://www.bl.uk/manuscripts/FullDisplay.aspx?ref=Cotton_MS_vitellius_a_xv> [accessed 23 July 2015]. All of my quotations are from the relevant volume of *Anglo-Saxon Poetic Records*, ed. G. KRAPP and E.V.K. DOBBIE, 6 vols. (New York, 1931-1942).

[6] E.G. STANLEY, "Review of K. O'B. O'Keeffe, *Visible Song: Transitional Literacy in Old English Verse* (Cambridge Studies in Anglo-Saxon England 4) Cambridge: Cambridge University Press, 1990", *Notes and Queries* 38.2 (1991), pp. 199-200, at p. 199.

Scribing as Sensory, Spiritual, and Mechanical

There can be no doubt that scribing was and is a sensory experience. Cheryl Jacobsen points out that palaeographers tend to describe scribal marks in terms of their appearance, where a scribe describes marks in terms of how they are made. So, for instance, "[w]hat the scribe calls a down-stroke the palaeographer calls a minim".[7] Even the sensory experiences of scribal tools can be sharply imagined. In the frontispiece to an early eleventh-century manuscript from Saint-Vaast, the scribe says:

> *Cum librum scribo, Vedastus ab aethere summo*
> *Respicit e caelis, notat et quot grammata nostris*
> *Depingam calamis, quot aretur pagina sulcis,*
> *Quot folium punctis hinc hinc laceretur acutis.*
>
> When I write a book, St Vedastus looks down
> From highest heaven and notes how many letters I depict
> With my pen, by how many furrows the page is ploughed,
> By how many sharp points the folio is punctured here and here.[8]

Such keen awareness is bound up with spirituality: in the process of wounding, the flesh of the folio starts to sound almost like the tortured flesh of Christ, an association which becomes stronger when Vedastus goes on to promise remission of sins to the same number as the letters, points, and furrows. The connection is spelt out in an early twelfth-century addition to a miscellany from Durham, where each tool has its own allegorical association. For instance:

> *Creta cuius minutiis dealbatur assiduam sanctarum cogitationum curam designat, que conscientiam splendidam reddit.*

[7] C. Jacobsen, "A modern scribe views scribes of the past", in: *Scraped, Stroked, and Bound: Materially Engaged Readings of Medieval Manuscripts*, ed. J. Wilcox (Turnhout, 2013: *Utrecht Studies in Medieval Literacy* 23), pp. 75-92, at p. 90.

[8] MS Arras, Médiathèque, 860 (530), f. 1r. Text and translation from E. Sears, "The afterlife of scribes: Swicher's prayer in the Prüfening Isidore", in: *Pen in Hand: Medieval Scribal Portraits, Colophons and Tools*, ed. M. Gullick (Walkern, 2006), pp. 75-96, at pp. 87-88. See R. Gameson, "'Signed' manuscripts from early Romanesque Flanders", in: *Pen in Hand*, pp. 31-73, for an alternative translation, pp. 72-73, with the manuscript page as Figure 21, p. 61.

> The chalk with whose fine particles it [the parchment] is whitened signifies an unbroken meditation of holy thoughts, which makes our conscience resplendent.[9]

Further, scribes could use their presence in the process of transmission to insert themselves into the commune that the copied texts created between readers and heaven. This applies to scribes working on volumes in the vernacular, and containing Old English poetry, just as it does to those working on Latinate and scriptural productions. The Nowell Codex ends with *Beowulf* and *Judith* but opens with three prose texts, the first of which is a version of the *Passion of Saint Christopher*. There, the saint's final prayer reads:

> *drihten min god sẏle gode mede þam þe mine þro ungaƿarite 7 þa ecean edlean þam þe hie mid tearum rǽde* .$_{7}$

> Lord my God, give a good reward to any who write about my suffering, and eternal reward to any who read it with tears.[10]

This mention of the scribe does not appear in all versions: it is not 'original' and was presumably introduced by a scribe at some phase of the text's reproduction,[11] as a more thoroughly embedded version of numerous scribal colophons which invite prayers for the scribe.[12] To some extent, as Fred Robinson argues, scribes could claim equivalence with authors in terms of spiritual significance, both "intermediaries through whom God speaks".[13]

[9] MS Durham, Dean & Chapter Library, B. IV.12, ff. 37v-38v. Transcription and translation from M.A. ROUSE and R.H. ROUSE, "From flax to parchment: A monastic sermon from twelfth-century Durham", in: *New Science Out of Old Books: Studies in Manuscript and Early Printed Books in Honour of A.I. Doyle*, ed. R. BEADLE and A.J. PIPER (Aldershot, 1995), pp. 1-13. I am grateful to Nick Baker for bringing this text to my attention.

[10] My transcription from MS London, British Library, Cotton Vitellius A. XV, f. 95 (97) (BL 98)r. 14-17. Translations from Old English are mine.

[11] See P. PULSIANO, "The Passion of Saint Christopher", in: *Early Medieval Texts and Interpretations: Studies Presented to Donald G. Scragg*, ed. E. TREHARNE and S. ROSSER (Tempe, AZ, 2002), pp. 167-199. As he notes, the prayer is similar in the unprinted BHL 1769.

[12] See R. GAMESON, *The Scribe Speaks? Colophons in early English Manuscripts* (Cambridge, 2002).

[13] F.C. ROBINSON, "Old English literature in its most immediate context", in: *The Editing of Old English*, ed. F.C. ROBINSON (Oxford, 1994), pp. 3-24, at p. 19.

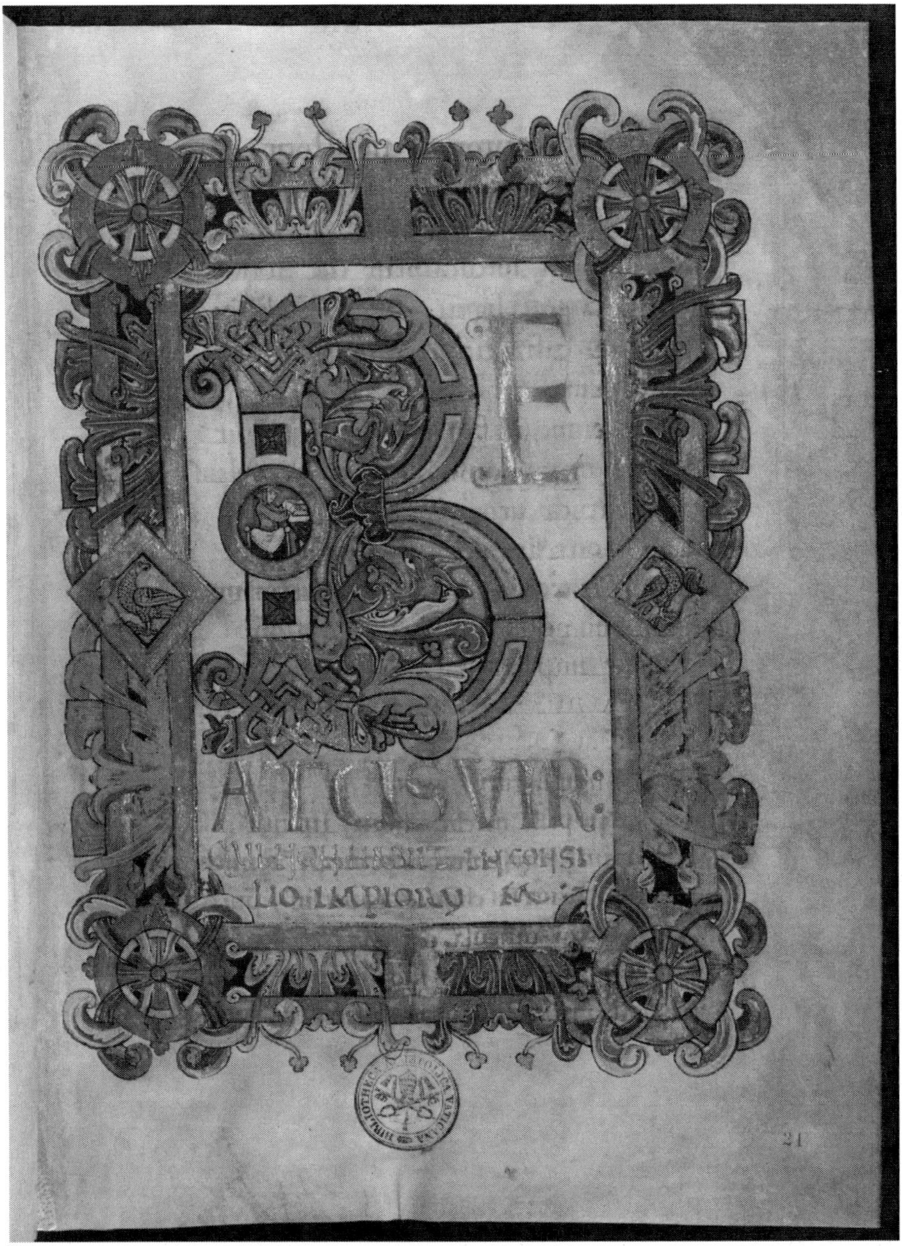

Fig. 6.1 MS Rome, Vatican Library, Reg. lat. 12, f. 21r. Reproduced by permission of the Vatican Apostolic Library, prot.15/1984-15R253.

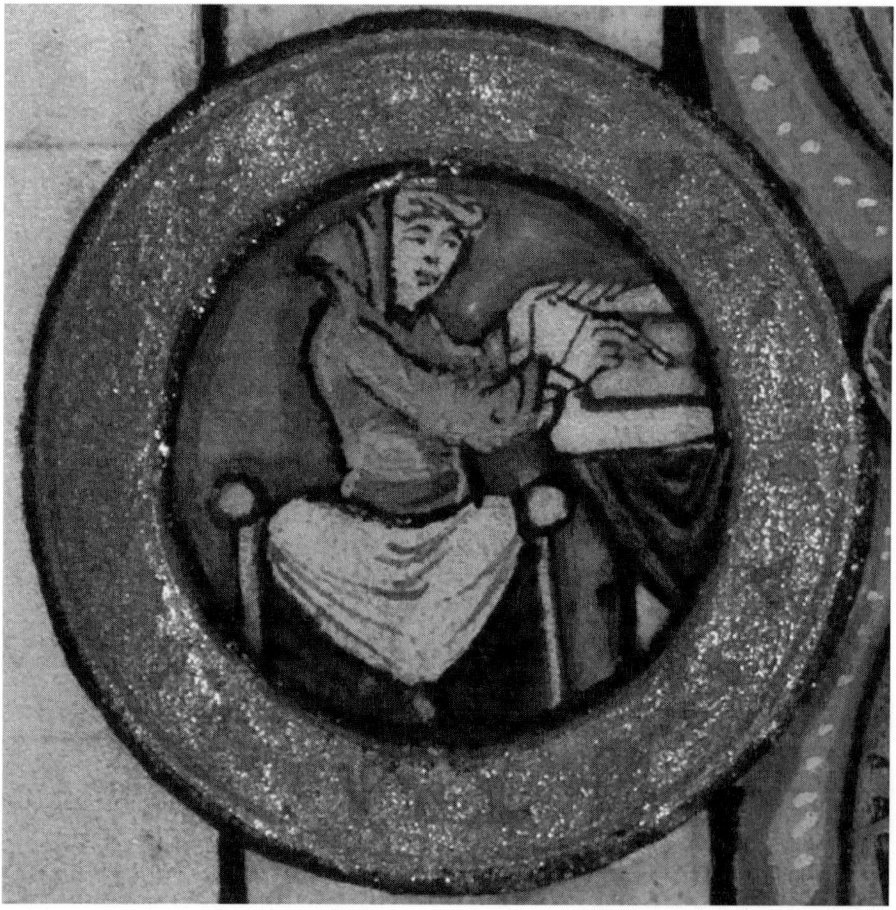

Fig. 6.2 MS Rome, Vatican Library, Reg. lat. 12, f. 21r, detail. Reproduced by permission of the Vatican Apostolic Library, prot.15/1984-15R253.

Anglo-Saxon illustrations of historical scribes emphasise this spiritual aspect of their work.[14] One example is that of St Matthew in the Lindisfarne Gospels, where the saint as scribe is shown sitting at ease, writing in his lap in relatively luxurious surroundings.[15] A haloed figure, half-hidden behind a cur-

[14] These images are widely printed and discussed. For full references and an alternative reading, see M. MICHAEL, "The birth of non-authorship: Interpreting the Lindisfarne Gospels St Matthew and the Codex Amiatinus Ezra", in: *Pen in Hand*, pp. 175-185.

[15] The Lindisfarne Gospels is MS London, British Library, Cotton Nero D. IV; this image f. 27r.

tain and holding a book, watches the evangelist, presumably figuring the divine word of God and true Book for which Matthew is an intermediary. Above the saint's head, his symbol of a winged man blows a trumpet in an act analogous to the scribal role, trumpeting forth the Gospel. The scribe is the author, and in both roles he channels truth, serenely receiving and delivering divine inspiration rather than struggling to reinterpret. Ezra is shown in a similar pose in the Codex Amiatinus, wearing colourful robes and eschewing the desk in front of him in favour of the more intimate process of writing on his lap.[16] The open bookcase behind him claims the scribe as possessor and transmitter of wisdom, performing a similar function to Matthew's angelic trumpet. As I have argued elsewhere, these images are part of an early conception of scribes as a passive conduit, serving the authorial voice by reproducing text.[17]

Either as a cause or result of this focus on scribing as a celebrated and meditative conduit, images of contemporary scribes are unusual in the Anglo-Saxon period. The only one of which I know is a small image in the initial *B* of a Beatus in the Bury Psalter, shown in Figs 6.1 and 6.2.[18] Unlike his more prestigious biblical counterparts, he works over a table and wears a simple, single coloured cowl, with a hood rather than a halo. Tiny, he is contained within the letter as a functional element, rather than occupying a full page like Matthew and Ezra. The green of his robe and blue background draw this small figure into the decorative scheme of the page rather than granting him individuality. This is the scribe as functionary rather than creator or interpreter, perhaps closer to scribes' self-perception as opposed to the creators of the texts they copied.

It may therefore not be surprising that the most attested sensory experience of scribing is the misery it induces. Richard Gameson has collected scribal colophons, the overwhelming majority of which, including all of those which mention sensory experience, record complaints. For instance:

[16] MS Florence, Biblioteca Medicea-Laurenziana, Amiatino I, f. V r. See also GAMESON, "The scribe speaks?", § 34, p. 47, who notes that there may have been an inscription around the image.

[17] S.C. THOMSON, "Scribes, sources, and readers: Using a digital edition to develop understanding of the *Beowulf* manuscript", *Poetica* 83 (2015), pp. 41-59, esp. pp. 41-42. See also M. FISHER, *Scribal Authorship and the Writing of History in Medieval England* (Columbus, OH, 2012), throughout, but e.g. pp. 20-21.

[18] MS Rome, Vatican Library, Reg. Lat. 12, f. 21r. The image is cited in this context in R. GAMESON, "Anglo-Saxon scribes and scriptoria", in: *The Cambridge History of the Book in Britain*, 1, *c. 400-1100*, ed. R. GAMESON (Cambridge, 2012), pp. 94-120, at p. 95.

> *Qui nescit scribere laborem esse non putat. Tribus digitis scribitur totum corpus laborat. Orate pro me qui istum librum legerit. F[init]. Per nomen sanctum filium tuum dominum nostrum Iesum Christum.*[19]
>
> He who does not know how to write does not think it is a labour. Writing is done with three fingers but the whole body labours. Pray for me whosoever shall have read this book. It is finished. Through the holy name, your son, our Lord, Jesus Christ.

Clearly, the potential sensory stimulation of an activity is not necessarily enough to render it exciting. I loved my first night shift in a factory: the slightly disjointed feel of sleeplessness and artificial light; smells of hot metal and grease; different languages around me; the feel of rapidly cooling plastic. But my excitement barely lasted the first shift; by the second night, the lack of autonomy took over. Possibly, scribes similarly experienced their work as passive parts of a machine, flawed facsimile-makers with no creative engagement of their own.[20]

Difficulty and Drudgery – Perceptions of Scribal Activity

Despite this self-presentation as miserable drudges, recent scholars have been keen to praise scribes, finding them "marvellously creative".[21] In his edition of the Exeter Book, Bernard Muir attributes the arrangement of texts and some adaptation to the scribe, whom he associates with the 'anthologist' who selected texts for inclusion, suggesting that "[i]n another manuscript context these same poems might have received different treatment at the hands of a different anthologist or scribe".[22] The same scribe has been argued to have adapted presentation by Winfried Rudolf, who found that marginal capitals

[19] MS Paris, Bibliothèque Nationale de France, lat. 9561 f. 81v. Text and translation from GAMESON, "The scribe speaks?", § 5, pp. 34-35. Cf. §§ 6, 19, 20, 31, 38 and perhaps 8, 23, 37.

[20] Cf. B. CERQUIGLINI, who argues for the making of facsimiles as a deadened process in *In Praise of the Variant: A Critical History of Philology*, trans. B. WING (London, 1999), first published as *Éloge de la variante: Histoire critique de la philologie* (Paris, 1989), p. 22.

[21] The quotation is from R. MCKITTERICK, "Glossaries and other innovations in Carolingian book production", in: *Turning Over a New Leaf: Change and Development in the Medieval Book*, ed. E. KWAKKEL, R. MCKITTERICK and R. THOMSON (Leiden, 2012), pp. 21-75, at p. 75.

[22] *Exeter Anthology*, ed. MUIR, p. 22.

support interpretation of the Riddles.[23] Andy Orchard has found the main scribe of Junius 11 to be fully engaged with *Genesis*, actively highlighting poetic repetition.[24] Elsewhere, Muir claims Anglo-Saxon texts as inherently "living, dynamic entities that were regularly adapted during the process of transmission".[25] Joyce Tally Lionarons makes a similar argument, but attributes the dynamism to scribing, arguing that "each rendition by an individual scribe represents a unique (re)performance of the work".[26] More cautiously, writing about the Nowell Codex, Josef Klegraf suggests that a scribe could "bring in features of his own 'style' as long as this practice does not interfere with a text's content or 'message'".[27] Considering the same manuscript, focussed on *Beowulf*, Kevin Kiernan has gone further, ascribing an authorial role to scribes,[28] supported recently by Helen Damico.[29]

However, earlier analyses have focussed on the mechanical aspect of scribal work. Scribes are castigated if they seem to have made changes, and admired if they have replicated their exemplars. The ideal scribe for early students of Old English poetry was thus one whose presence could not be detected: production of facsimiles, rather than editions, was the objective for scribes, if not for editors.[30] As Matthew Fisher has argued, this kind of judgement was and still is brought into a moral dimension, with scribes "suspected" of "corrupting" texts.[31]

[23] W. RUDOLF, "Riddling and reading: Iconicity and logographs in Exeter Book Riddles 23 and 45", *Anglia* 130 (2012), pp. 499-526.

[24] A. ORCHARD, "Intoxication, fornication, and multiplication: The burgeoning text of *Genesis A*", in: *Text, Image, Interpretation*, pp. 333-354, at pp. 339-340.

[25] B.J. MUIR, "Issues for editors of Old English poetry in manuscript form", in: *Inside Old English: Essays in Honour of Bruce Mitchell*, ed. J. WALMSLEY (Oxford, 2006), pp. 181-202, at p. 181.

[26] J.T. LIONARONS, "Introduction: Manuscript context and materialist philology", in: *Old English Literature in its Manuscript Context*, ed. J.T. LIONARONS (Morgantown, WV, 2004), pp. 1-10, at p. 5.

[27] J. KLEGRAF, "Testing faithful copying in the *Beowulf* manuscript", in: *Essays on the English Language and Applied Linguistics on the Occasion of Gerhard Nickel's 60th Birthday*, ed. J. KLEGRAF and D. NEHLS (Heidelberg, 1988), pp. 206-220, at p. 210.

[28] K. KIERNAN, *'Beowulf' and the 'Beowulf' Manuscript* (Ann Arbor, 1981, revised reprint 1999), esp. pp. 243-270.

[29] H. DAMICO, *'Beowulf' and the Grendel-Kin: Politics and Poetry in Eleventh-Century England* (Morgantown, WV, 2015).

[30] See e.g. D.G. SCRAGG, "Ælfric's scribes", in: *Essays for Joyce Hill on Her Sixtieth Birthday*, ed. M. SWAN (Leeds, 2006), pp. 179-189, at p. 185.

[31] FISHER, *Scribal Authorship*, e.g. p. 25. The language of suspicion and corruption is widely used, but see for instance *The Vercelli Homilies and Related Texts*, ed. D.G. SCRAGG (Oxford,

Michael Lapidge discusses this shift, considering the history of emending *Beowulf* and identifying a movement away from editorial "contempt for the transmitted text".[32] Lapidge supports this more critical approach to scribes' work, seeking to re-establish the distance between scribe and author, and placing the editor firmly in the latter's camp.[33] Douglas Moffat is similarly cynical about scribal capacity to "be like poets".[34] More recently, Lapidge has argued that the scribes of *Beowulf* failed to understand large parts of their exemplar, questioning their literacy in earlier forms of script.[35] Leonard Neidorf has followed him, suggesting that, with *Beowulf*, the scribes tried their best but bit off more than they could chew.[36] The Vercelli scribe is likewise found to show "little fluency" and "little intelligence" in copying the prose homilies which dominate the manuscript, and their editor is content to express "contempt" for him.[37] He is repeatedly guilty of "mechanical error" even though he seems to want to be "a slavish copyist at pains to reproduce his exemplar exactly".[38] This all follows Kenneth Sisam's claim that scribes simply cannot be trusted, because they freely altered wording and often did not understand what they were copying.[39] The truth is that scribes vary in their approach to their work, and some may have changed approach when working on different texts. To paraphrase Morrissey, some scribes were better than others; some scribes' projects had more scope for creativity than other scribes' projects. If later medieval practice is any guide, the same scribes may even have had different

1992), pp. LXXII and LXXIV; S. MORRISON, "What is scribal error, and what should editors do (or not do) about it?", in: *Probable Truth: Editing Medieval Texts from Britain in the Twenty-First Century*, ed. V. GILLESPIE and A. HUDSON (Turnhout, 2013), pp. 261-273, at p. 264.

[32] M. LAPIDGE, "On the emendation of Old English texts", in: *The Editing of Old English: Papers from the 1990 Manchester Conference* ed. D.G. SCRAGG and P.E. SZARMACH (Cambridge, 1994), pp. 53-68, at p. 57.

[33] LAPIDGE, "Emendation", pp. 54 and 66-67.

[34] D. MOFFAT, "Anglo-Saxon scribes and Old English verse", *Speculum* 67 (1992), pp. 805-827, at p. 814.

[35] M. LAPIDGE, "The archetype of *Beowulf*", *Anglo-Saxon England* 29 (2000), pp. 5-41.

[36] L. NEIDORF, "Scribal errors of proper names in the *Beowulf* Manuscript", *Anglo-Saxon England* 42 (2013), pp. 249-269.

[37] *The Vercelli Homilies*, ed. SCRAGG, p. LXXIII. His "contempt" was expressed at the International Medieval Congress in Kalamazoo 14-17 May 2015, in response to Catherine KARKOV's paper "The materiality of the cross in the Vercelli Book" in § 359.

[38] *Vercelli Homilies*, ed. SCRAGG, p. LXXI, the latter paraphrasing Celia Sisam in her facsimile, *The Vercelli Book: A Late Tenth-Century Manuscript Containing Prose and Verse: Vercelli Biblioteca capitolare CXVII*, ed. C. SISAM (Copenhagen, 1976), p. 29.

[39] K. SISAM, "The authority of Old English poetical manuscripts", in: *Studies in Old English Literature*, ed. K. SISAM (Oxford, 1953), pp. 29-44 throughout, esp. pp. 36-37.

attitudes to the same text when copying it in different contexts.[40] Scribal inconsistency is mirrored by scholars: as is apparent from this swift and incomplete survey, there is considerable variation in descriptions of scribal activity and what the criteria are for doing it well. And whether it is to be praised or reviled, it is clear that readers and editors of Old English poetry must engage with scribal activity. Such variation in terms used to describe individual scribal performances makes it difficult to analyse scribes, and still harder to access the context in which they worked. 'Mechanical' copying is, for instance, used by Klegraf to mean a scribe who writes in the patterns of his training, unconsciously converting orthography, layout, and script from exemplar forms to those with which he is comfortable. But Katherine O'Brien O'Keeffe, Leonard Neidorf, and perhaps Donald Scragg, use the same term to mean a scribe who reproduces what he sees in an exemplar without intellectually engaging with it or troubling to resolve it into sense.[41] I use it above to mean the process of reproduction without necessarily implying a lack of thought. How should we describe an eighth-century scribe who refreshes some parts of an old text in MS London, British Library, Additional 40165.A.1 to make it more readable?[42] And what is a scribe doing when he intentionally – rather than thoughtlessly – reproduces exemplar forms, such as the scribe who tried to write some phrases in the script of his exemplar in MS Würzburg, M.p.th.f.79,[43] or my findings about the scribes of the Nowell Codex, who varied the forms of initial capitals, apparently echoing those used in their exemplars?[44] What is the difference between this and Scragg's Vercelli scribe, who intended to reproduce his exemplar but utterly failed to do so?

It seems to be the case that a scribe's performance is judged by two criteria. First, what was the attitude to the exemplar(s): exact reproduction or remaking for some contextual reason? Secondly, did the process of the text

[40] FISHER, *Scribal Authorship*, e.g. pp. 41-45, 50-55.

[41] O'BRIEN O'KEEFFE, *Visible Song*, e.g. p. 164; NEIDORF, "Scribal errors"; D. SCRAGG, "Cambridge, Corpus Christi College 162", in: *Manuscript and Heritage*, pp. 71-83, at p. 77.

[42] W. SCHIPPER, "Textual varieties in manuscript margins", in: *Signs on the Edge: Space, Text, and Margin in Medieval Manuscripts*, ed. S.L. KEEFER and R.H. BREMMER Jr (Leuven, 2007), pp. 25-54, at p. 35.

[43] M.T. HUSSEY, "Anglo-Saxon scribal *habitus* and Frankish aesthetics in an early uncial manuscript", in: *Scraped, Stroked, and Bound*, pp. 15-37, esp. pp. 29-31.

[44] S.C. THOMSON, "Capital indications: How Scribe A thought readers should engage with the Nowell Codex", in: *Proceedings from the Fifth International Conference 'Language, Culture, and Society in Russian / English Studies'* (forthcoming).

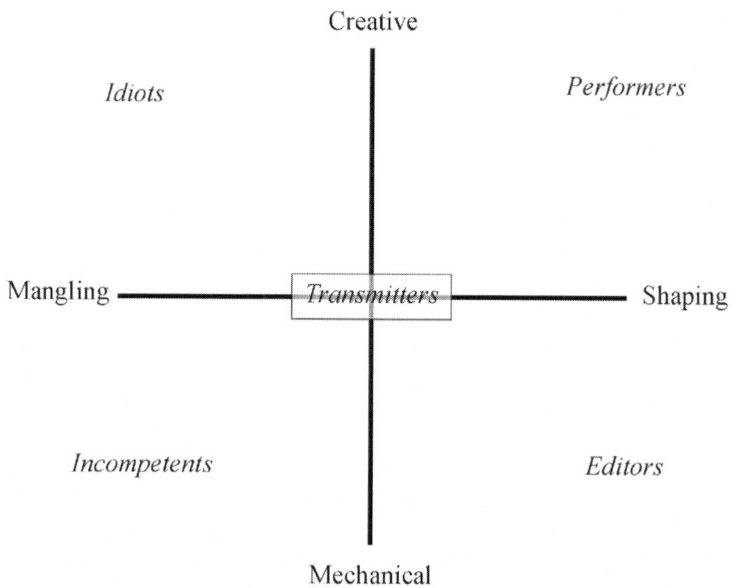

Fig. 6.3 Matrix of types of scribal performance

passing through their hands change that text for better or for worse? The first criterion assesses scribes on their own terms by asking what they thought they were doing in the process of copying. The second judges their results in the context of (intrinsically imperfect) modern understanding of their base text. It should be self-evident that both judgements are based on partial and subjective grounds. It is extremely difficult to assess what scribes thought they were doing with their texts; it is equally difficult to have any secure knowledge of their base texts. But, as I shall briefly suggest below, some such evidence can be gathered and analysed using some rather crude tools.

These two continua of assessing scribal performance can be placed together to produce a matrix, as shown in Fig. 6.3, which assesses both the degree of freedom scribes seem to take, and the extent to which they are improving or damaging their texts.[45] In the middle of the matrix are scribes who precisely recreate what they see: faithful 'transmitters' who create a facsimile

[45] Cf. Fisher's definition of "duplicative" and "replicative" copying in FISHER, *Scribal Authorship*, pp. 37-38.

copy. A scribe shaping his text creatively can be seen as a 'performer' of that text, akin to the scribal authors that Fisher and others have identified in the later period. A more mechanical 'shaper' works like a modern editor: seeking to present the source text accurately but re-shaped for a new context. A scribe who seeks to copy mechanically, but fails and mangles his text, is 'incompetent'; one who mangles the text while seeking to be creative with it is 'idiotic'. There is no space here to delineate the implications of these different types of activity, nor even to give examples of each case, but it is to be hoped that such a matrix will bring some clarity to discussions of scribal performance. I will, though, briefly explore some creativity that can be seen in codices containing Old English poetry before returning to the initial question of whether any of this activity indicates engagement with the rhythms of texts.

Some Instances of Scribal Creativity

It is clear that we do not yet fully understand what choices scribes made in the presentation of Old English verse. As Francis Newton puts it, "[t]he student of manuscripts must always be open to the possibility of form and artistry".[46] A possible area of scribal artistry is spacing. It has been clear to scholars for some time that word spacing in Old English is not random; it is equally clear that the inconsistency of spacing means that identifying any 'rules' is currently impossible. Thomas Cable noted this difficult situation, admitting that in *Beowulf* "there is spacing where I cannot explain it, and in other places no spacing where I would expect it to occur", but also noting that some of the use of spacing "forces on us unexpected perceptions of a complex and endlessly teasing aesthetic form".[47] Katherine O'Brien O'Keeffe has made similar, if more prosaic, observations about punctuation, noting "trends ... which suggest a deliberate and meaningful pattern" and repeatedly finding scribes making individual

[46] F. NEWTON, "A giant among scribes: Colophon and iconographical programme in the Eadui Gospels", in: *Writing in Context*, pp. 127-149, at p. 129.

[47] T. CABLE, "Review of Robert D. Stevick's *Beowulf: An Edition with Manuscript Spacing Notation and Graphotactic Analyses* (New York: Garland, 1975)", *Computers and the Humanities* 11 (1977), pp. 47-55, at p. 49.

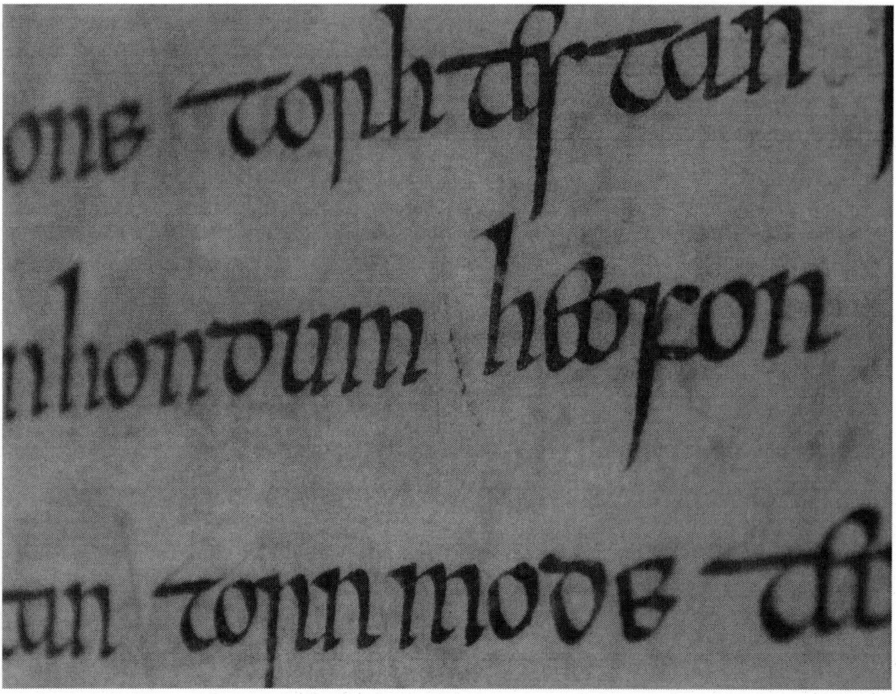

Fig.6.4 MS Exeter, Cathedral Libary, 3501 (the Exeter Book), f. 42r, lines 6-8, showing drypoint marking verse boundaries in *Guthlac A*. Reproduced by permission of the Dean and Chapter of Exeter Cathedral.

"expressive" choices.[48] A more recent assessment of punctuation follows the same line, finding it "not quite systematic, not quite random".[49]

The extent to which pointing should be used to mark separate verses certainly seems to have been an individual preference. In the Exeter Book, at least one later reader was clearly dissatisfied with the sparse pointing provided by the scribes. Marks, usually slashes, indicate verse boundaries through a number

[48] O'BRIEN O'KEEFFE, *Visible Song*, p. 72, here of capitalisation in MS Cambridge, Corpus Christi College, 422. 'Expressive' is used regularly throughout, e.g. pp. 75, 155, 187.

[49] D. DONOGHUE, "A point well taken: Manuscript punctuation and Old English poems", in: *Inside Old English*, ed. J. WALMSLEY (Oxford, 2006), pp. 38-58, at p. 57.

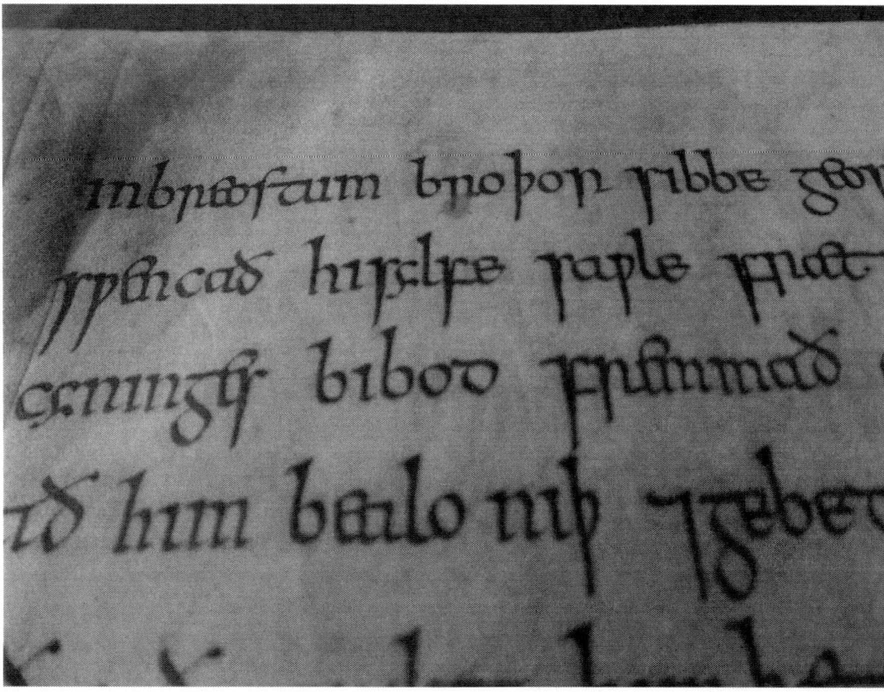

Fig.6.5 MS Exeter, Cathedral Libary, 3501 (the Exeter Book), f. 44v, lines 1-4, showing drypoint marking verse boundaries in *Guthlac A*. Reproduced by permission of the Dean and Chapter of Exeter Cathedral.

of texts, including *Guthlac* and *Juliana*.[50] They are used so regularly that they even occur where the scribe has pointed the verse ending. As shown in Fig.6.4, marks are repeated in the same site, with two lines at different angles between "*hondum*" and "*heofenum*"; sometimes they cross one another as in the first line of Fig. 6.5 between "*breostum*" and "*broþor*"; sometimes, marks contradict one another in their interpretation of metrical breaks as illustrated by Figure 6.6, where different readers have placed marks either side of "*ar*". This all suggests that more than one reader participated in this action and that some readers disagreed with one another about where verse boundaries lay. In Junius 11, diverse practice seems to have been read as incompetence rather than dif-

[50] The marks are discussed by D. McGovern, "Unnoticed punctuation in the Exeter Book", *Medium Ævum* 52 (1983), pp. 90-99. I am grateful to Jane Roberts for discussing them with me, and to Peter Thomas and the other staff at Exeter Cathedral for allowing me to examine them. Images reproduced by kind permission of the Dean and Chapter of Exeter Cathedral.

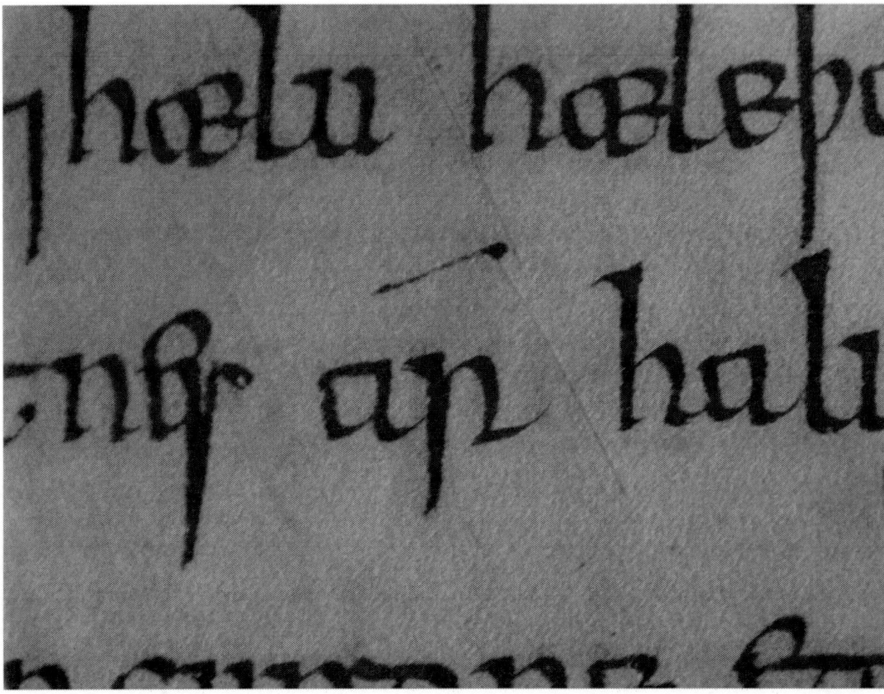

Fig. 6.6 MS Exeter, Cathedral Libary, 3501 (the Exeter Book), f. 42v, lines 7-8, showing drypoint marking verse boundaries in *Guthlac A*. Reproduced by permission of the Dean and Chapter of Exeter Cathedral.

ference of opinion: a proof-reader corrected *Christ and Satan*, including the addition of pointing in a number of places.[51] So, while scribes could make decisions about presentation, those choices were expected to fit within an overarching project. Junius 11 required metrical pointing, so failing to include it did not show admirable fidelity, but unthinking reproduction.

Scribes are generally identified and dated by the letterforms they use, and yet it is well known that they both could and did vary the forms they deployed. Kiernan suggests that palaeography "is not a test of dating but of chosen style".[52] An obvious instance is in the Exeter Book, where the scribe varies his Square Minuscule hand at key moments. This is particularly noticeable at the end of *The Phoenix*, lines 667-677, on f. 65v, where the b-verse, or second half

[51] O'BRIEN O'KEEFFE, *Visible Song*, pp. 183-184.

[52] KIERNAN, *'Beowulf' Manuscript*, p. 24.

of each poetic line, is in Latin. Whenever *a* appears in these words it is written in the half-uncial *oc* form, shifting back to the regular square topped minuscule *a* for Old English words.[53] Similar instances have been found elsewhere. Matthew Hussey showed that the scribe of MS Würzburg, M.p.th.f.79 was working hard to write in uncial script when he was more accustomed to writing in half-uncial.[54] Following Timothy Graham's work on MS Cambridge, Corpus Christ College, 57,[55] Julia Crick has identified a wide number of scribal attempts to archaise their hands, many of which are forgeries. Some, however, represent aesthetic choice rather than deception, demonstrating, as noted in the introduction to this piece, that "some texts needed to be seen as well as heard", and, further, that scribes were sophisticated in responding to their readers' multi-sensory expectations.[56] Patrick Conner, reviewing such instances, argues that "it is possible for scribes to call forth a hand" as required for a particular project.[57]

I have argued elsewhere that small capitals are another scribal feature which scribes used creatively.[58] The first scribe of *Beowulf* in the Nowell Codex uses minor, non-marginal, capitals quite consistently between two of the prose texts that he works on, differently in the poem *Beowulf* and differently again from the second scribe of *Beowulf*. Thus it seems likely that he saw himself as shaping the text of the poem and quite probably the other texts, too. There is, in fact, a quite remarkable degree of clustering of minor capitals in his portion of *Beowulf*. His average use is of one minor capital every 1.61 sides. It is, therefore, striking that seven occur within four sides at 1.75 per side from folio 163 (BL 166)r to 164 (BL 167)v.[59] These pages contain lines 1491b-1591a, from Beowulf's final words to Hrothgar before he dives into the mere

[53] Cf. *The Exeter Book of Old English Poetry*, ed. R.W. CHAMBERS, M. FÖRSTER and R. FLOWER (London, 1933), p. 83; see also the discussion in: *Exeter Anthology*, ed. MUIR, 1, pp. 25-27; J. ROBERTS *Guide to Scripts Used in English Writings up to 1500* (London, 2005) prints another page showing the same variation as § 11, p. 60.

[54] HUSSEY, "Anglo-Saxon scribal *habitus*", esp. pp. 29-31.

[55] GRAHAM, "CCCC 57", esp. pp. 29-30.

[56] J. CRICK, "Script and the sense of the past in Anglo-Saxon England", in: *Anglo-Saxon Traces*, ed. J. ROBERTS and L. WEBSTER (Tempe, 2011), pp. 1-30, at p. 28. Cf. M.P. BROWN, *The Book and the Transformation of Britain c. 550-1050: A Study in Written and Visual Literacy and Orality* (London, 2011), esp. pp. 36 and 57; PARKES, *Their Hands*, p. 133.

[57] P.W. CONNER, "On the nature of matched scribal hands", in: *Scraped, Stroked, and Bound*, pp. 39-73, at p. 50.

[58] THOMSON, "Capital indications".

[59] I use the same foliation system for the Nowell Codex as Kiernan's in *Electronic 'Beowulf'*.

up to the moment when blood from the decapitated monsters flows up through the lake and is seen by the waiting Danes and Geats. That is, the passage with more minor capitals than any other in the text is also the passage which contains the deaths of two monsters. As I have discussed elsewhere, some (but not all) other bursts of use also correspond with monstrous activity.[60] It seems likely that we are seeing a creative scribe responding to and re-presenting his text. It is worth noting in this context that I have not been able to discern any patterns of use in *Alexander's Letter to Aristotle*, the long prose text that precedes *Beowulf*, copied by the same scribe and probably coming from the same exemplar.[61] In this text, small capitals do cluster but apparently only around the start and end of the text, rather than across passages with particular meanings. It may, then, be the case, that scribes (or this scribe at least) were more inclined to engage creatively with poetry.

Throughout the four codices that contain the majority of extant Old English poetry, as George Krapp wrote of Junius 11, small capitals "are not systematically used, but when they appear it is almost always possible to see a definite purpose in their use".[62] In Fig. 6.7, I have laid out the frequency of minor capitals in some of the longer texts of the different manuscripts. Where different scribes are thought to have shared texts, I have also shown the frequency of use by the different scribes. I will not use most of the terms of comparison here, but have provided full data sets with figures per manuscript and poetic line as well as per manuscript side in the hope that more work can be done with them in the future.[63]

The simple points that I want to make here are, first, that the variation apparent within *Beowulf* is also apparent in *Christ and Satan*, the other shared text in this group, although the numbers of sides copied by the three scribes of the latter text vary too widely for this comparison to be secure. Secondly, there are some interesting variations and consistencies across the different manu-

[60] THOMSON, "Capital indications".

[61] A. ORCHARD, *A Critical Companion to 'Beowulf'* (Cambridge, 2003; paperback edition 2004), p. 35; K. SISAM, "The compilation of the *Beowulf* manuscript", in: *Studies*, ed. SISAM, pp. 65-96, at p. 94.

[62] *Junius 11*, ed. KRAPP, in: ASPR 1 (1931), p. XX.

[63] KLEGRAF, "Faithful copying", p. 206, discusses the value of numerical analysis in understanding scribal performance. The identification of a 'minor' capital is not always certain: frequently, the decision about whether to 'count' a letter is subjective. In the vast majority of cases, my counts agree with Krapp and Dobbie's.

Manuscript	Text	MS sides	MS lines	Poetic lines	Minor capitals (MC)	Per side	MS lines per MC	Poetic lines / MC	MS lines / poetic line	Poetic lines / MS page
Junius 11	Genesis	116	3,016	2,937	160	1.38	18.85	18.36	1.03	25.32
	Exodus	23	598	590	28	1.22	21.36	21.07	1.01	25.65
	Daniel	37	962	764	58	1.57	16.59	13.17	1.26	20.65
	Christ and Satan	17	446	730	32	1.88	13.94	22.81	0.61	42.94
	S.2. Christ and Satan	*3*	*81*	*124*	*12*	*4.00*	*6.75*	*10.33*	*0.65*	*41.33*
	S.3. Christ and Satan	*13*	*351*	*586*	*14*	*1.08*	*25.07*	*41.86*	*0.60*	*45.08*
	S.4. Christ and Satan	*1*	*14*	*20*	*6*	*6.00*	*2.33*	*3.33*	*0.70*	*20.00*
	Junius 11	**193**	**5,022**	**5,021**	**278**	**1.44**	**18.06**	**18.06**	**1.00**	**26.02**
Nowell Codex	Beowulf	141	2,896	3,182	67	0.48	43.22	47.49	0.91	22.57
	S.A. Beowulf	*88*	*1792*	*1,939*	*55*	*0.63*	*32.58*	*35.25*	*0.92*	*22.03*
	S.B. Beowulf	*53*	*1104*	*1,243*	*12*	*0.23*	*92.00*	*103.58*	*0.89*	*23.45*
	Judith	16	320	349	5	0.31	64.00	69.80	0.92	21.81
	Nowell Codex	**157**	**3,216**	**3,531**	**72**	**0.46**	**44.67**	**49.04**	**0.91**	**22.49**
Vercelli Book	Andreas	46	1,148	1,722	354	7.70	3.24	4.86	0.67	37.43
	Fates	4	100	122	34	8.50	2.94	3.59	0.82	30.50
	Soul and Body I	5	120	166	18	3.60	6.67	9.22	0.72	33.20
	Homiletic Fragment I	2	48	47	7	3.50	6.86	6.71	1.02	23.50
	Dream of the Rood	4	120	156	24	6.00	5.00	6.50	0.77	39.00
	Shorter poems	15	388	491	83	5.53	4.67	5.92	0.79	32.73
	Elene	26	832	1,321	222	8.54	3.75	5.95	0.63	50.81
	Vercelli Book	**87**	**2,368**	**3,534**	**659**	**7.57**	**3.59**	**5.36**	**0.67**	**40.62**
Exeter Book	Advent Lyrics	12	276	439	25	2.08	11.04	17.56	0.63	36.58
	Ascension	13	288	427	46	3.54	6.26	9.28	0.67	32.85
	Christ in Judgment	24	528	798	67	2.79	7.88	11.91	0.66	33.25
	Guthlac A	24	528	819	170	7.08	3.11	4.82	0.64	34.13
	Guthlac B	17	390	560	85	5.00	4.59	6.59	0.70	32.94
	Canticles of the Three Youths	5	110	191	17	3.40	6.47	11.24	0.58	38.20
	Phoenix	21	440	677	58	2.76	7.59	11.67	0.65	32.24
	Juliana	22	484	731	68	3.09	7.12	10.75	0.66	33.23
	Exeter Book	**138**	**3,044**	**4,642**	**536**	**3.88**	**5.68**	**8.66**	**0.66**	**33.64**

Fig. 6.7 Table with the frequency of minor capitals used by the scribes of selected texts in the four major codices of Old English verse.

scripts. In the first three texts of Junius 11, for instance, the use of minor capitals is broadly consistent, varying only between 1.22 and 1.57 per side, a negligible difference. In the Exeter Book, however, more variation is apparent. While most texts have around three minor capitals per side, the full range is from 2.79 per side in *Christ in Judgement (Christ* III*)* up to 7.08 per side in *Guthlac A*. Quite why the scribe used so many more minor capitals in the *Guthlac* texts is not revealed by this approach, but is worthy of further study. The general impression is that scribes have 'default' behaviours which vary under certain circumstances. This reinforces the idea of scribes who could be more or less engaged with the process of interpreting and re-presenting their texts. Scribe A in the Nowell Codex was certainly more engaged with a poetic than prosaic text, but more investigation into scribal behaviour across prose and poetry in, for instance, the Vercelli Book, is needed to know if this variation is frequent.

Manuscript	Text	Written sides	a verse	b verse	total no.	a %	b %	total %
Junius 11	Genesis	116	19	75	94	16.38%	64.66%	81.03%
	Exodus	23	1	18	19	4.35%	78.26%	82.61%
	Daniel	37	2	24	26	5.41%	64.86%	70.27%
	Christ and Satan	17	2	6	8	11.76%	35.29%	47.06%
	S.2 Christ and Satan	3	1	2	3	33.33%	66.67%	100.00%
	S.3 Christ and Satan	13	4	-	4	30.77%	0.00%	30.77%
	S.4 Christ and Satan	1	-	1	1	0.00%	100.00%	100.00%
	Junius 11	**196**	**24**	**123**	**147**	**12.24%**	**62.76%**	**75.00%**
Nowell Codex	Beowulf	140	36	22	58	25.71%	15.71%	41.43%
	S.A. Beowulf	87	17	12	29	19.54%	13.79%	33.33%
	S.B. Beowulf	53	19	10	29	35.85%	18.87%	54.72%
	Judith	16	3	6	9	18.75%	37.50%	56.25%
	Nowell Codex	**156**	**39**	**28**	**67**	**25.00%**	**17.95%**	**42.95%**
Vercelli Book	Andreas	46	7	10	17	15.22%	21.74%	36.96%
	Shorter poems	14	2	5	7	14.29%	35.71%	50.00%
	Elene	26	9	6	15	34.62%	23.08%	57.69%
	Vercelli Book	**86**	**18**	**21**	**39**	**20.93%**	**24.42%**	**45.35%**
Exeter Book	Advent Lyrics	12	1	1	2	8.33%	8.33%	16.67%
	Ascension	13	2	4	6	15.38%	30.77%	46.15%
	Christ in Judgment	24	6	8	14	25.00%	33.33%	58.33%
	Guthlac A	24	8	2	10	33.33%	8.33%	41.67%
	Guthlac B	17	4	3	7	23.53%	17.65%	41.18%
	Three Youths	5	1	2	3	20.00%	40.00%	60.00%
	Phoenix	21	7	5	12	33.33%	23.81%	57.14%
	Juliana	22	6	8	14	27.27%	36.36%	63.64%
	Exeter Book	**246**	**53**	**59**	**112**	**21.54%**	**23.98%**	**45.53%**

Fig. 6.8 Table with the coincidence of verse and side ending in selected texts in the four major codices of Old English verse.

Another presentational method that these scribes deploy to varying degrees is coincidence of the end of a manuscript side with the end of a poetic verse, as shown in Fig. 6.8.[64] Most scribes do this on more than half of the pages they copy, and some do it more frequently. This summary is a generalisation: the 'incompetent' scribe of Junius 11's *Christ and Satan*, and Scribe A of *Beowulf* do so only about 30% of the time; it is more frequent in the Exeter Book and Junius 11 than in the Nowell Codex and the Vercelli Book. More striking than these low incidences is the very high rate in Junius 11, where the main scribe made this happen on over 80% of pages through *Genesis* and *Exodus*. That

[64] Following Daniel Donoghue's definition in D. DONOGHUE, "Metre, OE", in: *The Blackwell Encyclopaedia of Anglo-Saxon England* ed. M. LAPIDGE, J. BLAIR, S. KEYNES and D. SCRAGG (Oxford, 1999, reprint 2001), pp. 310-311. As above in note 5, I have relied on the ASPR editions of poetic texts, but editorial definition of verse boundaries in Old English texts is not very variable.

even the most skilled scribe working hard at his presentation does not coincide verse and page endings on every occasion demonstrates that it was not absolutely necessary, or perhaps that it was challenging to achieve. It is also interesting that the main scribe of Junius 11, when he coincides verse and page ending, overwhelmingly does so for the b-verse, where there is less difference in verse treatment shown by scribes in other manuscripts. That is, in Junius 11 the coincidence of the end of a poetic line with the end of a manuscript page is almost as high as the coincidence of the end of a verse with that of a page. This is in line with the inconsistency in use of the other graphical features discussed above: the argument is not that every scribe was constantly thinking about how to present their text and working to do so in creative ways, but that many scribes sometimes did and that, therefore, these presentational devices had some value for readers.

Along with the general weight of statistical evidence of this phenomenon are a number of incidences where scribes have visibly worked hard to end their manuscript side at the end of a verse. At the end of God's speech to Lot in *Genesis*, line 2513, the scribe ends page 116, leaving enough space at the end of the line for most of line 2514a. At the end of line 385 of *Exodus* on page 161 of the manuscript, he does the opposite, writing the last three letters of "*stigon*" beneath the main ruling rather than splitting it across two pages. Another tactic can be seen at line 1866 of *Genesis*, page 89, where the last word of the poetic line, "*geðreadne*", is squeezed into the line, moving the right hand margin much further across than any of the preceding manuscript lines.

A significant weakness in this argument is that it may well be the case that many breaks relate to meaning rather than to metrics and are only "coincidentally metrical in shape".[65] It is certainly true that many pages are designed around meaning: in Junius 11 this is particularly noticeable when gaps are left at the foot of pages when the scribe clearly regarded the 'section' as complete.[66] However, it is also worth noting that in a number of instances, such as line 385 of *Exodus*, above, the break is not semantic. The sentence reads:

[65] O'Brien O'Keeffe, *Visible Song*, p. 164 uses this phrase in relation to pointing in the Exeter Book.

[66] See e.g. pages 3, 12, 13, 16, 40, 50, 116, and 151.

Siððan he gelædde leofost feora
haliges hæsum; heahlond stigon
sibgemagas, on Seone beorh.

Then he led the beloved people by holy command; the kinsmen climbed the hill to Mount Zion.

If meaning mattered above all other considerations, the scribe should have copied out line 386 beneath the ruled line; if neither meaning nor metrics mattered, he should have broken "*stigon*" across pages rather than using an additional line. The same is true of a number of other instances, including lines 270 and 1866 of *Genesis* noted above.

Another instance can be found in the Exeter Book, where f. 64v ends with line 623a of *The Phoenix*, concluding the side at the end of a verse but in the middle of a sentence. A hypothetical speech, a hymn of praise the author imagines being sung by the angels to God, has just started, with

Sib si þe, soð god, ond snyttrucræft,
ond þe þonc sy | þrymsittendum
geongra gyfena, goda gehwylces.[67]

Peace be with you, true God, and the strength of wisdom, and thanks to you, | seated in glory, for your fresh gifts and for every good thing.

In keeping with the fairly sparse punctuation policy of the Exeter Book, there are few points on the side. I count five before the final manuscript line, the others at manuscript lines 5 (twice), 8, 9, and 14.[68] In keeping with standard practice, a point precedes the start of the speech, which also starts with a minor capital. What is interesting here is that the manuscript line ends with line 623a and, where there would be space to write "*þrym*", the first part of the first word of 623b, the scribe instead places a point. There is no break of sense here: there can be little doubt that both the point and the break between pages relates to the coincidence of verse and side ending.

It is also worth noting that if scribes sought to bring sections of meaning to an end at the close of pages, they were not very good at it in prose. As noted

[67] *The Phoenix*, lines 622-624. Bars inserted in Old English and translation are mine, showing page breaks.

[68] Points follow poetic lines 596a and b, 600b, 602b, 610b. The last two are also punctuated by Krapp and Dobbie.

above, the first scribe of *Beowulf* also copied three prose texts. Excluding the final page of each text, there are strikingly few instances where a unit of meaning (a clause, or sentence, or section) comes to an end at the end of a page. It never happens in the fragment of *St Christopher*. There are three instances in *Wonders of the East*, one on the first page, possibly indicating that it was a desideratum.[69] There is not a single instance in fifty sides of *Alexander's Letter to Aristotle*.[70] *Wonders* is a highly structured text, divided into short sections mostly accompanied by images, which may have made it easier or more desirable to connect semantic breaks with page endings. However that may be, it remains the case that in seventy-three sides of prose, the scribe coincides the ending of just three with a break in a unit of meaning such as a sentence or a section, at a rate of 4.11%.[71] While the proportion of the end of poetic sides coinciding with a metrical or semantic break is hardly compelling in Scribe A's work, it is overwhelming in comparison with the rate of such breaks in his prose. Taken together with the evident intention to produce such breaks in Junius 11, it is clear that scribes sometimes organised their copying around the content of texts and that they seem to have found it easier to do so when those texts were structured metrically, and, further, that they sometimes (as in the example from *Exodus*, above) organised their copying on purely metrical criteria. Another way of putting this, in the context of the foregoing discussion, is that scribes were more inclined to creatively reshape their texts if they were poems.

Did Scribes "Whistle While They Worked"?

It is certain that some scribes thought about the process of copying, and that they found significance in their own role and the process of textual reproduction. It is also certain that at least some scribes actively understood the copying of Old English texts as the making of texts for aural reception. Scribing could be, and often was, a multi-sensory experience, engaged with the tools

[69] On ff. 95(97) (BL 98)v, 100(96) (BL 103)r, and 103 (BL 106)r.

[70] The modern editions make it look as though there is a sentence ending at the foot of f. 113(121) (BL 124)r, with a new sentence starting "*Eall* ..." on the next side. It is not marked by the scribe, who points before the editorial break, and the last letter of the first word on f. 113(121) (BL 124)v is not *l*.

[71] There are seventy-six prose sides, but three are the final sides of pieces and I do not include them here.

of the trade and with the process of book-making. And it is certain that, while some scribes conceived of their role and performed (more or less effectively) as mechanical reproducers of text, many did not and instead engaged creatively with their texts. But, to return to the questions asked at the start of this paper, is there evidence of scribes engaging with the metrical rhythms of Old English poetic texts? Is it possible to imagine a scriptorium where scribes whistled as they worked, hearing the words and verses they wrote? The short answer is that the evidence is inconclusive. Evidence of such individual and transitory experiences is sparse; proof is virtually impossible. But as work continues to consider the evidence for how scribes worked and what they expected readers to do with their texts, we draw closer to understanding some of the multiple contexts of scribal activity, and hence to appreciating the multiple sensory experiences provided by texts in Anglo-Saxon England.

Doing Things with Words: Language and Perception in Old English Riddles and Charms

VICTORIA SYMONS

Those who are wise must differentiate between "*worda ond worca*" ("words and actions"), so claims the coastguard who confronts Beowulf upon his arrival on the shores of Denmark (*Beowulf*, ll. 287-291a).[1] This assertion implies a straightforward dichotomy between language and reality: actions exist as objective facts, the perception of which can be either aided or clouded by one's use of words. The relationship between words and the world was one that preoccupied many early medieval writers, from Isidore of Seville and Gregory the Great to Ælfric of Eynsham, and is rarely as straightforward nor as binary as the coastguard's aphorism suggests. The Exeter Book riddles are, indeed, predicated upon a similar notion that "reality exists and is at the same time a mosaic of man's perception",[2] but in their focus on the role that language can play in mediating perception they demonstrate that, no matter how wise we may be, our sense of reality is inherently unreliable and open to

[1] "*Beowulf* and *Judith*, ed. E.V.K. DOBBIE, in: ASPR 4 (New York, 1953); unless otherwise specified, translations are my own.

[2] C. WILLIAMSON, *The Old English Riddles of the Exeter Book* (Chapel Hill, 1977), p. 25.

Sensory Perception in the Medieval West, ed. Simon C. THOMSON and Michael D.J. BINTLEY, *Utrecht Studies in Medieval Literacy*, 34 (Turnhout: Brepols, 2016), pp. 123-140.

BREPOLS PUBLISHERS DOI 10.1484/M.USML-EB.5.109507

manipulation. At the same time, the Old English charms conceptualise language not simply as a means of understanding reality, but of exerting control over it. This contribution will discuss the complex, nuanced, and at times contradictory relationship between perception, language and reality that informs the Old English riddles and charms, and the role that words can play as an alternative to the five senses as a means of understanding the world around us.

Isidore of Seville's *Etymologiae* was one of the most circulated works of the medieval period, with nearly a thousand surviving manuscripts or fragments attesting to its widespread popularity.[3] Its influence can also be seen, through quotations and allusions, in the works of many of the prominent thinkers of the early medieval period.[4] Over the course of its twenty volumes, Isidore's encyclopedia covers an exceptionally diverse range of material, including the seven liberal disciplines, the natural world, human history, the organisation of the Church, medicine, law, and architecture. The topic chosen to start this conspectus of learning is language, in a position that was by no means arbitrary. Rather than discuss a topic directly, Isidore more often prioritises explanations of the language with which that topic is associated. The result is a distinctive style and methodology that continues throughout the *Etymologiae* as a whole. The importance of meaning to this approach is explained, appropriately enough, in the entry for etymology itself:

> *Etymologia est origo vocabulorum, cum vis verbi vel nominis per interpretationem colligitur. ... Cuius cognitio saepe usum necessarium habet in interpretatione sua. Nam dum videris unde ortum est nomen, citius vim eius intellegis. Omnis enim rei inspectio etymologia cognita planior est.*[5] (I. XXIX)

> Etymology (*etymologia*) is the origin of words, when the force of a verb or a noun is inferred through interpretation ... The knowledge of a word's etymology often has an indispensable usefulness for interpreting the word, for when you have seen whence a word has originated, you understand its force more quickly. Indeed, one's insight into anything is clearer when its etymology is known.[6]

[3] *The Etymologies of Isidore of Seville*, trans. S. BARNEY, W.J. LEWIS, J.A. BEACH and O. BERGHOF (Cambridge, 2006), p. 24.

[4] For the influence of the *Etymologiae* on Anglo-Saxon writers, see L. LOCKETT, *Anglo-Saxon Psychologies in the Vernacular and Latin Traditions* (Toronto, 2011), pp. 225-226.

[5] All quotations from *Isidori Hispalensis Episcopi Etymologiarum sive originum libri XX*, ed. W.M. LINDSAY, 2 vols. (Oxford, 1911) [without pagination].

[6] All translations from *Isidore's Etymologies*, trans. BARNEY *et al.*

The fundamental connection between a thing's name and its meaning is further emphasised in Isidore's entry on nouns:

> *Nomen dictum quasi notamen, quod nobis vocabulo suo res notas efficiat. Nisi enim nomen scieris, cognitio rerum perit.* (I. VII)
>
> The noun (*nomen*) is so called as if it were 'denoter' (*notamen*), because by its designation it makes things known (*noscere*, ppl. *notus*), to us. Indeed, unless you know its name (*nomen*), the knowledge of a thing perishes.

In his work Isidore recognised and explored a clear and definite relationship between words and the world around him. For him, words and language act as direct signifiers of the world, and so the best way to understand the world, or any given topic in it, is to understand the meaning of the words that are used to describe it. As he puts it, knowledge of a thing "perishes" unless its name is known. This attitude affords a great deal of power to language. Even individual letters become:

> *indices rerum ... quibus tanta vis est, ut nobis dicta absentium sine voce loquantur.* [*Verba enim per oculos non per aures introducunt.*] (I. III)
>
> tokens of things ... and they have so much force that the utterances of those who are absent speak to us without a voice, [for they present words through the eyes, not through the ears].

Within the framework of the *Etymologiae*, words and language are so closely linked to understanding that they are even able to replace the fundamental human senses by which we navigate the world around us. Letters introduce information "through the eyes", while speech does the same by means of "ears". One does not need ever to have seen a cat, if one has a clear and accurate understanding of what the word means:

> *Musio appellatus, quod muribus infestus sit. Hunc vulgus cattum a captura vocant. Alii dicunt, quod cattat, id est videt. Nam tanto acute cernit ut fulgore luminis noctis tenebras superet. Unde a Graeco venit catus, id est ingeniosus,* ἀπὸ το καίεσθαι. (XII. II)
>
> The mouser (*musio*) is so called because it is troublesome to mice (*mus*). Common people call it the cat (*cattus*) from 'catching' (*captura*). Others say it is so named

because *cattat*, that is, 'it sees' – for it can see so keenly (*acute*) that with the gleam of its eyes it overcomes the darkness of the night. Hence, 'cat' comes from Greek, that is, 'clever', from καίεσϑαι ('lit up', i.e. the passive form of καίευ, 'kindle').

Key to this understanding of the function of language, of course, are the provisos 'clear' and 'accurate'. In order for language to replace sensory perception, both speaker and hearer need to share a common understanding of the meaning of the words they are using. In this context, Isidore's decision to structure his encyclopedia as an extended catalogue of definitions becomes inherently bound to his concept of the role of language in mediating reality. On one level, the *Etymologiae* as a whole becomes a sort of manifesto on the relationship between words and the world, with its ideology "rooted in the dream that language can capture the universe and that if we but parse it correctly, it can lead us to a proper understanding of God's creation".[7]

This same attitude towards language is also on display in the Exeter Book riddles, which are once again overwhelmingly concerned with definitions. Isidore's declaration that a name makes a thing known is echoed in the repeated refrain of the riddles to "*saga hwæt ic hatte*" ("say what I am called"). However, whereas the *Etymologiae* is predicated on the idea of mediating a clear and accurate view of the world through the use of clear and accurate language, the riddles more often focus on the implications of this dichotomy. If defining a thing in a certain way can allow one to perceive that thing's reality, then it stands to reason that shifting the definition allows the riddler to shift the way in which that reality is perceived. We can see this perceptual manipulation in action in *Riddle 86*:

Wiht cwom gongan þær weras sæton,
monige on mæðle, mode snottre.
Hæfde an eage ond earan twa
ond ii fet, xii hund heafda,
hryc ond wombe, ond honda twa,
earmas ond eaxle, anne sweoran,
ond sidan twa. Saga hwæt ic hatte.[8]

A creature came advancing to where men sat,

[7] P.K. MARSHALL, "Isidore", in: *Texts and Transmission: A Survey of the Latin Classics*, ed. L.D. REYNOLDS (Oxford, 1983), pp. 194-196.

[8] "The Exeter Book", ed. G.P. KRAPP and E.V.K. DOBBIE in: ASPR 3 (New York, 1936), p. 238. Riddles are numbered according to this edition.

> many at council, wise in mind.
> It had one eye and two ears
> and two feet, twelve hundred heads,
> a back and a stomach, and two hands,
> arms and shoulders, one neck,
> and two sides. Say what I am called.

Most likely this riddle would have left modern readers hopelessly perplexed, and perhaps done the same for their Anglo-Saxon counterparts, were it not for the fortunate survival of a Latin analogue complete with a solution.[9] Symphosius' *Enigma 95* appears to have provided the inspiration for this particular paradox:

> *cernere iam fas est quod uix tibi credere fas est:*
> *unus inest oculus, capitum sed milia multa.*
> *qui quod habet vendit, quod non habet unde parabit?*[10]

> Now might you see what you might scarcely believe: he has one eye but many thousands of heads. From where will he, who sells what he has, procure what he has not?[11]

Although both riddles explore a common conceit, it is immediately obvious that the author of the Old English version has made the source material his own.[12] Whereas Symphosius presents in his enigma a straightforward numerical conundrum, the Anglo-Saxon author quite literally fleshes out the paradox, bringing it to life through an extended description of the mysterious creature's various and contradictory body parts.[13]As he lingers over this description, the riddler infuses this poem with an unsettling undertone of horror. We all know, thanks to the title supplied with Symphosius' original, that the thing being described here is nothing more terrifying than a one-eyed seller of garlic.[14]And

[9] WILLIAMSON, *Riddles*, pp. 376-377.

[10] *Symphosius, The Aenigmata: An Introduction, Text and Commentary*, ed. T.J. LEARY (London, 2014), p. 51.

[11] *Symphosius*, ed. LEARY, p. 233.

[12] D. BITTERLI, *Say What I Am Called: The Old English Riddles of the Exeter Book and the Anglo-Latin Riddle Tradition* (Toronto, 2009), p. 69; J. WILCOX, "Mock-riddles in Old English: Exeter Riddles 86 and 19", *Studies in Philology* 93 (1996), pp. 180-187, at p. 182.

[13] For commentary on the Latin enigma see *Symphosius*, ed. LEARY, pp. 233-235.

[14] For other arguments concerning the riddle's potential solution or solutions, see WILCOX, "Mock-riddles", pp. 183-185; R. DI NAPOLI, "In the kingdom of the blind, the one-eyed man is

yet, until that reality is recognised, the riddle's speaker seems to be painting a very different sort of picture. There is an unsettling sense of unease that comes from imagining what sort of otherwise humanoid creature could possibly be possessed of twelve hundred heads and only one eye between them. As we read this poem, we are transported to a world populated by the more fantastical monsters of the medieval marvels tradition.[15] The *blemmyae*, for example, are said in the *Wonders of the East* to be

> *menn akende butan heafdum, þa habbaþ on heora breostum heora eagen 7 muð. Hi sindan eahta fota lange 7 eahta fota brade.*[16]

> men born without heads, who have in their breasts their eyes and mouths. They are eight feet long and eight feet wide.

By evoking a similarly monstrous image, Riddle 86 does something very clever with words. Its author does not simply use language to mediate the material world; instead, he uses it to manipulate how the material world is perceived. More specifically, he taps into the sense of the uncanny that accompanies a moment in which one's perception of the world suddenly shifts. The inability to rely on one's perception of reality is a staple of horror narratives, of course, and it is a situation often familiar from real life, too. We have all experienced something akin to the momentary horror of being confronted in the dead of night by some unidentifiable thing lurking in the shadows, only to realise that this is no axe-wielding murderer, but a towel dumped on a chair. It is this same effect that is created by the author of Riddle 86. The horror evoked by the impossible description of a multi-headed, single-eyed yet humanoid monster is rooted in the inability to rely on one's perception of reality, compounded by the sharp contrast of the eventual, mundane revelation. It is a testament to the skill of the author, and the power of his words, that this failure of sensory perception is experienced so viscerally not through a trick of the eyes, or the ears, but through the simple manipulation of language.

a seller of garlic: Depth-perception and the poet's perspective in the Exeter Book riddles", *English Studies* 81 (2000), pp. 422-455, at pp. 453-454.

[15] BITTERLI, *Say What I Am Called*, p. 71.

[16] A. ORCHARD, *Pride and Prodigies: Studies in the Monsters of the 'Beowulf' Manuscript* (Toronto, 1995), pp. 178 and 192-193.

The same technique that brings horror to Riddle 86 is used to comedic effect in the Exeter Book's so-called 'obscene' riddles.[17] The joke of these riddles relies on the reader coming to one conclusion, the obscene one, only for the riddler to supply the innocent interpretation:

Ic eom wunderlicu wiht, wifum on hyhte
neahbuendum nyt. Nængum sceþþe
burgsittendra nymþe bonan anum.
Staþol min is steapheah; stonde ic on bedde,
neoþan ruh nathwær. Neþeð hwilum
ful cyrtenu ceorles dohtor,
modwlonc meowle, þæt heo on mec gripeð,
ræseð mec on reodne, reafað min heafod,
fegeð mec on fæsten. Feleþ sona
mines gemotes seþe mec nearwað,
wif wundēn locc – wæt bið þæt eage.[18]

I am a wondrous creature, a joy to women,
useful to neighbours. I hurt none
of the town-dwellers, except my slayer alone.
My foundation is tall; I stand in bed,
hairy somewhere below. The peasant's daughter,
very beautiful, the proud maid,
sometimes dares to grasp me,
attacks my red skin, ravages my head,
holds me fast. She who seizes me,
the curly-haired woman, will very soon
feel our meeting – that eye will be wet.

In this riddle the reader is encouraged through suggestive language and explicit imagery to identify the thing described as male genitalia. From the subject's 'tall' and 'hairy' appearance to the tight grip of the peasant's daughter who seizes it, this is far from being a subtle piece of writing.[19] And yet, of course, the teller of this riddle is then able immediately to explain that the object in

[17] See P. MURPHY, *Unriddling the Exeter Riddles* (University Park, PA, 2011), pp. 175-220 and 221-234.

[18] *The Exeter Book*, ed. KRAPP and DOBBIE.

[19] On the existence of a "very recognisable lexicon of dirty riddling" in Old English see MURPHY, *Unriddling the Exeter Riddles*, pp. 176-177.

question is nothing more objectionable than an onion, plain and simple, and shame on anyone who thought otherwise.

What this riddle relies on is a delicate balancing act. In order for the joke to work, it is necessary for both interpretations of the riddle to be equally valid, with nothing to dissuade the reader from reaching the first conclusion, and nothing to undermine the validity of the second.[20] What is being described is not a particularly phallic onion, it is rather an onion that is simultaneously also a phallus. In relation to Riddle 12, another 'obscene riddle', Jennifer Neville argues that the solution itself is unimportant, with the point of such a text being instead its "dissolution of the categories through which we might have expected the Anglo-Saxon to define themselves".[21] Although Neville goes on to suggest that Riddle 25 does demand that its reader "choose correctly between 'penis' and 'onion'", I would argue that we are instead faced in this riddle with a similar deconstruction of oppositions. As with the 'One-Eyed Garlic Seller', the author of this poem takes Isidore's concept of words as definitions of reality and turns it on its head. Here, the same words are definitions not of one reality, but of two. These realities exist simultaneously, with neither one negated by the other. It is quite possible that readers of this riddle would never previously have considered the phallic aspects of onions, but they surely will now. And so, while this riddle is primarily a joke, it also demonstrates the power of words to change how reality is perceived. The connection between an onion and a penis is not altogether obvious but, once made, it certainly sticks in the mind, and it alters, however slightly, the reality of both objects in the eyes of the reader.

What these Old English riddles demonstrate is the ways in which words can be used to evoke, control, and manipulate sensory perception. The strict boundaries that delineate one thing from another, the definitions upon which Isidore's *Etymologiae* is predicated, begin to break down as the reader is shown how a single definition can in fact encompass a range of nuanced realities. The riddles serve to remind us repeatedly that the world as seen through our own eyes is not really the world as it is; perception is not only subjective,

[20] MURPHY, *Unriddling the Exeter Riddles*, p. 222; J.W. TANKE, "*Wonfeax wale*: Ideology and figuration in the sexual riddles of the Exeter Book", in: *Class and Gender in Early English Literature: Intersections*, ed. B.J. HARWOOD and G.R. OVERING (Bloomington, IN, 1994), pp. 21-42, p. 31; A.H. STEWART, "Double entendre in the Old English riddles", *Lore and Language* 3 (1983), pp. 39-52, at p. 39.

[21] J. NEVILLE, "Speaking the unspeakable: Appetite for deconstruction in *Exeter Book* Riddle 12", *English Studies* 93 (2012), pp. 519-528, at p. 520.

it is open to manipulation. Isidore's faith in human language to act as an alternative to sensory perception is turned upside down by the Anglo-Saxon riddlers, who demonstrate that our perception of reality, whether seen with our own eyes or perceived through language, should never be allowed to pass unquestioned.

Skilful as the Old English riddles are in their use of language, they nevertheless remain limited only to playing with perception. While these texts are able to alter the way their audience sees the world, the world itself remains the same. Certain Old English charms, however, go a step further. In these texts, we find a belief in the idea that the right words, used in the right way, can bring about a change not simply in the way that the world is perceived, but in the world itself. Before going further, a word should be said about the use of language in charms. It is tempting to interpret the idea that language can exert control over physical things as a form of superstition, magic, or perhaps even as lingering pre-Christian beliefs incorporated into the later Anglo-Saxon world view. W. Nöth, for example, identifies in these charms a form of magic reliant upon a "confusion of the dimensions of 'object' and 'sign'", in which "the sign and the 'thing' referred to are not considered as independent entities but as something forming an undifferentiated unity".[22] Moreover, "it is expected that a manipulation of the sign ... causes a simultaneous transformation of the 'thing'".[23] While this conflation of 'sign' and 'thing', or 'word' and 'reality', is indeed the process upon which various Old English charms operate, it is far from necessary that this is an expression of magic. This is an attitude towards language that is entirely in agreement with a Christian world view.[24] Prayers, after all, are simply words spoken with the hopes of bringing about a change in the world around us.[25] The biblical relationship between words and the world is indicated in the opening lines of St John's Gospel:

> In the beginning was the Word, and the Word was with God, and the Word was God. The same was in the beginning with God. All things were made by him; and

[22] W. NÖTH, "Semiotics of the Old English charm", *Semiotica* 19 (1977), pp. 59-83, at p. 66.

[23] NÖTH, "Semiotics of the Old English charm", p. 66.

[24] See T.D. HILL, "The *Æcerbot* charm and its Christian user", *Anglo-Saxon England* 6 (1977), pp. 213-221.

[25] HILL, "The *Æcerbot* charm", pp. 220-221. On the relationship between prayer and the physical world in medieval theology see B. WARD, *Miracles and the Medieval Mind: Theory, Record and Event 1000-1215* (Aldershot, 1987), pp. 3-19.

without him was not anything made that was made. In him was life; and the life was the light of men. (John 1:1-4)

Here, the world is not simply mediated through words; rather, words are used to create the world. This affords words themselves a great deal of power, above and beyond the potency of definitions explored in the *Etymologiae*. Isidore's writing demonstrates the use of language to mediate reality. If reality is not simply mediated by words, but created from words, then it follows that reality can also be changed through words. What we find in the charms, then, is nothing more than the logical conclusion of the concept of language presented in St John's Gospel. It is perhaps no coincidence that this passage is one of the most frequently cited biblical texts in the surviving corpus of Anglo-Saxon charms.[26]

Anglo-Saxon charms are usually short texts, both vernacular and Latin, which contain directions for curing ailments and other misfortunes such as barren fields, lame horses and lost property.[27] Most textual charms, those written in manuscripts, are a combination of prescribed actions, words, and physical ingredients. While a number of these charms survive in the margins of other manuscripts, there are also three volumes of charms, written in two manuscripts known as the Lacnunga and Bald's Leechbook.[28] These were probably medical handbooks, and they preserve for us a rich collection of several hundred Anglo-Saxon and Latin charms. Manuscript margins provide a further source of written charms. The brief metrical charm *Wið wen* ("Against a Wen") comes from the margins of MS London, British Library, Royal 4 A. XIV:

Wenne, wenne, wenchichenne,
her ne scealt þu timbrien, ne nenne tun habben,

[26] On the use of St John's Gospel in medieval charms see M. MACLEOD and B. MEES, *Runic Amulets and Magic Objects* (Woodbridge, 2006), p. 134; R.A. BANKS, *The Place of the Liturgy in the Literature of Anglo-Saxon Magic and Medicine* (unpublished doctoral thesis, Queen Mary, London University, 1968), pp. 395 and 411.

[27] For definitions of the term 'charm' as applied to Anglo-Saxon texts see L.K. ARNOVICK, *Written Reliquaries: The Resonance of Orality in Medieval English Texts* (Amsterdam, 2006), p. 28; K. RUPP, "The anxiety of writing: A reading of the Old English *Journey Charm*", *Oral Tradition* 23 (2008), pp. 255-266, at pp. 255-256; L. OLSAN, "The inscription of charms in Anglo-Saxon manuscripts", *Oral Tradition* 14 (1999), pp. 401-419, at pp. 401-402.

[28] *Bald's Leechbook: British Museum Royal Manuscript 12 D. XVII*, ed. C.E. WRIGHT and R. QUIRK (Copenhagen, 1955: *Early English Manuscripts in Facsimile* 5); A.N. DOANE, *Anglo-Saxon Manuscripts in Microfiche Facsimile* 1 (New York, 1994: *Medieval and Renaissance Texts and Studies* 136), No. 265.

ac þu scealt north eonene to þan nihgan berhge,
þer þu hauest, ermig, enne broþer.
He þe sceal legge leaf et heafde.
Under fot wolues, under ueþer earnes,
under earnes clea, a þu geweornie.
Clinge þu alswa col on heorþe,
scring þu alswa scerne awage,
and weorne alswa weter on anbre.
Swa litel þu gewurþe alswa linsetcorn,
and miccli lesse alswa anes handwurmes hupeban,
and alswa litel þu gewurþe þet þu nawiht gewurþe.[29]

Wen, wen, wen-chicken,[30]
here you shall not build, nor have your abode.
But you shall go north to the nearby hill
where, miserable one, you have a brother.
He shall lay a leaf at your head.
Under the wolf's foot, under the eagle's wing,
under the eagle's claw, may you wane forever.
Shrivel like a coal on the hearth,
shrink like slime on the wall,
and waste away like water in a bucket.
Become as little as a grain of linseed,
and much less than a hand-worm's hip-bone,
and become so very little that you become nothing.

At first glance it would seem that this poem, like the riddles discussed above, is concerned with the manipulation of perception. On one level, this charm is all about how the patient sees the tumour that is afflicting them. Over the course of thirteen lines, the patient is encouraged to visualise the tumour growing progressively smaller and more distant, with comparisons made to coals cooling in the hearth and water pouring from a bucket. Finally, at the charm's conclusion, the tumour has grown so small and so distant that it has become "*nawiht*" ("nothing") at all.

It should be noted that perception can itself be a powerful thing, with the potential ability to effect material changes in a patient's physical condition. A

[29] "The Anglo-Saxon Minor Poems", ed. E.V.K. DOBBIE, in: ASPR 6 (New York, 1942).

[30] The word *wenchichenne* is variously translated as either 'wen-chicken' or 'little wen'. See J.A. VAUGHAN-STERLING, "The Anglo-Saxon 'metrical charms': Poetry as ritual", *Journal of English and Germanic Philology* 82 (1983), pp. 186-200, at p. 195.

number of modern medical studies indicate that a patient's state of mind can play a significant role in his recovery.[31] Encouraging a patient to think of a tumour not as a life-threatening affliction, but as a little "wen-chicken" may well have had a positive effect on his mental fortitude, translating into tangible improvements in the patient's condition. As Thomas Hill points out, many of the medical charms deal with problems "amenable to the power of suggestion".[32] The effect that such manipulation of perception has on an illness itself is still, however, only indirect. I would argue that a primary purpose of this charm was to use words to bring about a direct change in the patient's physical condition, beyond the positive effects that may come from an improved state of mind. Such physical change would be achieved through the poem's use as a focus for meditative hypnosis.

The use of hypnosis as a form of pain control has been explored in recent years by various medical practitioners as an alternative to conventional anaesthesia. Hypnotic techniques are taught by some midwives as a method for dealing with labour pains, for example.[33] Closer to the situation presented by this charm is a case report detailing the experience of a patient whose allergies to regular anaesthetic necessitated the use of hypnosis as pain relief during an operation to remove a tumour in the knee.[34] In certain instances, the report concludes, hypnosis can be used to block "not only pain perception but also surgical stress as a whole", rendering it "a valuable tool as an adjunct to pharmacological anaesthesia".[35]

I would suggest that the Wen charm was composed for use in similar circumstances. With no knowledge of pharmacological anaesthesia in medieval medicine, such a text could be used to bring about a meditative state in order to relieve a patient's experience of pain. To that end, this charm is notable for

[31] B. FREDRICKSON, "The value of positive emotions", *American Scientist* 91 (2003), pp. 330-335; C.D. RYFF and B. SINGER, "The contours of positive human health", *Psychological Inquiry* 9 (1998), pp. 1-28; B. FREDRICKSON and R.W. LEVENSON, "Positive emotions speed recovery from the cardiovascular sequelae of negative emotions", *Cognition and Emotion* 12 (1998), pp. 191-220; S. FOLKMAN, "Positive psychological states and coping with severe stress", *Social Science & Medicine* 45 (1997), pp. 1207-1221.

[32] HILL, "The *Æcerbot* charm", p. 219.

[33] A.M. CYNA, G.L. MCAULIFFE and M.I. ANDREW, "Hypnosis for pain relief in labour and childbirth: A systematic review", *British Journal of Anaesthesia* 93 (2004), pp. 505-511.

[34] E. FACCO, S. PASQUALI, G. ZANETTE and E. CASIGLIA, "Hypnosis as sole anaesthesia for skin tumour removal in a patient with multiple chemical sensitivity", *Anaesthesia* 68 (2013), pp. 961-965.

[35] FACCO *et al.*, "Hypnosis as sole anaesthesia", p. 964.

its use of sound. This becomes obvious in its very first line, with the triple repetition of both the elements *wen-* and *-enne*. This emphasis on verbal repetition continues throughout the poem, sometimes complemented by the use of rhyme (see ll. 8-10).[36] Similarly, Marie Nelson draws attention to the accumulation of assonance in the poem's closing lines, through the repeated use of the vowel 'i':[37]

> *Swa litel þu gewurþe alswa linsetcorn,*
> *and miccli lesse alswa anes handwurmes hupeban,*
> *and alswa litel þu gewurþe þet þu nawiht gewurþe.* (ll. 11-13)

The poem slips into hypermetric lines as it draws to an end, with the result that the lines themselves grow longer as the wen grows repeatedly smaller.[38] The expansion of these lines serves to focus attention on the imagery they contain, as the reading pace necessarily slows to accommodate the additional vocabulary. It is here that we encounter some of the poem's most engaging similes. Who could help but be charmed by the image of a hand-worm's hip-bone?

These linguistic and thematic features combine to render the poem a suitable focus for meditation, whether it be spoken aloud by the patient or listened to in recital.[39] This is no longer simply using words to alter someone's perception of the world, although there is plenty of that going on in these lines as well. What we have here, rather, is the use of words – and nothing but words – to bring about a direct change in a patient's physical condition. This charm presents the use of words not simply to manipulate a patient's perspective of their illness: it uses words to combat the physical symptoms of the illness itself.

There are other practical ways in which words may have been put to use in the charms. One regular feature of the Anglo-Saxon charms is the inclusion of the *Pater Noster*, often to be repeated a specified number of times in conjunc-

[36] VAUGHAN-STERLING, "Metrical charms", p. 195.

[37] M. NELSON, *Structures of Opposition in Old English Poems* (Amsterdam, 1989), p. 59.

[38] NELSON, *Structures of Opposition*, p. 59, suggests that a similar counterbalance is achieved through the use of the intensifier *micel* 'great', 'large' to describe the wen's diminishing size.

[39] On the ability of a skilled poet to make use of "rhythmical poetry" in order to involve the "whole personality of his hearers to the point of readiness for muscular and motor response", or to exert varying degrees of hypnosis over his audience, see D. THOMPSON, *The Uses of Poetry* (Cambridge, 1978), pp. 6-11.

tion with other words or actions.[40] A particular charm for carbuncles found in the Leechbook, for example, calls for the prayer to be repeated no fewer than twelve times.[41] Cameron suggests that the presence of the *Pater Noster* in these charms may have been designed to instill confidence in the patient by lending an air of divine authority to the person performing them, in a similar manner to the white coat, framed diplomas and "professional detachment" sported by more recent doctors.[42] In the case of the charm against carbuncles, he also suggests a more practical function for the prayer: as a form of time-keeping. Repeating the prayer a set number of times whilst boiling herbs, as instructed in the text, would ensure that the remedy which the charm prescribes had been allowed to simmer for the necessary length of time.[43] Whatever the practical applications of these charms, and regardless of the results they may have achieved, the fact that these charms were composed at all, and then continued in circulation for several centuries before being written in costly manuscripts, demonstrates a confidence in their effectiveness.[44] The survival of these charms attests to a belief in the ability of words, and words alone, to physically change the world around us.

As outlined above, this understanding of language as a means of exerting control over physical things is inherently rooted in a biblical world view, and a similar attitude towards language extends beyond the charms into the writing of many early medieval Christian thinkers. In his *Homily on St Bartholomew's Day*, Ælfric of Eynsham admonishes those who use the wrong words whilst collecting medicinal herbs:

[40] See BANKS, "Place of the liturgy", pp. 386-405; R.J. MENNER, *The Poetical Dialogues of Solomon and Saturn* (New York, 1973), pp. 40-42.

[41] O. COCKAYNE, *Leechdoms, Wortcunning, and Starcraft of Early England*, 2 (London, 1864: *Rolls Series* 35), p. 358.

[42] M.L. CAMERON, *Anglo-Saxon Medicine* (Cambridge, 1993), p. 157.

[43] CAMERON, *Anglo-Saxon Medicine*, pp. 38-39.

[44] See L.A. GARNER, "Anglo-Saxon charms in performance", *Oral Tradition* 19 (2004), pp. 20-42, p. 20; HILL, "The *Æcerbot* charm", p. 221; an investigation into the practical effects of Anglo-Saxon remedies is currently being led by Christina Lee and Freya Harrison at the University of Nottingham. For preliminary results, see C. LEE and F. HARRISON, "Ancient biotics – a medieval remedy for modern day superbugs?" (University of Nottingham Press Release, March 2015) <http://www.nottingham.ac.uk/news/pressreleases/2015/march/ancientbiotics–a-medieval-remedy-for-modern-day-superbugs.aspx> [accessed 23 July 2015]; see also CAMERON, *Anglo-Saxon Medicine*, pp. 117-158.

> *Ne sceole we urne hiht on læcewyrtum besettan: ac on þam ælmihtigum scyppende þe ðam wyrtum þone cræft forgeaf; Ne sceal nan man mid galdre wyrte besingan ac mid godes wordum hi gebletsian 7 swa þicgan.*[45]
>
> We should not place our hope in medicinal herbs, but in that Almighty Creator who gave those herbs their power. No man shall sing over herbs with charms, but with God's words bless them, and so eat them.

Likewise an anonymous homilist, writing at about the same time as Ælfric, warns:

> *Nis na soðlice nanum cristenum men alyfed þæt he ... wyrta gaderunga mid nanum galdre butan mid pater noster ond mid credo, oððe mid summon gebede þe goda belimpe.*[46]
>
> It is truthfully not permitted to any of Christian men that he ... gather herbs with any charms except with the *Pater Noster* and with the Creed, or with some other prayer that pertains to God.

These prohibitions are interesting because they focus not only on the power of words to be beneficial to a patient, but also on the use of words to define, and therefore alter, the nature of a physical object. In both cases, medicinal herbs can be rendered either acceptable or forbidden depending not on the nature of the herbs themselves, but on the words that are chosen to accompany them. Herbs that are gathered or used whilst reciting "*galdre*" ("charms") are forbidden, but replace those charms with the words of the *Pater Noster* and the use of the same herbs is transformed from a prohibited act into one of Christian worship. Although the physical object is the same in both instances, its nature has been altered simply by changing the words associated with it.

This use of language to define, control, or change the physical world can be seen in the very beginnings of the Anglo-Saxon Church. In the early seventh century, a decade or two before Isidore of Seville began compiling the *Etymologiae*, Pope Gregory the Great composed a letter to Bishop Mellitus concerning the organisation of the newly established English Church. A key challenge faced by the Augustinian mission, it would seem, was the disposal of

[45] *Ælfric's Catholic Homilies: The First Series*, ed. P. CLEMOES (London, 1997: *Early English Texts Series* 17), p. 450.

[46] R. FOWLER, "A late Old English handbook for the use of a confessor", *Anglia* 83 (1965), pp. 1-34, at pp. 16-34.

the cultural trappings left behind by the now superseded pagan beliefs. Gregory addressed these concerns in his letter, in which he famously advised the appropriation of heathen temples for Christian worship although, pragmatically, only the ones that were sturdily built.[47]

In the same letter, Gregory also considered the issue of sacrifices still being practised amongst the Anglo-Saxons:

> *Et quia boues solent in sacrificio daemonum multos occidere, debet eis etiam hac de re aliqua sollemnitas inmutari: ut die dedicationis uel natalicii sanctorum martyrum, quorum illic reliquiae ponuntur, tabernacula sibi circa easdem ecclesias, quae ex fanis commutatae sunt, de ramis arborum faciant, et religiosis conuiuiis sollemnitatem celebrant, nec debil iam Animalia immodest, et ad laude Dei in eu suo Animalia occident et donator omnium de satietate sue gratias referant.*[48] (*Historia Ecclesiastica*, I. 30)

> And because they are in the habit of slaughtering much cattle as sacrifices to the devils, some solemnity ought to be given them in exchange for this. So on the day of the dedication or the festivals of the holy martyrs, whose relics are deposited there, let them make for themselves huts from the branches of trees around the churches which have been converted out of shrines, and let them celebrate the solemnity with religious feasts. Do not let them sacrifice animals to the devil, but let them slaughter animals for their own food to the praise of God, and let them give thanks to the Giver of all things for His bountiful provision.[49]

At first glance, the process that Gregory advises here appears to be syncretism, or the reinterpretation of the beliefs of one religion to co-exist with those of another.[50] Thus, during the Roman occupation of Britain, the inhabitants of Bath were not prohibited from worshipping the native goddess Sulis.[51] Instead, as part of the phenomenon termed by Tacitus as *interpretatio Romana*, Sulis

[47] See G. DEMACOPOULOS, "Gregory the Great and the pagan shrines of Kent", *Journal of Late Antiquity* 1 (2008), pp. 353-369.

[48] *Bede's Ecclesiastical History*, ed. and trans. B. COLGRAVE and R.A.B. MYNORS (Oxford, 1969), pp. 106-108.

[49] *Bede's Ecclesiastical History*, ed. and trans. COLGRAVE and MYNORS, pp. 107-109.

[50] R.A. MARKUS, "Gregory the Great and a papal missionary strategy", *Studies in Church History* 6 (1970), pp. 29-38; R. GAMESON, "Augustine of Canterbury: Context and achievement", in: *St. Augustine and the Conversion of England*, ed. R. GAMESON (Stroud, 1999), pp. 1-40, at pp. 31-33; DEMACOPOULOS, "Pagan shrines", p. 367.

[51] On the sanctuary to Sulis Minerva in Bath see L. REVEL, "Religion and ritual in the western provinces", *Greece and Rome* 54 (2007), pp. 210-228, at pp. 215-222.

was simply interpreted as an apparition of the Roman goddess Minerva, leaving both populations free to worship their chosen aspect of the deity.[52] Syncretisms relies on the same attitude towards words and definitions that Isidore espouses and the Old English riddles exploit: that the world exists as an objective reality, and words can either aid or alter our perception of it. Just as an onion can simultaneously be seen as a phallus, so Sulis in another light becomes Minerva.

In fact, what Gregory advises in his letter is not syncretism at all, but a process that entails an even more subtle and wide-reaching use of language. Gregory leaves no room for the reinterpretation of these sacrifices; he is adamant that the killing of oxen under such circumstances is an act of pagan sacrifice, and he is equally adamant that such acts cannot be allowed to continue. What is permissible in their place, however, is the act of killing oxen as a part of Christian feasting. The act itself appears to be largely the same: even the repurposed temples can continue to serve as the venue. But by changing the language used to describe the act, Gregory is able to change not simply the perception of the act, but the nature of the act itself. Like the patient's tumour, or the medicinal herbs, the objective reality of the ox's death is transformed by doing nothing more than changing the words associated with it.

The significance of language is a central conceit upon which both the Old English charms and the riddles are predicated. Both groups of texts are concerned, in different ways, with the relationship between words and the world as we perceive it. In the riddles, this relationship is often centred upon the power of definitions as demonstrated in Isidore's *Etymologiae.* For Isidore, the relationship between words and the world is concrete and direct; reality is an objective fact, and it can be understood simply by obtaining a clear and accurate knowledge of the words used to define it. This conceit is thoroughly exploited by the Exeter Book's riddles. If reality can be perceived through the use of the right words in the right order, then it follows that an even more judicious use of well-chosen words can alter that perception. Thus an onion defined carefully can also be perceived as a penis, or the subjective nature of sensory perception can be evoked through a well-crafted description of a garlic seller.

[52] M. ALDOUS-GREEN, "Gallo-British deities and their shrines", in: *A Companion to Roman Britain*, ed. M. TODD (Oxford, 2004), pp. 193-219, at p. 201; against this view see J. WEBSTER, "Interpretation: Roman word power and the Celtic gods", *Britannia* 26 (1995), pp. 153-161, at p. 153.

Like the *Etymologiae*, these riddles still rely on the existence of an objective reality, but they use language to alter how that reality is perceived.

A number of Anglo-Saxon charms take this conceit a step further. Here, it is not one's perception of reality that is being altered through the use of words, but reality itself. Regardless of how successful they may have been, and they were perhaps more effective than modern prejudices suggest, the very fact that such charms were preserved for posterity in written form is evidence for the strength of the notion that the right words, used in the right way, could bring about tangible changes in the physical world. Furthermore, as demonstrated in Pope Gregory's letter to Mellitus, and in Ælfric's homily some four centuries later, this attitude towards the power of language was thoroughly woven into the world view of early medieval Christians. For the Anglo-Saxons, then, the relationship between language, perception, and the physical world was very much one of give and take. The power of language was such that it could function as a rival to the physical senses, and it provided Anglo-Saxon authors with the ability to exert control over both how their world was perceived, and how it really was.

Sight, Sound, and the Perception of the Anglo-Saxon Liturgy in Exeter Book *Riddles 48* and *59*

FRANCESCA BROOKS

Neither *Riddle 48* nor *59* end with the more familiar formulation of the vernacular riddling tradition, "*saga hwæt ic hatte*" ("say what I am called"). Instead, both pose the question of how the riddle has been produced in the first place. By questioning the aural phenomena produced by a ritual – the giving of voice to an inanimate object – the riddles demand not just verbal response, but also theological interpretation.

Riddle 48

Ic gefrægn for hæleþum hring endean,
torhtne butan tungan, tila þeah he hlude
stefne ne cirmde, strongum wordum.
Sinc for secgum swigende cwæð:
"Gehæle mec, helpend gæsta".
Ryne ongietan readan goldes

Sensory Perception in the Medieval West, ed. Simon C. THOMSON and Michael D.J. BINTLEY, *Utrecht Studies in Medieval Literacy*, 34 (Turnhout: Brepols, 2016), pp. 141-158.

BREPOLS PUBLISHERS DOI 10.1484/M.USML-EB.5.109508

guman galdorcwide, gleawe beþencan
hyra hælo to gode, swa se hring gecwæð.[1]

I heard of a ring that was a messenger to gathered men. Beautiful but tongue-less, though it did not loudly voice its cry, this treasure spoke strong words. Keeping silent, it said: "Save me, helper of souls". Men may grasp the meaning of this mysterious speech, the red-gold of an incantation. Those wise in thought should trust their salvation to God, just as the ring has told.[2]

Riddle 59

Ic seah in healle hring gylddenne
men sceawian, modum gleawe
ferþþum frode. Friþospede bæd
god nergende gæste sinum
se þe wende wriþan; word æfter cwæð
hring on hyrede, hælend nemde
tillfremmendra. Him torhte in gemynd
his dryhtnes naman dumba brohte
ond in eagna gesihð, gif þæs æþelan
goldes tacen ongietan cuþe
ond dryhtnes dolg, don swa þæs beages
benne cwædon. Ne mæg þære bene
æniges monnes ungefullodre
godes ealdorburg gæst gesecan,
rodera ceastre. Ræde, se þe wille,
hu ðæs wrætlican wunda cwæden
hringes to hæleþum, þa he in healle wæs
wylted ond wended wloncra folmum.[3]

I saw in the hall a gilded ring. Men looked upon it with wise minds and sharp spirits. God, the Saviour, offered peace and salvation to all who sought it in the turning of the ring. A word after it spoke, the ring to the gathering – it named the Saviour of worthy men. Mute, it brought the name of the Lord to eyes' sight, bright in their minds. If one could grasp the meaning of the gold token, the wounded Lord, do as the wounds of the ring have said. Not every man may, the lost soul, seek God's royal dwelling, the city of the heavens. Advise, if you will, how the wrought

[1] All references to the *Riddles* are from "The Exeter Book", ed. G.P. KRAPP and E.V.K. DOBBIE, in: ASPR 3 (London, 1936); *Riddle 48* is at pp. 205-206.

[2] Translations from Old English are my own.

[3] "Exeter Book", pp. 209-210.

wounds spoke to the gathering, when in the hall this ring was twisted and turned in the hands of the people.

Presented from the alternative perspective of a witness who enables the reader to view the miracle of the chalice speaking, *Riddle 59* challenges our interpretative skills as we are asked to unravel both the identity of the religious ring and to 'read' (or *rædan*) this liturgical episode. Criticism of the *Dream of the Rood* has often focussed upon the connections between the poem and Anglo-Saxon liturgical practices, while Éamonn Ó Carragáin has also explored the ways in which imagery from Psalm 18 has infused the poem.[4] More recently, Christopher Jones has explored the "enmeshment of the liturgy, devotion and literary invention" in the vernacular, arguing that we should look beyond liturgical poetry to the ways in which vernacular poetry "paraphrased" liturgical materials.[5] Similarly, Bruce Holsinger has explored the ways in which *Caedmon's Hymn* is a special example of "the dynamic and dynamically changing relationship between liturgical cultures and vernacular writing" in the shaping of Old English literary form.[6] While critical attention has largely focussed on solving *Riddles 48* and *59*, with a consensus that 'chalice' is the solution, they have only rarely been the focus of closer scrutiny and literary analysis.[7] When Okasha writes, "[i]t may be that ... the riddler is less concerned to make the answer difficult to guess than to encourage the audience to ponder the religious significance of the inscribed *hring*", she gestures towards one way

[4] For an example of this see J. BOLTON HOLLOWAY, "*The Dream of the Rood* and liturgical drama" *Comparative Drama* 18 (1984), pp. 19-37; S. CHAGANTI, "Vestigial signs: Inscription, performance and *The Dream of the Rood*", *Proceedings of the Modern Language Association of America* 125 (2010) pp. 48-72; E. Ó CARRAGÁIN, *Ritual and the Rood: Liturgical Tradition and the Old English Poems of the Dream of the Rood Tradition* (London, 2005).

[5] C.A. JONES, "Performing Christianity: Liturgical and devotional writing", in: *The Cambridge History of Early Medieval Literature*, ed. C.A. LEES (Cambridge, 2013) pp. 427-445, at p. 427.

[6] B. HOLSINGER, "The parable of Caedmon's 'Hymn': Liturgical invention and literary tradition", *Journal of English and Germanic Philology* 106 (2007), pp. 149-175.

[7] Craig Williamson sums up the various attempts to solve *Riddle 48*, with solutions usually suggesting some kind of sacramental vessel, in C. WILLIAMSON, *The Old English Riddles of the Exeter Book* (Chapel Hill, NC, 1977), p. 287. Both Dieter Bitterli and Patrick Murphy refer to *48* and *59* only in passing in their studies of the Exeter Book, and Elizabeth Okasha's essay largely serves to propose an alternative solution, that of a 'finger-ring'. D. BITTERLI, *Say What I Am Called: The Old English Riddles of the Exeter Book and the Anglo-Latin Riddle Tradition* (Toronto, 2009); P. MURPHY, *Unriddling the Exeter Riddles* (Pennsylvania, 2011); E. OKASHA, "Old English '*hring*' in *Riddles 48* and *59*", *Medium Aevum* 62 (1993), pp. 63-69.

of moving forward.[8] Grounding these riddles within their liturgical context and recent critical work on the Anglo-Saxon liturgy, I read the chalices as the "*hælu calic*" ("cup of salvation"), and recognise the riddles as drawing on familiar verses from Psalms 113 and 115 in an engagement with contemporary Anglo-Saxon perspectives on liturgical practice.[9]

M.J. Toswell describes Anglo-Saxon England as a "memory culture", "in which every monk and nun engaged in a process of rumination that would have every word of every psalm always habitually at the tip of the tongue" so that the psalms become "a kind of background murmur in the structure and content of Old English poetry".[10] The tenth-century Exeter Book is recorded in 1072 amongst the books listed by Bishop Leofric at Exeter Library alongside thirty-one liturgical books including "two psalters, presumably of the Gallican type" which would have contained the psalms.[11] Exeter was rich in liturgical materials for the composers of *Riddles 48* and *59* to draw upon. The voices of the liturgy are already present in the silent speech of the cryptic codes of *Riddles 48* and *59*, and can be activated by the eyes and ears of its audience for whom the liturgy (and its mnemonic symbols, gestures, rituals, and songs), would have formed a crucial part of cultural and aural memory. I will argue that the exploration of the highly sensory experience of the liturgy in *Riddles 48* and *59* invites the reader to move from physical, sensory perception to a spiritual perception. These riddles teach their readers how to grasp the deeper meaning of a central part of theology and of the liturgy – that is, the chalice's symbolic status as salvation and the blood of Christ – by asking them to ruminate on some familiar verses from the psalms.

[8] OKASHA, "Old English '*hring*'", p. 67.

[9] My source for the psalms are the vernacular metrical translations of the Latin found in *The Paris Psalter*. M.J. Toswell writes that "[m]ost of the surviving Old English versions of the psalms appear to date from the mid- to late tenth century", roughly contemporary with the Exeter Book, and writes that the occurrence of the metrical psalms in multiple manuscripts suggests that "the metrical psalter was a well-known version of this book of the Bible in late Anglo-Saxon England" (M.J. TOSWELL, *The Anglo-Saxon Psalter* (Turnhout, 2014), pp. 304 and 307). For recent critical work on the liturgy see C.A. JONES, "The book of the liturgy in Anglo-Saxon England", *Speculum* 73 (1998), pp. 659-702; M. BRADFORD BEDINGFIELD, *The Dramatic Liturgy of Anglo-Saxon England* (Woodbridge, 2002); H. GITTOS, *Liturgy, Architecture and Sacred Places in Anglo-Saxon England* (Oxford, 2013).

[10] TOSWELL, *Anglo-Saxon Psalter*, pp. 4, 263.

[11] R.W. PFAFF, *The Liturgy in Medieval England: A History* (New York, 2009), p. 73; M. LAPIDGE, "Surviving booklists from Anglo-Saxon England", in: *Learning and Literature in Anglo-Saxon England: Studies Presented to Peter Clemoes on the Occasion of his Sixty-Fifth Birthday*, ed. M. LAPIDGE and H. GNEUSS (Cambridge, 1985), pp. 33-89, at p. 67.

The Anglo-Saxon liturgy offers critics an "enigmatic body of evidence" due to the nature of existing sources and the many remaining unedited liturgical manuscripts.[12] However, recent critical studies have uncovered the richness of the late Anglo-Saxon interest in the liturgy which spurred "a period of national liturgical experiment and innovation".[13] Helen Gittos argues that "[f]rom the late tenth century ... it is evident that parts of the liturgy were being carefully and repeatedly reworked" by figures such as Cuthbert, Ælfric, and Archbishops Dunstan and Wulfstan: although earlier textual sources do not survive it is likely that change had already been in progress for some time.[14] Jones suggests that the greatest change came with a new approach which "read all elements of the liturgy as 'texts' and, in their divine totality, as a 'book'".[15] His argument is illustrated by Ælfric in a letter to Wulfstan:

> *Nu gyf hwa nyte hwæt þis getacnige, he leornige æt oðrum men on leden oððe on englisc.*
>
> Now, if anyone does not know what this [ceremony] signifies, let him learn it from somebody else, in Latin or in English.[16]

Jones explains that Ælfric's use of the verb *getacnian* ('to betoken') is a means of "urging on [his secular priests] a new way of perceiving, rather than of performing their liturgical duty", promoting a 'reading' of the book of the liturgy which focuses on the spiritual perception of liturgical signs and tokens.[17] The word *tacen* is as rich in its etymology and cultural usage as *ræde* ('sign, symbol, evidence') and is also related to *tæcen* ('to show, explain, teach'); a *tacen* is a sign which teaches us some deeper truth. *Riddle 59*'s request that we "*ræde, se þe wille*" ("advise if you will") echoes the liturgical concern for perceiving the liturgy, for as Nicholas Howe has explored, the Old English *rædan* "denoted a variety of necessary functions within Anglo-Saxon culture" including "to give advice or counsel", "to explain something obscure" to mean "the interpretation of ordinary writing", as well as being used to describe a

[12] M. BRADFORD BEDINGFIELD, "Ritual and drama in Anglo-Saxon England: The dangers of the diachronic perspective", in: *The Liturgy of the Late Anglo-Saxon Church*, ed. M. BRADFORD BEDINGFIELD and H. GITTOS (Woodbridge, 2005), pp. 291-318, at p. 302.

[13] BRADFORD BEDINGFIELD, *Dramatic Liturgy*, p. 1.

[14] GITTOS, *Liturgy, Architecture and Sacred Places*, p. 9.

[15] JONES, "Book of the liturgy", p. 660.

[16] Quoted in JONES, "Book of the liturgy", p. 660.

[17] JONES, "Book of the liturgy", p. 702.

'riddle'.[18] The riddles, with their objectified solutions, offer the perfect means of addressing liturgical innovation; here, like the liturgy, the meaning of a resonant representational act is focussed into the single symbolic token of the golden chalice, or, as *Riddle 59* calls it, the "*goldes tacen*" ("gold token", line 10). Ælfric's insistence that interpretation can be learnt in language, that language can explicate and demystify whether this language be Latin or the vernacular, also valorises these texts: *Riddles 48* and *59* can be culturally located within the efforts of Ælfric and others to teach the Anglo-Saxons exactly how to read the tokens of the liturgy.

The words spoken by the chalices in each of these riddles invoke 'salvation': with the chalice in *Riddle 48* imploring "*Gehæle mec*" ("Save me", line 5) and in *Riddle 59* it names the Saviour, "*hælend nemde*" ("named the Saviour", line 6). The moment at which the chalice is raised in the liturgy corresponds to a verse in Psalm 115, quoted here in Old English:

> *Ic her hælu calic hæbbe befangen,*
> *and naman dryhtnes neode cige.*
> *Beorht ys and fæger beacen dryhtne*
> *on his gesyhðe swylt haligra.*[19]

> I have taken up the cup of salvation and call out to invoke the name of the Lord. Bright and beautiful to the eye is this token of the Lord and the sight of the death of his servants.

Much like *Riddles 48* and *59*, visual and verbal elements are woven together in the liturgy's enactment in the psalm. The visual presentation of the chalice, a splendid sight in itself, and the visible gesture of raising it, are combined with the verbal invocation of the name of the Lord. These elements are also illuminated by the naming of the chalice as the "*hælu calic*", offering a linguistic explication of the signification of the token, a focus which the riddles also share in their drive towards a solution. The words of the psalm become a verbal accompaniment to the visual spectacle of the ceremony: both sight and sound are invoked as a means for its audience to perceive and engage with the meaning of the chalice held up before them.

[18] N. Howe, "The cultural construction of reading in Anglo-Saxon England", in: *The Ethnography of Reading*, ed. J. Boyarin (Berkeley, CA, 1993), pp. 58-75, at p. 61.

[19] "The Paris Psalter and the Meters of Boethius", ed. G.P. Krapp, in: ASPR 5 (New York, 1933), line 8-11, verse 4-5, pp. 100-101.

There is a clear echo of the words of the psalm in the vocabulary of the riddles. In *Riddle 48*, the shared focus is in the use of the personal pronouns *ic* and *mec*, which invite the individual to relate to the ritual's actualisation by taking on an active role. Both riddles and ritual require this immersive and participatory perspective, and this might be read as a moment at which the riddle appears particularly suited, as a form, to the exploration of liturgical ritual.[20] In *Riddle 59*, the actualisation comes through 'naming', giving the token a verbal realisation of its signification and addressing the need to explicate in language. According to Toswell's taxonomy of the ways in which Old English poetry used the psalms, I read the riddles' psalmic play as falling into the final category in which

> there are formal and thematic similarities to the psalms, similarities in structure, word choice, or imagery in the surviving Old English poetry. At times, this amounts almost to adaptation of a psalm or psalm verse; at other times, the linkage seems simply to reflect a psalmic thought structure.[21]

The shared focus and the overlap in vocabulary in the psalm verse and the riddles suggests that we have an example of psalm adaptation.

The riddles' psalmic thought structure is particularly evident in the vernacular concern for reading the liturgy's symbolic tokens. Unlike its Latin source, the Old English psalm refers to the chalice as a "*beacen dryhtne*" ("token of the Lord", line 10).[22] Frequently used in collocation with *tacen*, *beacen* broadly means 'sign' or 'portent' but often occurs in specifically religious contexts where it is used to refer to "the miracles performed by Christ", "an idol", a "significant gesture", and the "*beacen rodes*" ("sign of the cross").[23] The Old English directly addresses the chalice's superficial visual beauty ("*beorht*" and "*fæger*"), but also the object's status as a signifier. This same concern is also present in the riddles: in *Riddle 48* the chalice is described as *torhtne*, a word

[20] Elisa Miller Mangina has explored the influence of the first-person voice of the psalms on Old English poetry more generally. E. MILLER MANGINA, *Selfhood and the Psalms: The First-Person Voice in Old English Poetry* (unpublished doctoral thesis, Cornell University, 2002).

[21] TOSWELL, *Anglo-Saxon Psalter*, p. 285.

[22] In the Latin the chalice is simply referred to as "*calicem salutaris*" ("the cup of salvation"). For a more detailed analysis of the ways in which the Old English metrical psalms translate the Latin originals see TOSWELL, *Anglo-Saxon Psalter*, pp. 283-339.

[23] According to a search of the *Online Dictionary of the Old English Corpus*, <http://tapor.library.utoronto.ca.libproxy.ucl.ac.uk/doecorpus/simple.html> [accessed 13 May 2015], hereafter *DOEC*.

which like *beorht*, denotes both a literal and figurative beauty and brightness, yet there is also a deeper "mystery" ("*ryne*") to be "grasped" ("*ongietan*"); likewise in *Riddle 59* the ring is "gilded" ("*gylddenne*"), but is also a "*tacen*" to be interpreted and read for its signification.

While the riddles seem to echo the words of Psalm 115, the chalices' ability to keep silent whilst speaking is a playful distortion of the words of Psalm 113, where the participants of the liturgy are warned against the superficial seductions of gold and silver idols:

þa wæron deofulgild deorce hæþenra
golde and seolfre, þa her geara menn
worhtan wigsmiðas wræste mid folmum.
þa muð habbað, and ne magon hwæþere
wiht hleoðrian ne word sprecan;
beoð onforan eagan, ne magon feor geseon.
...
Ne cleopigað hi care, þeah þe hi ceolan habban.[24]

Their gold and silver idols are obscure and heathen, beautifully wrought by the hands of idol-smiths. They have mouths but they cannot cry out with their voices, or speak words; they have eyes, but cannot see ... And neither can they call out in sorrow, even though they have throats.

The psalm reminds the listener of the limits of human creation: these idols may be beautiful but they are bound to the earthly and the fleshly. If they have anthropomorphic or zoomorphic features these are purely decorative: man is unable to bestow animism on the things he makes. These idols do not 'signify' in the way that the chalice does. Even so, there is considerable semantic overlap between the riddles and the psalm. *Riddle 59*'s use of *wrætlican* echoes Psalm 113's emphasis on the idols as handmade objects. Although *wrætlic*'s primary meaning is 'wondrous, curious', throughout the riddling corpus it is used almost exclusively in reference to objects which have been hand-crafted and are highly-wrought.[25] The golden ring in *Riddle 49* is "*butan tungan*" ("tongue-less", line 2), and we must assume both mouth and throatless too, but makes sounds nevertheless. In both texts, the chalices speak despite the psalm's negation of their capacity to do so and the riddles' own agreement that

[24] "Paris Psalter", p. 99, verses 12-16, lines 37-48.
[25] *DOEC*.

the chalices keep "silent" ("*swigende*") and are "mute" ("*dumba*"). Recalling the psalm, the riddles encourage their audience to ruminate on the symbolic status of the chalice, which elevates it above the limits placed upon the handiwork of man and allows it to speak though mute, just as interacting with the chalice takes its audience beyond their mere sensory perceptions and into a spiritual world.

Editors and critics have offered an easy answer to the final challenge of *Riddle 59*, noting that the chalices in both riddles appear to be inscribed with a message: the "*readan goldes guman galdorcwide*" (lines 6-7) in *Riddle 48* and the speaking "*benne*" (line 12) in *Riddle 59*.[26] It is inscription which facilitates the silent speech of these inanimate objects – the riddles are locked in a circle of self-reference and repeat a familiar trick of the corpus by leading us to the realisation that we have animated the riddle subject with speech in the process of reading aloud. However, the liturgical context of *Riddles 48* and *59* makes the miraculous speech of these chalices more complex. The inscriptions are just one element within the resonant space of ritual and the riddles' exploration of this ritual, which contribute towards the communication of a message that defies the silent setting.[27] As Joan Branham notes:

> Ritual depends on ... a wide spectrum of ingredients such as symbolic objects, consecrated time, specific gestures, and appropriate personages. Only the merging and 'emplacement' of these complementary items can transform and qualify a space, rendering it sacred.[28]

The contextual setting of the chalices within the "*healle*" of *Riddle 59* and before the gathered "*hæleþum*" in *Riddle 48*, and the combination of object, gesture, silent inscription, and voiced prayer, all imbue the riddling objects with a resonance that enables a message which exceeds human speech. The interpretative work required of the reader is more complex than a simple act of naming; all of this sensory data must be perceived and understood for its greater spiritual meaning.

[26] See for example WILLIAMSON, *Riddles of the Exeter Book*, pp. 288 and 213.

[27] In using the term 'resonance' I draw on Stephen Greenblatt's definition in which the "object" has a power "displayed to reach out beyond its formal boundaries to a larger world, to evoke in the viewer the complex, dynamic cultural forces from which it has emerged"; S. GREENBLATT, "Resonance and wonder", *Bulletin of the American Academy of Arts and Sciences* 43 (1990), pp. 11-34, at pp. 19-20.

[28] J. BRANHAM, "Sacrality and aura in the museum: Mute objects and articulate space", *The Journal of the Walters Art Gallery* 52-53 (1994-1995), pp. 33-47, at p. 41.

Filled with sensory verbs and visual and verbal data, *Riddles 48* and *59* alert us to the fact that a deeper spiritual perception is necessary through the "paradoxical theme" of "silent speech".[29] The chalice in *Riddle 48* "*swigende cwæð*" ("speaks although silent", line 4) and in *Riddle 59* "*his dryhtnes naman dumba brohte in eagna gesihð*" ("Mute it brought the name of the lord to eyes' sight", line 8-9), challenging our easy classification of sight and sound and our sensory perception of speech. The aural state of silence creates a space in which we realise that it is, in fact, an impossibility, as Susan Sontag notes:

> one must acknowledge a surrounding environment of sound or language in order to recognize silence. Not only does silence exist in a world full of speech and other sounds, but any given silence takes its identity as a stretch of time being perforated by sound.[30]

Silence, paradoxically, allows us to take note of the sounds which are usually drowned out by everyday cacophonies, or which fade into the background of our experience. Within religious thought silence is also a form of eloquence: for Thomas Merton, "the mercy of God is not heard in words unless it is heard, both before and after the words are spoken, in silence".[31] The aural state of silence creates a space, in the absence of everyday stimuli, which demands the attentions of our spiritual rather than our physical senses.

The chalice which "*tila þeah he hlude stefne ne cirmde*" ("did not loudly voice its cry", lines 2-3) requires an intensified and exalted attention to be heard. It might be worth noting that this kind of inaudible speech may have struck a familiar chord with a congregation used to experiencing the liturgy at a distance. Jungmann explains that, in the Frankish liturgy for example, "each step of the activity was joined by a significant word, spoken by the *liturgus* not aloud, but only softly to himself".[32] For the majority of the congregation, kept at a distance from the ritual they were witnessing, spoken words may have been seen but not heard. The riddles playfully address this sense of perspective and the sensory mix-up involved in experiencing the liturgy through the media-

[29] M. NELSON, "The paradox of silent speech in the Exeter Book riddles", *Neophilogus* 62 (1978), pp. 609-615, at p. 609.

[30] S. SONTAG, *Styles of Radical Will* (London, 1969), p. 11.

[31] T. MERTON, *The Monastic Journey* (New York, 1977), p. 200.

[32] J.A. JUNGMANN, *Missarum Sollemnia: Eine genetische Erklärung der römischen Messe*, 2 vols. (Vienna, 1948), trans. *The Mass of the Roman Rite: its Origins and Development*, trans. F.A. BRUNNER, 2 vols. (New York, 1950), 2, p. 41.

tion of the *liturgus*. The silence of *Riddle 48* sharpens and hones its audience's own abilities to listen. While lines 2-3 quieten the sound of the chalice by negating the words related to sound and voice used, they leave behind the aural trace of its religious signification – a resonance, an echo. The negating *ne* is counterbalanced by the emphasis upon sound in the line: "*hlude*" ("loud") is reinforced and echoed by "*cirman*" ("to cry out, or make a loud noise"). Both *hlude,* which Bosworth-Toller notes is frequently used "with reference to the voice, with verbs of calling, speaking, laughing" and therefore implies vocal sound, and "*stefn*" ("voice") compound the miraculous nature of the chalice's ability to speak.[33] *Stefn* and *cirman* appear several times throughout the Exeter Book riddles but usually only in the context of birds, or zoomorphic objects given the characteristics of bird song and animal calls.[34] The chalice's ability to speak without reference to an anthropomorphised or zoomorphic voice suggests the object's status beyond the animal and fleshly. The patterning of descriptors for the voice focuses our auditory attention on this miracle.

The weaving of visual and verbal in the riddles is enriched by the distinct sensory focus in each: while *Riddle 48* focuses on sound, *Riddle 59*'s attentions are primarily on sight. *Riddle 48* begins "*Ic gefrægn*" ("I heard", line 1), and it returns to its focus on hearing at its close with the verb "*hyran*" ("to hear of / to exalt", line 8), completing the ring-like circle of sound.[35] Riddle 59 shifts the sensory perspective by beginning "*Ic seah*" ("I saw", line 1); verbs of looking are also combined with the visual gestures which give the ceremony meaning. It is the turning of the ring which activates its speech:

Friþospede bæd
god nergende gæste sinum
se þe wende wriþan; word æfter cwæð

God, the saviour, offered peace and salvation to all who sought it in the turning of the ring. A word after it spoke (lines 3-5).

[33] Definitions are taken from the online edition of *The Bosworth-Toller Anglo-Saxon Dictionary*, <http://bosworth.ff.cuni.cz> [last accessed 10 April 2014].

[34] DOEC. *Stefn* also appears in *Riddles 8* and *24*, two bird riddles, and in *Riddle 14*, the horn gifted a zoomorphic voice. *Cirm* also appears in *Riddle 8*, and *57*, also a bird riddle.

[35] Martin Foys suggests that critical readings of the two riddles have remained "deaf" to the "complicated sensory network" and performs a "sonic reading" in which "[m]utely speaking rings compound visual, auditory and soundless expression"; M. Foys, "A sensual philology for Anglo-Saxon England", *postmedieval* 5 (2014), pp. 456-472, at p. 467.

Wendan ('to turn, to change the direction of') suggests both the turning of the ring by the individual, and the circulation of the ring amongst the people – a gesture which shifts between communal performance and a private act of reflection.

Wriþan means 'to twist' or to 'give a curved form to', but it also contains a word for ring, *wriþa*: the gesture holds the object within it, suggesting the way in which communal engagement and ritual performance make the object meaningful. *Wendan* can also mean 'to alter' and 'change from one condition to another', evoking the transformative processes by which ritual and gesture transform the liquid of the chalice. Again, physical gestures and communal engagement with an object appears to unlock its miraculous potential: transforming symbolic token into symbolic realisation. John Harper reminds us that the singing of the psalms "developed as a shared practice": in the riddle the shared gestures of twisting and turning and their transformative powers seem to reflect upon the ways in which communal engagement with these riddle-texts similarly activates their performative potential.[36]

If the sounds in *Riddle 48* facilitate an intensified kind of spiritual hearing, then in *Riddle 59* it is the ritual's sights which attune its readers to higher spiritual modes of perception. In a world from which sound is entirely absent, the visual becomes an eloquent mode of perceiving the chalice's meaning: it is the act of looking, *sceawian,* which allows the "*modum gleawe*" ("the spirit to discern wisely", line 2) the meaning of the spectacle. In the sacred space of religious silence the true resonance of ritual is illuminated; silence draws our attention to the alternative modes of spiritual perception enabled by the sensory data of the liturgy.

Riddle 59's verbs of looking are combined with references to spiritual faculties of perception. By invoking the "*mod*" ("heart, mind", line 2), "*ferhþ*" and "*gæst*" ("soul, spirit, mind", lines 3 and 4/14), and "*gemynd*" ("mind-memory", line 7), the riddler gestures beyond an earth-bound perception of the sensory. However it is the verb *ongietan* ('to understand', 'to grasp', or 'to perceive'), used in both texts, which enables the sensory experience of the liturgy and its symbolic focus upon the golden chalice to be fully understood by the riddles' readers. Bosworth-Toller lists eight distinct meanings for *ongietan* which move through perception by sensory means – perception through seeing, hearing and feeling – before listing the perception, knowing, and recognition

[36] J. HARPER, *The Form and Orders of Western Liturgy from the Tenth to the Eighteenth Century: A Historical Introduction and Guide for Students and Musicians* (Oxford, 1991), p. 67.

of a 'thing to be what is really is'. In the *Riddles*, *ongietan* is used at the pivotal moment when the audience are seeing and hearing the chalice, but in a mirroring of the fluid connotations of *ongietan,* the word works to move the reader beyond sensory perception to a spiritual knowledge. In *Riddle 59*, we are told "*gif þaes æþelan goldes tacen ongietan cuþe*" ("if one could grasp the meaning of the gold token", lines 9-10); in *Riddle 48*, "*Ryne ongietan readan goldes guman galdorcwide*" ("Men may grasp the meaning of this mysterious speech, the red-gold of an incantation", lines 6-7). *Ongietan* is the perceptual means by which the audience sees beyond the purely visual surface of the "*readan-goldes*" ("red-gold", line 6) and the "*goldes tacen*" ("gold token", line 10), or even the aural "*galdorcwide*" (literally "sound-saying" line 7), to an intangible, incorporeal spiritual signification, which we must grasp figuratively rather than literally.

These are the only two riddles in which the verb *ongietan* is found, although it appears seventy-eight times in Alfred's translation of Gregory's *Pastoral Care*; it is in this context that the spiritual significance of *ongietan* is illuminated.[37] In the *Pastoral Care*, *ongietan* is the means by which spiritual concepts such as divine peace, sin, and the teachings of the Bible are understood by the clergy.[38] While *Riddles 48* and *59* are not the only riddles in the Exeter Book with Christian themes and interests, they do appear to be unique in being liturgical riddles: *Riddles 30* and *55,* which present the rood, invoke ritual contexts for the cross but are more secular in focus and certainly don't offer a lens onto liturgical practice in the way the chalice riddles do. In light of this, and the broader interest of the Exeter riddle collection in perception and interpretation, it is striking that *ongietan* has been reserved for *Riddles 48* and *59* and their explication of spiritual perception. In the *Pastoral Care*, *ongietan* also enables people to see beyond "*flæslican weorc*" ("the work of the flesh") to spiritual "*soðfæstnesse*" ("truth"):

> *Swæ eac be ðæs modes eagum, gif ðæt* ondgit *ðæs mennescan ge ðohtes* ongit *þæt hit self dysig hið [sie] & synfull, ðonne gegripð hit ðurh ðone wenan ... he* ongiet *þa bierhto ðæs soðan leohtes.*

[37] *DOEC.*

[38] *King Alfred's West-Saxon Version of Gregory's Pastoral Care*, ed. H. Sweet (London, 1871), pp. 362, 417, and 370.

> So also it is said of the mind's eyes that if the *understanding* of human thought *perceives* itself foolish and sinful, through that idea ... he *understands* the brightness of the true light.[39]

Here, the successive acts of grasping, understanding and perceiving, all expressed by *ongietan*, eventually lead to the recognition of the true light of Christian faith. The Alfredian mind's eye illuminates the meaning of lines 8-9 in *Riddle 59*. Before the gold token is grasped, it is "*dumba brohte ond in eagna gesihð*" ("speechlessly brought to the eyes' sight", line 8-9). These are simultaneously the physical eyes of the witnesses of the ceremony and an inner, spiritual mind's eye which exceeds the human function of speech – in this inner eye, verbal and visual data are superseded. The gold token is seen by the soul's eye which grasps not the brightness of the chalice's gold, but the brightness of its true spiritual light.

In *Riddles 48* and *59*, sensory modes of perception centre on a reading of the material surface of the chalices and what can be perceived beyond this materiality. The surfaces of the chalices communicate primarily through the inscriptions, which have two lives as 'speech'. The first is interior, silent, and visual, an inscription privately read for the visual form of the letters or its inscribed iconographic programme, like the more figurative "*benne*" or "*wunda*" of the chalice of *Riddle 59*; the second is a verbal utterance which is activated by being voiced aloud. Although few Anglo-Saxon chalices survive, we might look at the eighth-century copper, silver, and niello gold Tassilo Chalice for comparison, which is inscribed with both an iconographic programme depicting Christ with the initials *I* and *S* (for *Iesus Salvator*), and a written dedication to Tassilo, Duke of Bavaria, and his wife, Liutpirc.[40] The letters present a message of salvation which closely echoes that of *Riddles 48* and *59*, but the chalice primarily speaks through its visual narrative. Participants would initially have been drawn by the gleam of gold to engage visually with this object; as the viewer continued to look upon the chalice they would have been encouraged to read both its iconographic programme and its prayer to Christ in honour of the Duke and his wife. The act of looking becomes a more complex process of interpretation as visual and verbal programmes are read. The silent act of looking would eventually be accompanied by the verbal reading of the inscription, and the gestures of twisting and turning required to facilitate such

[39] Emphases are mine; *Gregory's Pastoral Care*, ed. SWEET, pp. 69-70.

[40] D.M. WILSON, *Anglo-Saxon Art: From the Seventh Century to the Norman Conquest* (London, 1984), pp. 135-136.

a reading, with the participant ultimately being drawn into a spiritual performance through the use of the senses. Like the Tassilo Chalice's inscribed dedication and prayer, the inscription in *Riddle 48* invites its own vocalisation in the use of the personal pronoun: "*Gehæle mec helpend gæsta*" ("Save me, helper of souls", line 5). By transforming the voice of the chalice into a spoken act, the reader is taught how to engage in the performance of ritual and to understand his own access to salvation.

Each inscription in *Riddles 48* and *59* gestures simultaneously beyond the material surface towards a deeper religious signification. By engaging the participant, the riddle reflects on the "dramatic ritual" of the Anglo-Saxon liturgy, in which participants are encouraged to see themselves engaging in "a re-enactment, a usurpation of voice and action" which renders the events of the passion present.[41] As Calvin Kendall writes, "[inscriptions] were performatives that took effect not once in the past, but always and continually in the present, at the moment the receptive worshipper out of fear or hope accepted the role of 'you'".[42] Kendall is referring to paraliturgical materials here, such as inscriptions found in the masonry of church architecture rather than liturgical objects, but his comment draws our attention to the way in which the sacred space and setting of the liturgy presented its congregation with a rich display of visual and verbal elements that continually required reading and interpretation. The self-identification of the inscription in *Riddle 48* allows the activating voice to understand that the chalice represents his own access to salvation as a mediating token.

In *Riddle 59*, the inscribed "*benne*" ("wounds", line 12) of the chalice are paired with the "*dryhtnes dolg*" ("wounded lord", line 11), the wounded physical body of Christ. The inscribed wounds remind the viewer that the wine held by the chalice is the true blood of Christ's wounds. As Chaganti notes in her study of inscribed reliquaries:

> The interaction among the object's many forms of representation – text, image, enshrining shape – all contribute to the constitution of a sacred experience through the object's inscriptional features existing in a dialectical relationship to its performance context.[43]

[41] BRADFORD BEDINGFIELD, *Dramatic Liturgy*, p. 11.

[42] C.B. KENDALL, *The Allegory of the Church: Romanesque Portals and their Verse Inscriptions* (New York and London, 1998), p. 96.

[43] S. CHAGANTI, *Medieval Poetics of the Reliquary: Enshrinement, Inscription, Performance* (New York, 2008), p. 12.

Material surface and inscription demonstrate the extent to which visual and verbal languages are intertwined in the ritual object, and are invoked in its ritual usage within wider ceremonial practice. Both the visual and verbal dimensions of inscription come to be seen and are heard to speak when the participants of the liturgy 'read' them for their symbolic meaning. The riddle's role as a verbal representation of a material object adds an extra layer of complexity and play, as the riddle must be heard before the chalice can be seen.

In *Riddle 59*, the chalice is described as a "*goldes tacen*" ("gold token", line 10), immediately signalling its representational status, and in *48* the chalice can be taken to be gold as its inscribed message is of "*readan goldes*" ("red-gold", line 6). Gold has its own expressive force and eloquence afforded by its expense and its cultural significance. There are numerous scriptural references to the material; in the context of this argument, however, it is worth noting that it is often used to describe the sacramental vessels kept at the altar and other offerings made to God.[44] In his *Pastoral Epistle*, Ælfric writes: "Understand that each chalice shall be made of molten material, gold or silver, glass or tin; never shall it be of horn nor wood".[45] Most surviving historical and ecclesiastical references to chalices in the Anglo-Saxon Church attest to the fact that gold was generally the material of choice.[46] When *Riddle 59* invokes "*godes ealdorburg*" and the "*rodera ceastre*" which the "*gæst gesecan*" ("God's royal dwelling", "the city of the heavens", "the soul seeks" lines 14-15), the gold comes to recall the heavenly city in the book of Revelation which is "itself pure gold, like to clear glass".[47] The gold of the chalice gestures beyond its material surface to its symbolic salvific status and the promise of the heavenly city. The transparency of the gold in Revelation is also a reminder to look beyond and to read into the material surface to elucidate what it conceals or represents. In *Riddle 48*, it is the use of the formula "*readan goldes*" ("red-gold", line 6) which resonates with deeper symbolic meaning: *read* evokes both the wine the chalice holds and the freshly spilt blood of Christ, connecting the exterior surface of the chalice with its transubstantiated substance. The

[44] See for example Exodus 39 and Numbers 7.

[45] "Aelfric's Pastoral Epistle", ed. in: *Ancient Laws and Institutes of England: Comprising Laws Enacted under the Anglo-Saxon Kings from Æthelbirht to Cnut*, 2, *Containing the Ecclesiastical Laws*, ed. B. THORPE (London, 1840; reprint 2012), pp. 364-389, at p. 385.

[46] For a detailed list of references to chalices in the Anglo-Saxon records see C.R. DODWELL, *Anglo-Saxon Art: A New Perspective* (Manchester, 1982), p. 203.

[47] Revelation 21:8.

decorative surface articulates the substance and its transformation within, reminding us to read beyond the superficial materiality of the object.[48]

By sampling Psalm 113, which addresses heathen idols, and Psalm 115, which sanctifies the signifying token of the chalice, the riddles push their readers and listeners to move beyond the sensory perception of verbal psalm and visual token. This focus on interpretation and the understanding of a deeper spiritual perception can be located within the broader context of vernacular liturgical innovation and the teaching of the liturgy during the tenth century. Geoffrey Shepherd writes:

> [t]here can be no surprise in finding that so many psalm passages were adapted into the vernacular. The influence is pervasive, often in phrase but also in form. The style and construction of many semi-lyrical, semi-elegiac pieces in the Exeter Book testify to this influence.[49]

As this paper has demonstrated, psalmic influence in the vernacular, in phrase and in form, is not just found in the semi-lyrical and semi-elegiac poems of the Exeter Book. The recalling of verses from the psalms enables the exploration and subversion of the riddles as a sacred linguistic space. Everything from weaponry, to musical instruments and birds is given the gift of speech in the Exeter Book's riddling world. *Riddles 48* and *59*, however, move beyond this playfulness. The prosopopoeia of these chalices is not just a literary or rhetorical device that facilities the linguistic mechanisms of riddling exchange, but is rather its own internal interpretative riddle which enables a more holistic engagement with key theological issues.[50] Sightless vision is a defining feature of reading and hearing and the riddle is a form particularly suited to encouraging its audience to consider the liturgical and cultural contexts which surround the object and give it meaning – to move beyond the sensory to a spiritual perception. The setting of the ritual – gesture, spoken word, and sights of the liturgy – all are present in the riddles, while the chalices themselves remain invisible, existing only in the space between words and waiting for the audi-

[48] E.R. ANDERSON, "The semantic puzzle of red gold", *English Studies* 81 (2000), pp. 1-14, at p. 10.

[49] G. SHEPHERD, "Scriptural poetry", in: *Continuations and Beginnings: Studies in Old English Literature*, ed. E.G. STANLEY (London, 1966), pp. 1-36, at p. 23.

[50] For more on prosopopoeia in Old English poetry see M. SCHLAUCH, "*The Dream of the Rood* as prosopopoeia", in: *Essays and Studies in Honor of Carleton Brown*, ed. C. FAIRCHILD BROWN (New York, 1940), pp. 23-34.

ence's performative engagement to bring the true meaning of this token to life in our inner perceiving eye.

All that Glitters: The Role of Pattern, Reflection, and Visual Perception in Early Anglo-Saxon Art

MELISSA HERMAN

The act of engaging with art almost always begins with viewing, regardless of whether the artwork under consideration is a painting, sculpture, or performance installation, contemporary or classical; art is mediated by the visual experience. The understanding of visual perception (how sensory information about the world is gathered by the eyes and processed by the brain) is the subject of on-going study in the fields of psychology and neurology, and has perhaps unsurprisingly found its way into art history.[1] Indeed, most museums and gallery spaces in the modern world are designed around a visually dominant interaction between viewer and work of art, as visitors are actively-separated from the pieces by boundaries, barriers, cases, and, quite often, stern-

[1] The scientific and art historical bibliographies of works examining the mechanics and function of visual perception are extensive, but for further discussion see e.g. J.J. GIBSON, *The Perception of the Visual World* (Boston, MA, 1950); J.J. GIBSON, *The Senses Considered as Perceptual Systems* (Boston, MA, 1966); R. ARNHEIM, *Visual Thinking* (Berkeley, CA, 1969); R. ARNHEIM, *Art and Visual Perception: A Psychology of the Creative Eye* (Berkeley, CA, 1974, revised and expanded from the original edition published in 1954); R. GREGORY, *The Intelligent Eye* (London, 1970); D. MARR, *Vision* (San Francisco, CA, 1982).

Sensory Perception in the Medieval West, ed. Simon C. THOMSON and Michael D.J. BINTLEY, *Utrecht Studies in Medieval Literacy*, 34 (Turnhout: Brepols, 2016), pp. 159-180.

BREPOLS PUBLISHERS DOI 10.1484/M.USML-EB.5.109509

faced museum guards.[2] The physical distance between a viewer and an artwork denies or at least severely limits the use of any other senses and prioritises visual perception to dictate viewer experience. The result of this type of viewing is twofold: firstly modern viewers are conditioned to give precedence to visual perception when approaching artwork in any context, and secondly this visual information is used to supplement the missing sensory data not provided by the other senses. In essence, visual perception can simulate a fuller engagement with the art, providing a viewer with the impression of a rough textured surface against fingertips or the sound of fabric brushing over smooth marble in the absence of physically engaging with the work.

The privileged status of the visual is indisputably lessened outside of modern gallery spaces and their strictly prescribed viewing practices. This primacy of visual engagement over other sensory experiences further wanes when analysing artwork from historical periods when, although decoration was utilised, most objects had a functional purpose. Despite their functionality, decorated artefacts demanded a visual engagement from their contemporary audience by the very presence of their ornamentation, on the part of both those who bore them and those who viewed them. Moreover, the intricacy of the ornamental designs found on some historical artefacts, such as those found on the metalwork of seventh-century Anglo-Saxon England, suggest that there was a nuanced understanding of the way the ornament would be viewed, and a deliberate manipulation of the viewing experience through both material and decorative scheme.

The first step in approaching early Anglo-Saxon metalwork is to avoid the assumption that the highly decorated and patterned objects are simply expressions of a society that appreciated the aesthetic of complex ornament on the surface of an object.[3] There may be minimal documentary evidence to explain the significance of the patterns, or why they were chosen, but the choices made in the material used and decorative programme were deliberate and served an important role as part of the object and its function.[4] The limited nature of the

[2] J. CRARY, *Techniques of the Observer: On Vision and Modernity in the Nineteenth Century* (Cambridge, MA, 1990), esp. p. 16.

[3] R. DESHMAN, "Anglo-Saxon art after Alfred, 1974", in: *Eye and Mind: Collected Essays in Anglo-Saxon and Early Medieval Art by Robert Deshman*, ed. A.S. COHEN (Kalamazoo, MI, 2010), pp. 12-34, at pp. 31-32; D.M. WILSON, *Anglo-Saxon Art from the Seventh Century to the Norman Conquest* (London, 1984), p.10; H. GEAKE, *The Use of Grave-goods in Conversion-Period England, c. 600-c. 850* (Oxford, 1997), p. 125.

[4] There are three distinct parties involved in the contemporary viewing experience of an Anglo-Saxon metalwork artefact: the viewer or audience, who sees the object; the craftsman /

material record ensures that whatever conclusions are drawn from the artwork and the decoration concerning its function in Anglo-Saxon society must to some degree be speculative. That being said, however, it is still possible to recognise deliberate choices and preferences behind the type of decoration employed on a specific kind of object.

There is an underlying aesthetic in early Anglo-Saxon metalwork for covering most of the surface of an object, filling the decorative field with intricate, detailed, and highly complex ornament. Whether the visual elements are recognisably zoomorphic, abstracted, purely geometric, or some combination of the three, it is very rare to find objects with much empty space or minimal ornament.[5] Instead, most of the available space is covered with complex and sometimes overlapping patterns. What is not often noted, however, is the manner in which these create a dense visual field that the eye must traverse in order to see and absorb the imagery presented, despite the fact that recent scholarship has begun to raise questions about early Anglo-Saxon ornament as a deeply symbolic and often deliberately ambiguous visual language.[6] This understanding makes it possible to consider the extensive and complex decoration of Anglo-Saxon objects as far more significant than simply illustrating *horror vacui*. It

artist who technically created and possibly designed the object; and the patron or bearer who wears and displays the object and might have commissioned and possibly designed it. However, any specific provenance for individual objects that might clarify these roles is absent. For discussion of artistic patronage in the Anglo-Saxon period see: M. LAPIDGE, "Artistic and literary patronage in Anglo-Saxon England", in: *Comitenti e produzione artistico-letteraria nell'alto medioevo occidentale*, 2 vols. (Spoleto, 1992: *Settimane di Studio del Centro Italiano di Studi sul'Alto Medioevo* 39 (1992), 1, pp. 137-191. There is documentary evidence that artists and craftsmen were employed during the Anglo-Saxon period, although the line between the two would have been far less clearly defined (if it existed at all) than in modern times. For discussion of this evidence see: C.R. DODWELL, *Anglo-Saxon Art: a New Perspective* (Manchester, 1982), pp. 44-83 and WILSON, *Anglo-Saxon Art*, pp. 13-15. For a discussion of the role of the goldsmith in Anglo-Saxon England see: E. COATSWORTH and M. PINDER, *The Art of the Anglo-Saxon Goldsmith* (Woodbridge, 2002). For the purposes of this paper the terms 'craftsman' and 'artist' can be seen as interchangeable, although 'craftsman' will be used for the sake of consistency.

5 To say that objects with minimal decoration are rare does note mean that they did not exist. Items like the triangular belt buckle found at Prittlewell, Essex, with no decoration, or the triangular buckle found in Faversham, Kent, with a single dominant decorative element, are present in the material record but are vastly outnumbered by the more heavily ornamented and patterned objects.

6 J. HAWKES, "Symbolic lives: The visual evidence", in: *The Anglo-Saxons from the Migration Period to the Eight Century: An Ethnographic Perspective*, ed. J. HINES (Woodbridge, 1997), pp. 311-337, at pp. 312-318; EAD., "Anglo-Saxon sculpture: Questions of context", in: *Northumbria's Golden Age*, ed. J. HAWKES and M. MILLS (Stroud, 1999), pp. 204-215, at pp. 204-208.

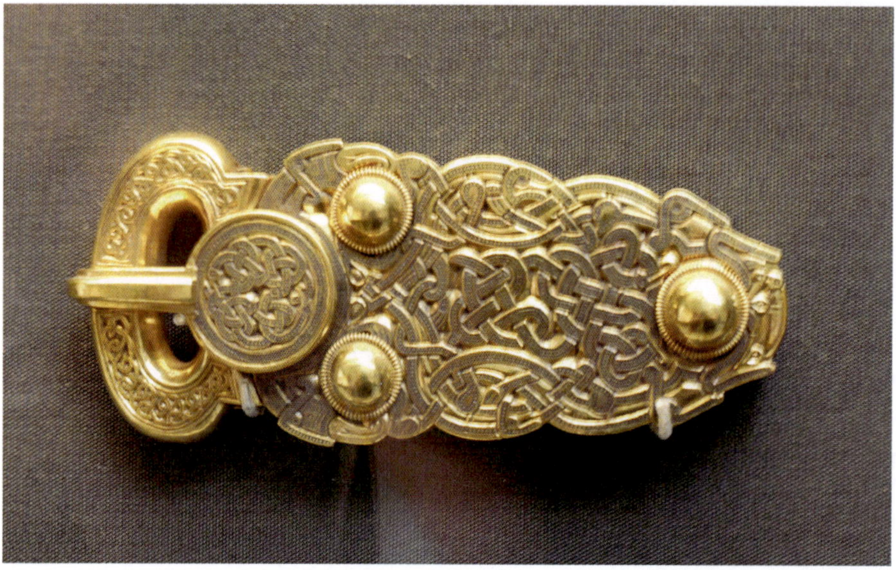

Fig. 9.1 Gold belt buckle, seventh century, Mound 1, Sutton Hoo, Suffolk. Photo by the author courtesy of the Trustees of the British Museum.

means it is possible to focus on the transformative properties of the complex patterns; an approach which prioritises shifting experience as the eye moves over this dense decoration, uncovering successive shapes which can be focussed on in turn.[7]

The great gold buckle from Sutton Hoo is an ideal object to exemplify this process (Fig. 9.1).[8] It has long been recognised as incorporating thirteen discrete zoomorphs, each of which can be deciphered with close attention, and through familiarity with the conventions governing the presentation of beasts in Anglo-Saxon art – picking out eyes, hip and / or shoulder joints and paws from the sinuous pattern. However, without such traditional knowledge, or the time to examine the object, it is unlikely that much would be perceived beyond stylised patterning. As a consequence, engagement with the ornamentation on the buckle involves a process of viewing and uncovering, rather than a momen-

[7] E.H. GOMBRICH, *The Sense of Order: A Study in the Psychology of Decorative Art* (Ithaca, NY, 1979).

[8] *The Making of England: Anglo-Saxon Art and Culture AD 600-900*, ed. L. WEBSTER and J. BACKHOUSE (London, 1991), No. 15, pp. 31-33.

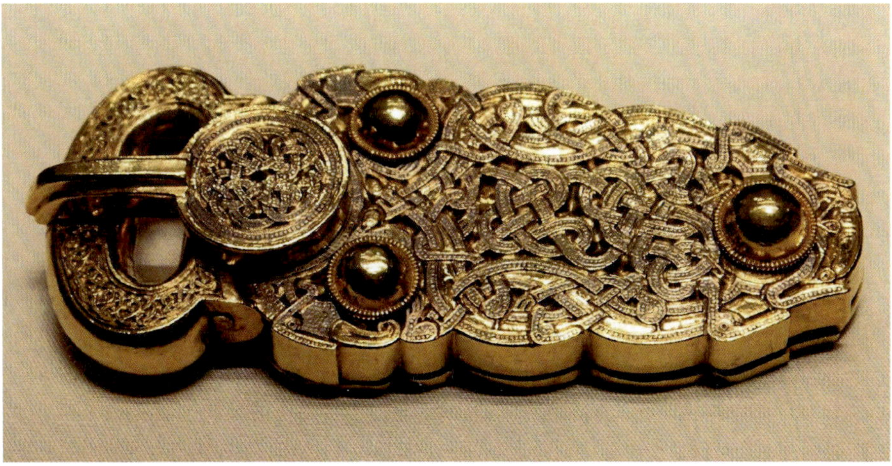

Fig. 9.2 Gold belt buckle, seventh century, Mound 1, Sutton Hoo, Suffolk. Photo by the author courtesy of the Trustees of the British Museum.

tary, passing impression; time is required to explore and unravel its complexities.

At first glance (Fig. 9.2), perhaps the most important glance for present purposes, the buckle presents a shining mass of lines and variegated surfaces. Upon closer inspection the confusion resolves into a complex but orderly and geometric sinuous pattern. And upon even closer examination the pattern becomes clearly zoomorphic with eyes, limbs, jaws, and beaks emerging into focus. The effective confusion or ambiguity of the buckle's decoration would have been enhanced whenever it was worn.[9] The placement of the buckle at waist level, surrounded by moving fabrics and other pieces of jewellery, would have made close viewing of the design impossible, leaving an observer with little more than a series of transitory impressions.

The play of light on this highly reflective object (be it sunlight or firelight), would have further challenged observation and understanding of the decorative

[9] The question of whether the Sutton Hoo buckle was an object that could be functionally worn as a buckle or was a symbolic object is divisive within the scholarship. For the purposes of this study it will be assumed that the buckle was worn on a belt, even if it was done so only ceremonially, and would therefore have been viewed in that context. For more comprehensive arguments about the role of the belt buckle see: R.L.S. BRUCE-MITFORD, *The Sutton Hoo Ship Burial*, 2, *Arms, Armour and Regalia* (London, 1978), pp. 556-558; W. FILMER-SANKEY, "The 'Roman Emperor' in the Sutton Hoo ship burial", *Journal of the British Archaeological Association* 149 (1996), pp. 1-9.

scheme. The polished gold of the buckle would have glinted and shone when exposed to light, even at low levels. The variegated, textured surface, marked by the rounded golden curves of the zoomorphs and the dark, niello hollows between them, would reflect the light from different points and at different angles. If the light source itself was moving at the time of viewing, either being provided by flickering candle, torch, or firelight, or if the bearer of the buckle himself was moving through the lit space, the effect of fractured light reflecting off the buckle would be enhanced.

The manipulation of light, reflection, shadow, and the decorative ornament on the surface of the buckle is made possible by the nature of the material used. Gold can be polished to a high gleam, reflecting the light and dazzling the eye. The black niello serves the opposite purpose, absorbing the light and defining the edges of the glittering forms undulating across the surface. However, there is also a tactile quality to the buckle's appearance that is created by the combination of material and decorative elements. The shine of the gold where it is left unadorned, as on the three rivets or the tongue, conjures up the sensation of smoothness and perhaps even that of the coolness of polished metal. The areas where the gold is more heavily worked (either by the zoomorphic forms or the collars of the rivets) give the visual sensation of texture, bumps and ridges, or even roughness. This evocation of an additional sensory experience through visual perception adds another layer of sensory manipulation and nuance to the work. This movement of light and reflection across the myriad planes of the buckle's surface would create a sense of fluidity, as though the shapes on the buckle were moving, rather than the light passing over them. This movement would enhance the zoomorphic qualities of the ornament, giving it a sense of life and motion, which would increase the depth of the viewing experience. Thus, the need for the viewer to contemplate, giving time and attention to the buckle, does not negate the experience of a less considered engagement with the object; rather it offers multiple experiences that alter with every encounter.

The idea of patterns within patterns creating a complex visual experience is also readily apparent on a late sixth- or early seventh-century disc brooch (Fig. 9.3), found at King's Field in Faversham,[10] although the ornament differs significantly from the decoration found on the great gold buckle from Sutton Hoo. This gilt silver-plated brooch with cabochon and cloisonné garnets repre-

[10] R. Avent, *Anglo-Saxon Garnet Inlaid Disc and Composite Brooches* (Oxford, 1975), p. 159.

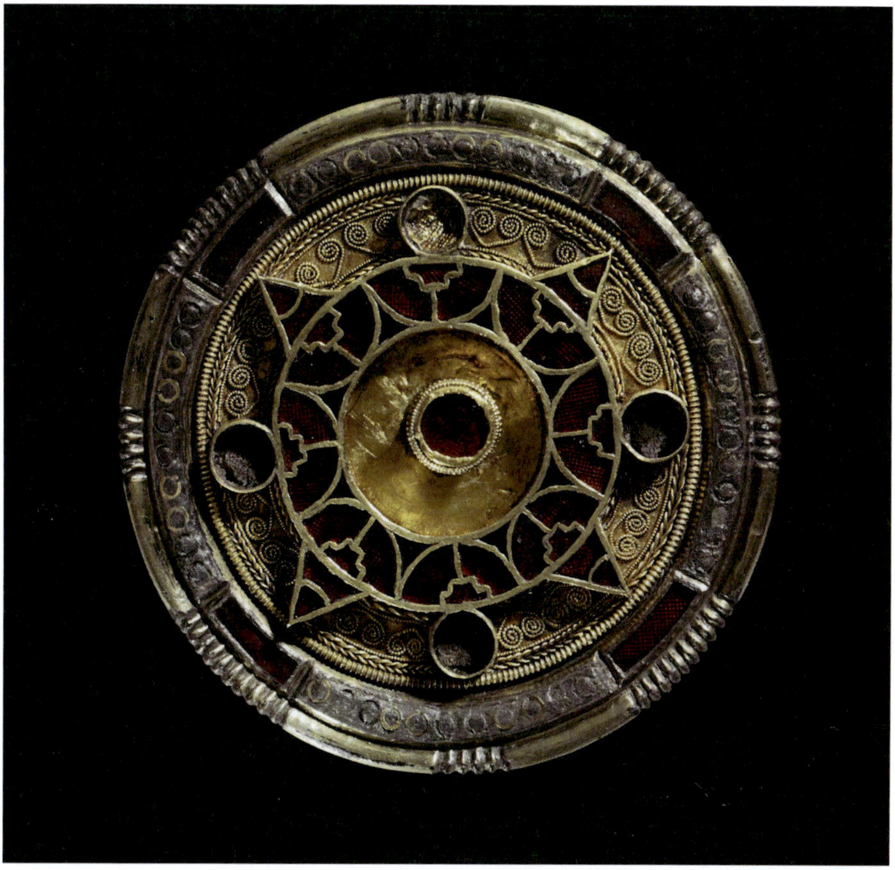

Fig. 9.3 Gold and garnet disc brooch, late sixth or early seventh century, King's Field, Faversham. Photo © The British Museum.

sents a significant number of similarly ornamented disc brooches with geometric patterns in garnet and filigree that were produced during the sixth and seventh centuries.[11] The brooch has four distinct fields of ornamentation with different patterns in each. The outermost field comprises a narrow circular band decorated with a pattern of grooves arranged in alternating numbers of five and eleven which creates the subtle impression of rings or hoops along the

[11] For the corpus of early Anglo-Saxon disc brooches see: AVENT, *Anglo-Saxon Brooches*; *Making of England*; T.R. BLURTON, *Enduring Image: Treasures from the British Museum* (London, 1997).

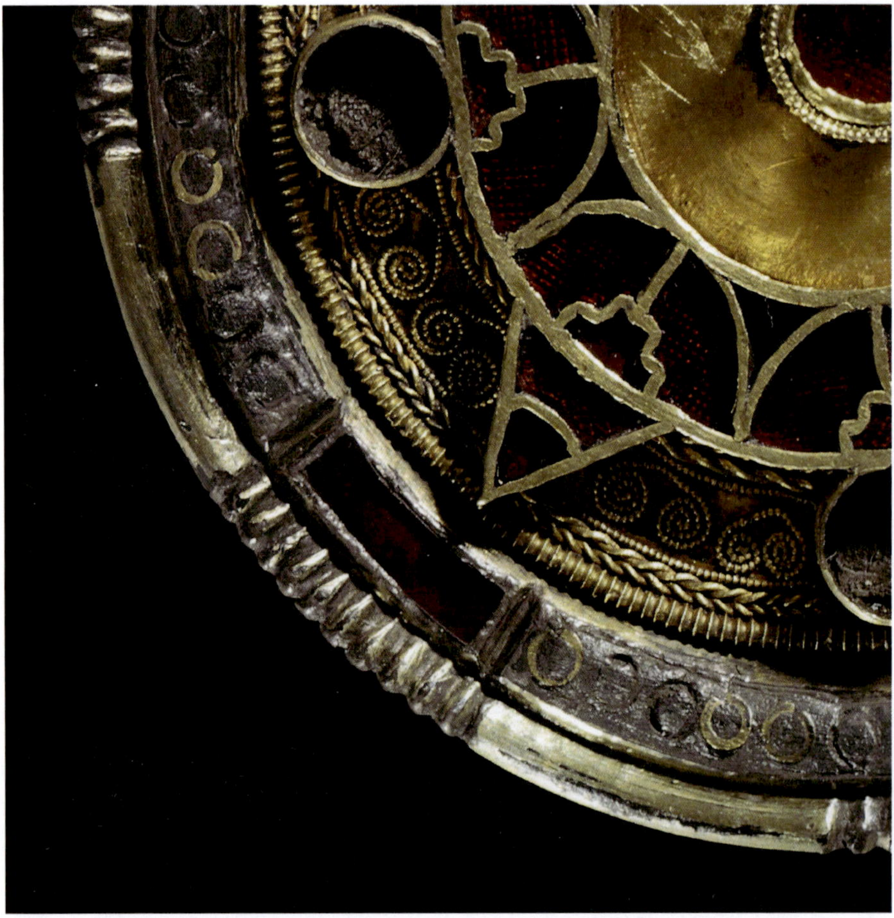

Fig. 9.4 Detail, King's Field brooch. Photo © The British Museum.

edge of the brooch, in groups of four or ten respectively. The next band is slightly wider and interspersed with four rectangular cabochon garnets set equidistant from each other, with the intervening spaces articulated by carved panels of silver filled with incised circles, which were originally emphasised by inlaid gilt. The inner edge of this band is lined by a beaded wire, which frames the outer edge of that abutting it, a flat band of silver gilt. This is bounded by thin twists of wire, single on the inner edge and doubled to form a herringbone pattern on the outer edge, next to the beaded wire. Enclosed by these is a repeated filigree pattern of paired 'spiral hearts'. Overlying the filigree and containing the pairs of spiral hearts are a series of cloisonné cells, alternately triangular and circular. These extend from a band of garnet cloisonné arranged in a complex geometric pattern of stepped T-shaped cells, half circles, and triangles. Between the outer bands and the central cloisonné garnet stud, framed by a beaded wire, is a band of plain, unadorned silver gilt. This represents the field on which the garnet cells and filigree 'spiral hearts' are placed, and so may have originally held a contrasting material, like shell.

The decoration of this brooch, while intricate, lacks the dense and transformative arrangement characterising the ornament on the Sutton Hoo buckle. Nevertheless, it presents a precision and intricacy of design that invites an analogous viewing experience. While a viewer's eye does not move along sinuous shapes, resolving them into recognisable forms, the multiple decorative fields formed by the different materials, colours, textures, and patterns similarly force the eye to move from one to another (Fig. 9.4). The entirety of the design draws attention first to one section, perhaps the cloisonné, but as the eye rests on that point, other areas shift into focus, such as the more subtle filigree which leads the eye along the intricate lines and swirls of beaded wire to the gilt circles set into the silver of the penultimate ring, which draw attention towards the inset garnets. These, in turn, highlight the incised outer ring, and so on. The decoration overall creates a sense of patterns within larger patterns which interrelate despite the seemingly discrete nature of each decorative element. In order to view the brooch, as with the buckle, a viewer must contemplate it, allowing the eye to move across the surface as the patterns resolve and dissolve and the whole becomes fractured parts, which then coalesce once again into a whole. In this way the intricate patterns appear to encourage the act of viewing, and the process of examining and understanding these complexities, rather than just presenting one view of the object as whole.

Again, while the experience of the brooch is overwhelmingly visual, embedded within the visual perception is a tactile one as well. The brooch utilises two reflective metals – silver and gilt – and deliberately contrasts them by both texturing the outer ring and inlaying gilt into the decoration of the penultimate ring. The relative smoothness of these reflective outer rings is in sharp contrast (both visually and in terms of perceived texture) with the inner field of filigree, which appears rough and woven, almost like textile. The glassiness of the garnets offers another visual and textural contrast, appearing smooth and bright and catching the light more subtly than the polished metal rings or the broken surface of the filigree. The material around the central boss of the brooch (now lost) would have provided an additional layer of visual contrast both in terms of interaction with light and perceived textural sensation. Finally the brooch provides a sense of differing heights between the different fields of decoration, particularly between the filigree background and the inset garnets in their cells, which encourages the eye to traverse across and the fingertips to imagine. Like the buckle, the visual perception of the complex and multi-layered ornament is both enhanced and influenced by the materials with which it was made, dictating the way in which the viewer engages with the brooch.

With both objects, the buckle and the brooch, the viewing of the object is driven and directed by the use of colour, texture, and the employment of light and shadow. There is, of course, an overall pattern to the decoration in the form of thirteen interlacing beasts on the buckle and the symmetrical geometric shape formed by the garnet cloisonné on the brooch. However, the overall complexity of both examples makes it difficult for a viewer to process it in its entirety. Instead, the viewer's eye is led through a range of surfaces and levels of understanding; visually processing the different textures of smooth metal, slick polished stone, and textured filigree, moving along the different heights, depths and channels created by the variegated surface of the design, and forced to process both the intricate detail and the composition of the decorative scheme. This intentional manipulation of the visual process to dictate a viewing experience is accomplished by the skilful use of the materials of the artwork, the overall decoration down to its most minute detail, and an adroit understanding of visual perception.

In creating this directed viewing experience the decorative pattern or iconography on the metalwork are intended to complement and utilise the specific nature of the materials from which it is made, making analysis of the materiality as important as iconographic study. Materials can be understood to have significance independent of their use in specific types of objects. In early Anglo-Saxon England certain materials were imbued with significance and meaning, which they, in turn, conferred to the object into which they were incorporated.[12] The use of material embedded with such significance can be

[12] In contemporary scholarship, across many disciplines, materiality has come to infuse any number of critical and analytical approaches to everything from objects to texts to historical narratives. For a more comprehensive discussion of materiality, art, and culture see: G. DOY, *Materializing Art History* (Oxford, 1998); I. WOODWARD, *Understanding Material Culture* (Los Angeles, CA, 2007); K. ROBERTSON, "Medieval things: Materiality, historicism and the premodern object", *Literature Compass* 5 (2008), pp. 1060-1080; C. KNAPPETT, *Thinking Through Material Culture: An Interdisciplinary Perspective* (Philadelphia, 2011); M. YONAN, "Toward a fusion of art history and material culture studies", *West 86th: A Journal of Decorative Arts, Design History and Material Culture* 18 (2011), pp. 232-248.

interpreted as an effort to incorporate those symbolic and cultural associations into the finished object, be it brooch, buckle or sword. Therefore it is necessary to understand the significance of the material in order to understand how it enhanced the function of the object itself as well as the decorative scheme, aside from the visual role it may have played in dictating the viewing experience. It is certainly the case that some materials were considered especially valuable and desirable in early Anglo-Saxon England. Dominic Janes has shown that precious metals were widely used to indicate power and wealth throughout the ancient world among disparate societies, but that the metals deemed sufficiently precious in one culture were not always considered so in others; value was greatly influenced by rarity and the resulting restriction and control of a metal's use by a society's elites.[13]

Gold is a material that seems to have been almost universally deemed precious and valuable and thereby worthy of conveying status, largely because of its scarcity, which led to its being monitored and controlled by social elites.[14] It was obtained in various ways in the early medieval world, though only rarely by local mining, and however it was obtained (by looting, tribute demands, grave robbing, or confiscation), its circulation remained restricted to the highest social circles.[15] In addition to its rarity value, gold is also highly malleable, which means that it can be worked with a high degree of dexterity and relative ease and thus used to great effect.[16] Finally, it has a brilliance which reflects light and catches the eye and, most importantly, does not diminish with rust or discolouration.[17] Given its enduring brilliance and the widespread associations between gold and socio-economic power, it is perhaps unsurprising that gold also came to be associated with supernatural or divine power.[18] The Greco-Roman pantheon is described as possessing a myriad of golden objects ranging

[13] D. JANES, *God and Gold in Late Antiquity* (Cambridge, 1998), p. 18; see also E.W. HERBERT, *Red Gold of Africa: Copper in Pre-Colonial History and Culture* (Madison, WI, 1984), p. XIX; I. MORRIS, 'Circulation, deposition and the formation of the Greek Iron Age', *Man* 24 (1989), pp. 502-519, at p. 515.

[14] HERBERT, *Red Gold*, p. XIX; JANES, *God and Gold*, p. 18.

[15] L. WEBSTER, "Ideal and reality: Versions of treasure in the early Anglo-Saxon world", in: *Treasure in the Medieval West*, ed. E.M. TYLER (Woodbridge, 2000), pp. 49-60, at p. 50; COATSWORTH and PINDER, *Anglo-Saxon Goldsmith*, p. 6.

[16] JANES, *God and Gold*, p. 19; C. BEHR, "The symbolic nature of gold in magical and religious contexts" (2010) <http://finds.org.uk/staffshoardsymposium/papers/charlottebehr> [accessed 17 August 2014].

[17] JANES, *God and Gold*, p. 19.

[18] For an extensive discussion of this relationship in the antique period, see JANES, *God and Gold*. See also BEHR, "Symbolic nature of gold".

from items of clothing, tools and weapons, even to means of transportation.[19] The gods of early medieval Scandinavian world were also tied to gold, and are described in twelfth-century Eddic poetry as living in a golden hall and using golden objects.[20] Gold was used to decorate temples, palaces, and eventually churches, with the intention of inspiring awe and wonder.[21] Eventually, the ritual objects used in the observation of Christian worship came to be made of gold and other precious materials,[22] suggesting that the potency of gold as a material was so deeply embedded that it could transcend major ideological, cultural, and religious shifts. This link between gold and divinity inflates the value and significance of the use of gold in ornamentation, doubly reinforcing its associations with power and preciousness. Thus the significance of gold becomes cyclical: gold is used to indicate and ornament the divine because it is precious and denotes power, and is viewed in this way (in part) because it is associated with the divine.

Like gold, silver was also commonly valued as precious and used to convey status. It was also difficult to obtain directly and, in the early medieval period, often obtained through the reuse of pre-existing objects, like silver Roman coins, or imported from distant regions.[23] Silver is also highly reflective when polished, giving it an even brighter appearance than gold, as suggested by Pliny the Elder's comparison of silver with daylight.[24] Unlike its precious metal counterpart, silver tarnishes if not handled and maintained properly, losing its brilliance and becoming dull and discoloured.

[19] JANES, *God and Gold*, p. 19.

[20] BEHR, "Symbolic nature of gold". For specific references in the *Vǫluspá* (from the Codex Regius, MS Reykjavik, Árni Magnússon Institute for Icelandic Studies, GKS 2365 4to) see *Völuspá: the Sybil's Prophecy*, ed. H. PÁLSSON (Edinburgh, 1996): pp. 63-65, at stanzas 60 and 61.

[21] JANES, *God and Gold*, pp. 43-44, 52-54; S. LA NIECE, *Gold* (London, 2009), pp. 92-96; BEHR, "Symbolic nature of gold".

[22] JANES, *God and Gold*, pp. 42-44; LA NIECE, *Gold*, pp. 92, 102-103; BEHR, "Symbolic nature of gold".

[23] K. LEAHY, *Anglo-Saxon Crafts* (Stroud, 2003), pp. 153-154.

[24] "*praecipuam gratiam huic materiae fuisse arbitror non colore, qui clarior in argento est magisque diei similis*" ("the chief popularity of this substance has been won not by its colour, that of silver being brighter and more like daylight"); Pliny the Elder, *Historia Naturalis*, 33, c. 19, in: *Pliny, Natural History*, ed. D.E. EICHHOLZ, trans. H. RACKHAM and W.H.S. JONES, 10 vols (Cambridge, MA, and London, 1938-1962: *Loeb Classical Library*), 9, pp. 46-47.

Garnet, a deep red stone with distinctive light refractive properties,[25] was the dominant gemstone used for jewellery throughout Europe in the early medieval period, from the fourth to the seventh centuries.[26] Although minerals identified as garnet are relatively more common than other gemstones,[27] the regions that produced garnets of the appropriate colour and quality were significantly far removed from western Europe, some as far away as India.[28] This meant that they were a limited resource in the north and so were regarded as valuable and exotic.[29] Thus, as with the silver and gold, the rarity of garnets meant that access could be controlled and restricted, making their use a sign of wealth and status. The colour of garnet was also significant in this respect, ranging from a bright red to a deep, dark burgundy that can appear almost purple, depending on the refractive qualities of the individual stone and the way in which a craftsman manipulates it. Red and purple were both long associated with imperial status in the Roman world and by royalty in the early medieval period, lending further significance and status to stones of those colours.[30] Complex and nuanced Christian meanings were also invested in these colours, especially red.[31] The most obvious association here was with the blood of Christ.[32]

Garnet cloisonné, occasionally offset with stones or inlay of other colours, seems to have prevailed in the ornamentation of late fourth- or early fifth-cen-

[25] N. ADAMS, "The garnet millennium: The role of seal stones in garnet studies", in: *'Gems of Heaven': Recent Research on Engraved Gemstones in Late Antiquity c. AD 200-600*, ed. C. ENTWHISTLE and N. ADAMS (London, 2011), pp. 10-24, at p. 10.

[26] T. CALLIGARO, S. COLINART, J-P. POIROT and C. SUDRES, "Combined external-beam PIXE and µ-Raman characterisation of garnets used in Merovingian jewellery", *Nuclear Instruments and Methods in Physics Research Section B: Beam Interactions with Materials and Atoms* 189.1 (2002), pp. 320-327, at p. 320.

[27] ADAMS, "The garnet millennium", p. 10.

[28] CALLIGARO, COLINART, POIROT and SUDRES, "Combined external-beam PIXE", p. 326; ADAMS, "The garnet millennium", pp. 10, 19-21.

[29] J.W. HUGGETT, "Imported grave goods and the early Anglo-Saxon economy", *Medieval Archaeology* 32 (1988), pp. 63-96, at pp. 88-89, 91.

[30] JANES, *God and Gold*, p. 84.

[31] P. KITSON, "Lapidary traditions in Anglo-Saxon England, part I: The background: The Old English lapidary", *Anglo-Saxon England* 7 (1978), pp. 9-60, at p. 27.

[32] P. KITSON, "Lapidary traditions in Anglo-Saxon England: part II, Bede's *Explanatio Apocalypsis* and related orks", *Anglo-Saxon England* 23 (1983), pp. 73-123, at p. 86; E. COATSWORTH, "The pectoral cross and portable altar from the tomb of St. Cuthbert", in: *St. Cuthbert, His Cult and His Community to AD 1200*, ed. G. BONNER *et al.* (Woodbridge, 1989), pp. 287-302, at pp. 295-296; JANES, *God and Gold*, p. 75.

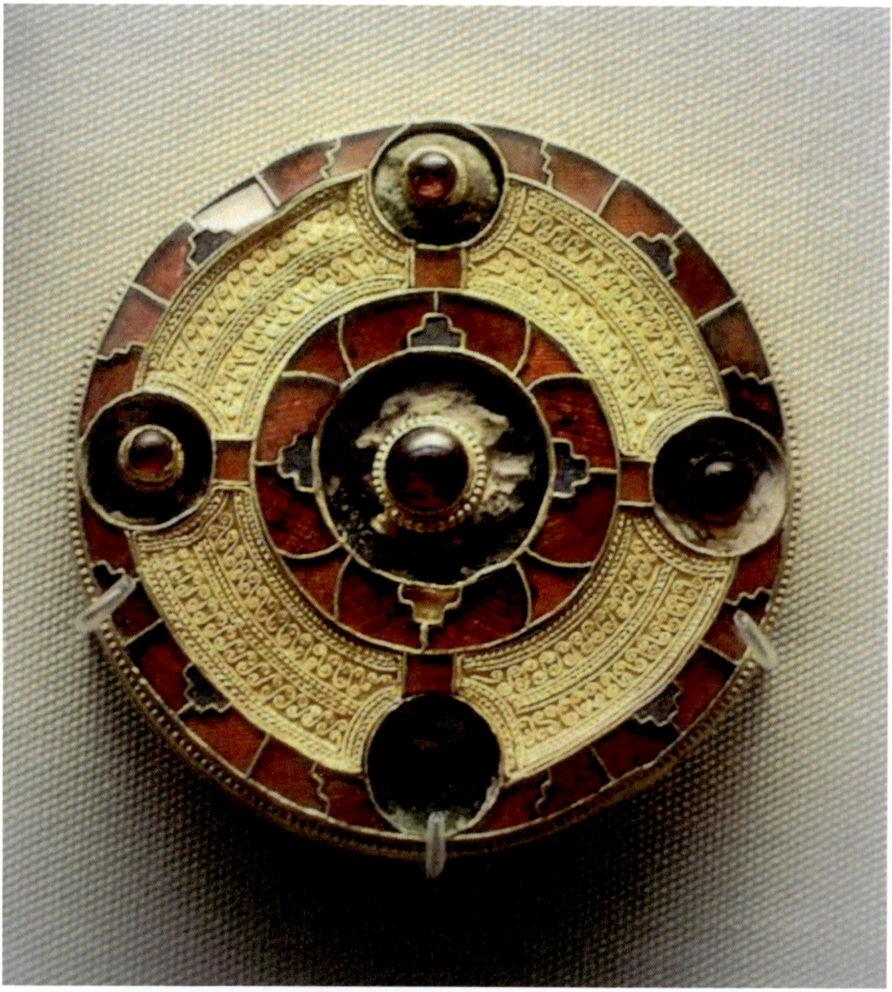

Fig. 9.5 Gold and garnet disc brooch, early seventh century, Priory Hill, Dover. Photo by the author courtesy of the Trustees of the British Museum.

tury Germanic gold, or more rarely silver, and the type of jewellery it was used to create, cloisonné brooches, buckles, weapon fittings and pendants.[33] The pervasiveness of the style was so entrenched among Germanic societies that by

[33] D.N. ADAMS, *Late Antique, Migration Period and Early Byzantine Garnet Cloisonné Ornaments: Origins, Styles and Workshop Production* (unpublished doctoral thesis, University College London, 1991), pp. 81-83.

the sixth century a law forbidding the use of jewels on buckles for military personnel was enacted throughout the Roman Empire.[34] The significance of this law, preserved in the Codex Justinianus, lies in the prohibition itself: the need to discourage the wearing of such highly ornamented jewellery indicates just how pervasive the practice was.

Within this longstanding Germanic tradition, gold and garnet jewellery was both the fashionable and the traditional form of expressing status in personal ornamentation in seventh-century Anglo-Saxon England.[35] These materials were used on a myriad of objects, from dress ornaments, like pendants, brooches, buckles and pins, to armaments such as seax fittings and sword pommels. The garnets used were either rounded and polished cabochon stones, or cut flat stones that were shaped and inset into cloisonné cells. There is some discussion about the origins of the supply of each type of garnet, with the flat garnets considered to have emerged from Bohemia, in East Central Europe, while the cabochon type was probably from a more distant source, like Afghanistan or India.[36] The cabochon stones, being thicker, tend to appear darker and deeper in colour, while the flat garnets are generally cut into thin, transparent slices and set over reflective foils to increase the brightness of the red tones.[37] The two types of garnet were used both independently and in conjunction with each other and could be set alongside other stones or materials, such as glass or shell, but the aesthetic of red and yellow, gold and garnet, remained dominant.

The intentional manipulation of the viewer's sensory engagement with early Anglo-Saxon metalwork was not limited to reflection, shadow, or perceived texture within a complex pattern, but could also be achieved by the additional use of colour. An early seventh-century disc brooch (Fig. 9.5) found at Priory Hill near Dover combines both types of garnet with composite gold. This piece has two rings of garnet cloisonné accented by T-shaped glass cells. The first ring borders the entire brooch while the second encircles the central boss. The space between the two is filled with dense gold filigree, divided into four quadrants by four round bosses, each connected to the inner cloisonné ring

[34] ADAMS, *Garnet Cloisonné Ornaments*, p. 326.

[35] J. SPIER, *Byzantium and the West: Jewelry in the First Millennium* (London, 2012), pp. 3237.

[36] B. ARRHENIUS, *Merovingian Garnet Jewellery* (Stockholm, 1985); LEAHY, *Anglo-Saxon Crafts*, p. 160; D.A. HINTON, *Gold and Gilt, Pots and Pins: Possessions and People in Medieval Britain* (Oxford, 2005), p. 53.

[37] LEAHY, *Anglo-Saxon Crafts*, pp. 160-161; HINTON, *Gold and Gilt*, pp. 53-54.

by a single square inset garnet. The filigree ornamentation forms five bands of alternating patterns, three creating a herringbone effect, interspersed by two with elaborate scrolling. The five bosses are each made by round cabochon garnets collared by beaded gold wire and set onto shaped white paste. One of the small bosses and most of the paste is now missing. The central boss and the cavity that would have been filled with white paste are significantly larger than the four satellite bosses, each of which is accented by a border of filigree. A distinctive cruciform is formed by the pattern of bosses within the overall disc shape. The pairing of the cabochon and cut garnets accentuates the different colouration of the stones, deep but dark as opposed to bright, while the use of gold filigree creates a more fragmented reflective effect in contrast to the smooth polish of the cloisonné garnets.

The attention paid to the colour, tone, and reflective quality in the creation of these objects indicates the importance embedded in these visual effects. The manipulation and mixing of the sensory experience must be seen as deliberate and significant, as a conscious effort on the part of the craftsmen or designer to control the experience of the viewer. Nigel Barley suggested that Anglo-Saxons probably perceived colours as inextricably attached to objects, as opposed to abstract concepts of description, meaning that their 'red' is not equivalent to our modern conception of 'red'.[38] Here, it is worth noting Barley's argument, following Mead and Lerner, that Anglo-Saxon colour terms referred more to brightness than colour gradient, meaning that hue or saturation is prioritised in Old English colour terminology.[39] In the light of this, it is particularly interesting that Anglo-Saxon goldsmiths, adept at modifying the thickness of the stones being set, could manipulate the brightness and hue of the garnets used, employing thinner stones to achieve lighter effects, and thicker stones to present darker tones, while the hatch-marked gold foils set behind the stones reflected more light, making the backed stones brighter.[40]

In addition to offering, through technical manipulation, the means to control the perceived brilliance, the red and purple tones of the garnets were also,

[38] N.F. BARLEY, "Old English colour classification: Where do matters stand?", *Anglo-Saxon England* 3 (1974), pp. 16-18.

[39] W.E. MEAD, "Color in Old English poetry", *Publications of the Modern Language Association of America* 14 (1899), pp. 169-206; L.D. LERNER, "Colour words in Anglo-Saxon", *Modern Language Review* 46 (1951), pp. 246-249; BARLEY, "Colour classification", pp. 16-18.

[40] COATSWORTH and PINDER, *Anglo-Saxon Goldsmith*, pp. 132-148.

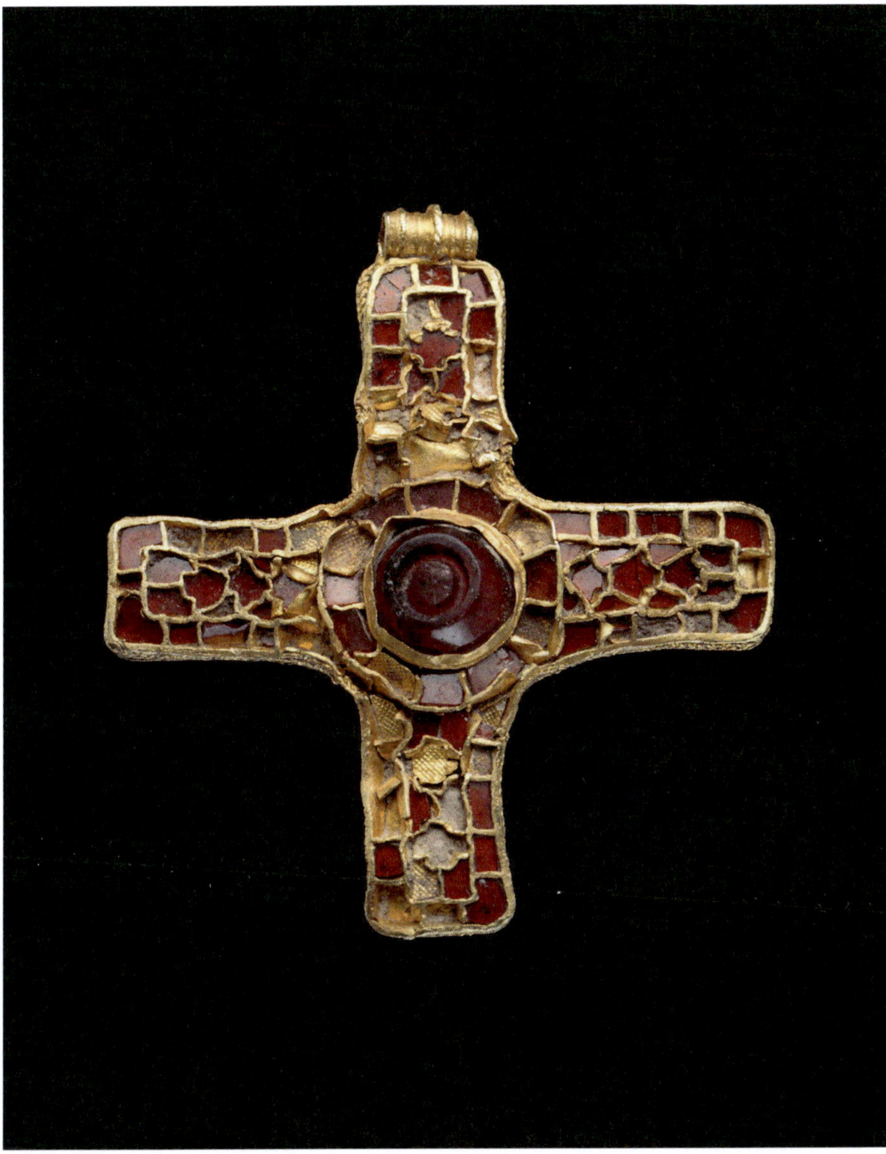

Fig. 9.6 Gold and garnet cross pendant, seventh century, Holderness, East Yorkshire. Photo © Ashmolean Museum, University of Oxford.

as noted, associated with imperial frames of reference throughout the late antique and early medieval world. Furthermore, the early Anglo-Saxon exegetical work of Bede linked the colour red with four of the twelve stones of the Apocalypse, describing two as related to blood and two as related to fire – a set of associations established in early Christian exegesis.[41] Such detailed exegetical engagement with the colours articulated by gold and garnet metalwork, as well as the technical skill involved in achieving the different colours, together provide strong indications that the colours as well as the stones and materials used were capable of exemplifying deeply symbolic meanings and significances in early Anglo-Saxon society.

In this respect it is perhaps not coincidental that the early to mid seventh-century pendant cross found in Holderness, East Yorkshire, is composed entirely of gold and garnet cloisonné (Fig. 9.6), not unlike the brooch found at Priory Hill. This equal-armed cross is bordered by a frame of square set garnets, while the arms are filled with more arrow-shaped, albeit roughly carved, stones. The central boss is set with a large cabochon garnet, darker in colour than the surrounding ring of square-set cloisonné, and drilled with a ring that was likely to be set with contrasting glass or gold infill. Despite its somewhat battered state, the materials and their settings again demonstrate how colour and light could be manipulated to create a richly evocative viewing experience, while additionally playing on exegetical frames of reference in its design. But, here again, the flat inset garnets are much brighter and more reflective than the central garnet, which appears very dark by comparison. Such manipulation of the colour and the reflectiveness of the stones illustrates another example of a deliberate effort to control the viewer's visual experience in order to evoke responses to a specific set of symbolic associations, perhaps making a specific reference to the lifeblood of Christ on the cross,[42] or the apocalyptic flames promised of the Day of Judgment.[43]

[41] Bede, *Apocalypseos*, ed. R. Gryson, *Bedae Presbyteri Expositio Apocalypseos*, (Turnhout, 2001: *Corpus Christianorum Series Latina* 121A), p. 543; Bede, *Commentary on Revelation,* trans. F. Wallis, (Liverpool, 2013: *Translated Texts for Historians*), p. 154. See also Kitson, "Lapidary traditions part ii", p. 88.

[42] Nennius, *Annunciatio S, Mariae*, ed. and trans. in: Nennius, *British History and the Welsh Annals*, ed. and trans. J. Morris (London, 1980), pp. 8-11. See also: Mead, "Color in poetry", p. 186; Kitson, "Lapidary traditions part ii", p. 76.

[43] Mead, "Color in poetry", p. 186; Kitson, "Lapidary traditions part ii", p. 76; M. Bradford Bedingfield, "Anglo-Saxons on fire", *Journal of Theological Studies* 52.2 (2001), pp. 658-677.

In studying these pectoral crosses, or any of their counterparts, it becomes clear that the distinctive gold and garnet cloisonné is so pervasive that it must have been the preferred ornamentation of the form. The effect of bright red hues, darker red pools, and bright gold shining through is evocative in a manner distinct from the traditional significance and potency. The lines of *The Dream of the Rood* which describe a visionary cross both dripping with blood and shining with treasure, seem to articulate this aesthetic exactly:

Geseah ic þæt fuse beacen
wendan wædum ond bleom; hwilum hit wæs mid wætan bestemed,
beswyled mid swates gange, hwilum mid since gegyrwed.

I saw that doom-beacon
turn trappings and hews: sometimes with water wet,
drenched with blood's going; sometimes with jewels decked.[44]

Anyone familiar with the verse could not help but recall the shining yellow gold and deep red garnets of the Anglo-Saxon crosses.[45] Indeed, the poem has long been linked to the pectoral cross discovered in Cuthbert's coffin, and by extension the other gold and garnet pectoral crosses recovered from this period, both for the combination of red and gold as for the effect of the gold shining through the translucent garnets.[46]

It becomes clear that the early Anglo-Saxon craftsmen used specific materials, worked in a precise manner, and formed a distinctive design, in order to influence the way in which a viewer perceived and engaged with the art of the time. The complexity and multilayered effect of the design on such objects was undoubtedly intended to encourage the viewer to actively engage with the imagery and contemplate all the visual experiences presented by it. The artists have created a dense and complex visual maze, prioritising a shifting and transitory view that moves across the surface of any object over the logical focus point of a coherent image, in order to allow a viewer to decipher the patterns

[44] *The Dream of the Rood*, ed. M. SWANTON (New York, 1970), lines 21-32, pp. 1-2; S.A.J. BRADLEY, *Anglo-Saxon Poetry* (London, 1982), p. 160.

[45] E. COATSWORTH, "The decoration of the Durham Gospels", in: *The Durham Gospels, Durham Cathedral Library A. II. 17*, ed. C.D. VEREY, T.J. BROWN and E. COATSWORTH (Copenhagen, 1980), pp. 50-63, at p. 59; COATSWORTH, "Cross and altar", p. 296; COATSWORTH and PINDER, *Anglo-Saxon Goldsmith*, pp. 161-162.

[46] COATSWORTH, "Cross and altar", p. 296; C. KARKOV, *The Art of Anglo-Saxon England* (Woodbridge, 2011), pp. 31-32.

and details hidden within.[47] This sense of resolving and dissolving patterns creates a sense of ambiguity in the viewer, suggesting that there was a value given to uncertainty, both of the image and of the meaning. This ambiguity created by the Anglo-Saxon craftsmen offers a multivalency or fluidity of meaning regardless of whether the pattern is composed of traditional zoomorphs, geometric shapes, decorative elements or crosses. The viewer contemplates the decoration, moving his eye over the composition as directed by shape, colour, reflection and iconography, and bringing his own interpretive context to the piece.

It is necessary to understand that there was a tangible sense of importance and significance attached to the materials themselves in Anglo-Saxon society, especially when those materials were rare or precious. Wealth and treasure were prized commodities, necessary to establish a place in Anglo-Saxon society through their display and distribution, and holding an importance that went well beyond whatever monetary value they embodied. Information about status and hierarchy was embedded in the aesthetic created by the traditional materials of gold, silver and garnet. However, the decorative effects of personal ornamentation, and therefore its transmission of information to a viewer depended upon imagery as much as materiality, with all being mediated by the visual perception of the artwork. Indeed, the technical proficiency and intricacy shown in the decorative choices made in these objects suggests that the type of decoration and the manner in which it was executed were important in establishing the value and preciousness of the object. Part of that technical facility was the ability to manipulate both materials and intricate decoration in order to create the desired visual effect – not just as a single finished impression, but in the creation of an active, involved, and mobile way in which to view it. The ornamentation produced by these craftsmen also embodied preciousness in its own right, a tangible representation of value embedded in its intricacy and articulation of fine detail.

The ambiguity of the anonymous zoomorphs and geometric shapes, which create the most intricate and visually confusing pattern, enhances the mysterious and contemplative nature of viewing them. The manipulation of visual perception by the material and ornament of early Anglo-Saxon metalwork disrupts the viewer's engagement with the art, using light, reflection, texture,

[47] E. PIROTTE, "Hidden order, order revealed: New light on carpet-pages", in: *Pattern and Purpose in Insular Art: Proceedings of the Fourth International Conference on Insular Art, Held at the National Museum & Gallery, Cardiff 3-6 September 1998*, ed. M. REDKNAP *et al.* (Oxford, 2001), pp. 204-207, at pp. 203-204.

and colour to limit the eye to transitory impressions and disparate views. There is no way to identify the creatures or understand the shapes, and there is no need to do so: the pattern and the way it moves becomes the primary focus. However, the pattern is awash with meaning and purpose beyond aesthetically pleasing decoration. This artistic tendency to utilise symbolic imagery in apotropaic and talismanic ways, and to delight in ambiguous and spatially disconcerting pattern, persists throughout the seventh century and well beyond, appropriating and being appropriated by the late antique artistic conventions imported into England by the Augustinian mission as part of the conversion to Christianity.

Taking Out the Eye of a One-Eyed Man and Other Hypothetical Moments of Sensory Impairments in Early Medieval Law

PATRICIA SKINNER

Medieval law codes from the sixth to the ninth centuries have long been mined for the information they contain on bodily injury and compensation, the recent work of Lisi Oliver again bringing them into prominence.[1] Irina Metzler, Edward Wheatley, Joshua Eyler and Wendy Turner have also drawn closer attention to the position of the sensory-impaired in medieval society, demonstrating how historians of pre-modern health and medicine have fruitfully mined non-medical texts for information.[2] A recent collection on

[1] In particular L. OLIVER, *The Body Legal in Barbarian Law* (Toronto, 2011); EAD., "Protecting the body in early medieval law", in: *Peace and Protection in the Middle Ages*, ed. T.B. LAMBERT and D. ROLLASON (Durham, 2009), pp. 60-77; EAD., "Sick maintenance in Anglo-Saxon law", *Journal of English and Germanic Philology* 107 (2008), pp. 303-326; EAD., "Genital mutilation in medieval Germanic law", in: *Capital and Corporal Punishment in Anglo-Saxon England*, ed. J.P. GATES and N. MARAFIOTI (Woodbridge, 2014), pp. 48-73.

[2] I. METZLER, *Disability in Medieval Europe: Thinking about Physical Impairment during the High Middle Ages,* c.*1100-1400* (London and New York, 2006); EAD. *A Social History of Disability in the Middle Ages: Cultural Considerations of Physical Impairment* (London and New York, 2013); E. WHEATLEY, *Stumbling Blocks before the Blind: Medieval Constructions of a*

Sensory Perception in the Medieval West, ed. Simon C. THOMSON and Michael D.J. BINTLEY, *Utrecht Studies in Medieval Literacy*, 34 (Turnhout: Brepols, 2016), pp. 181-194.

BREPOLS PUBLISHERS DOI 10.1484/M.USML-EB.5.109510

medicine and the law, whilst largely focussing on the later Middle Ages, reminded us again that legal texts are a fruitful source for the topic of physical impairment and therapy, whilst the rich seam of Anglo-Saxon sources on law and punishment continues to be mined and set against other regulatory material such as penitentials and sermons.[3] What is less well-studied, however, is the diversity of sensory impairment in the medieval past. Not all 'blind' people were / are 'blind', levels of hearing might vary from person to person, and the completely deaf might or might not enjoy the power of speech, depending on when they had become deaf. Moreover, the law codes' consideration of the aftermath of injury focuses not so much on the physical well-being of the victim as on the compensation (and possible contribution to doctors' fees) payable by the perpetrator. This is why it is necessary to widen any survey to other types of source material. Although doctors' fees and 'sick maintenance' were envisaged in some legal texts, they seem only to relate to a finite period as a serious wound healed, rather than supporting an incapacitated person indefinitely.[4] There was a point at which cure for the immediate injury would have to be replaced by care for the permanently-changed victim. The actual profession of the 'learned men' who were called in to assess such matters is not described: were these doctors, lawyers or simply local dignitaries? We are not told, although the fact that *medici* were often asked to sign legal documents that had nothing to do with medical matters suggests that perceived 'professional' status in the early medieval community was fluid and transferable between tasks.[5] Nor do we have any early medieval court cases to set alongside the early medieval laws to determine what might have happened in practice, although injury cases brought before thirteenth- and fourteenth-century courts, complete with vivid narrative testimony as to the circumstances and serious-

Disability (Ann Arbor, MI, 2010); *Disability in the Middle Ages: Reconsiderations and Reverberations*, ed. J. EYLER (Aldershot, 2010); *The Treatment of Disabled Persons in Medieval Europe*, ed. W. TURNER and T. VANDEVENTER PEARMAN (Lampeter, 2010).

[3] *Medicine and the Law in the Middle Ages*, ed. W. TURNER and S. BUTLER (Leiden, 2014); *Capital and Corporal Punishment*.

[4] D.A. BINCHY, "Sick maintenance in early Irish law", *Ériu* 12 (1934), pp. 78-134; OLIVER, "Sick maintenance"; a revisionist view of the provisions is offered by S. JURASINSKI, "'Sick maintenance' and earlier English law", in: *Capital and Corporal Punishment*, pp. 74-91.

[5] C. PILSWORTH, "'Can you just sign this for me John?': Doctors, charters and occupational identity in early medieval northern and central Italy", *Early Medieval Europe* 17 (2009), pp. 363-388. Dr Luca Larpi at Manchester is currently investigating the definition of the 'professional' in early medieval Europe.

ness of the wound, hint at the fluidity of what was, and what was not, considered an 'impairment'.[6]

In this contribution I should like to reflect on the *gradations* of sensory impairment visible in earlier medieval law codes and other sources. Metzler has suggested that the material considerations of impairment may well have been uppermost in the Middle Ages, where the ability to contribute to the economic work of the family or community was determined by the level of mobility or dexterity. Drawing upon somewhat later sources, ranging from hagiography to guild statutes and manorial rolls, she illustrates the ambivalence with which those unable to work and support themselves were viewed. The language of the 'deserving poor' replaced the previous categorisation of poor people as a group, and sensory and mobility impairments were scrutinised more closely by those responsible for charitable assistance.[7] This did not, however, necessarily bring with it full social acceptance.[8] Sensory loss obviously contributed to the ability (or not) to work: sight impairment limited distant or close work; deafness and / or speech impediment may have restricted effective communication.

Early medieval law codes, from Ireland to Byzantium, envisage impairment in a number of different ways, and in fact do recognise the heterogeneous nature of disabling injuries. Illicit, interpersonal violence resulting in physical injury was usually punished with financial penalties, and is often presented in a series of detailed clauses relating to the specific parts of the body injured, and sometimes to the social status of the victim. At the same time, however, some legal codes feature physical injury and impairment (mutilation of limbs and / or disfigurement) as punishments for criminality: these form part of the claim to authority of the ruler, but might, in their turn, be averted by a financial payment to avoid the shame and humiliation of a missing body part or disfigured face. In this respect, as William Ian Miller has so perceptively indicated, medieval rulers acted in almost exactly the same manner as hostage-takers who also threatened mutilation – and engaged in it – to extract a faster and larger pay-

[6] In England: P. SKINNER, *Living with Disfigurement in the Early Middle Ages* (New York, forthcoming 2016), especially Chapter 2; in France: H. SKODA, *Medieval Violence: Physical Brutality in Northern France, 1270-1330* (Oxford, 2013); in Italy: T. DEAN, *Crime and Justice in Late Medieval Italy* (Cambridge, 2007).

[7] METZLER, *Social History*, pp. 36-91 on 'work'. And see S. FARMER, *Surviving Poverty in Medieval Paris: Gender, Ideology and the Daily Lives of the Poor* (Ithaca, NY, 2002).

[8] METZLER, *Disability*, pp. 25-26.

ment.[9] Blinding did not, as a general rule, feature in legislation, but it was certainly threatened and used as a tool of punishment (and political manoeuvring) in the early medieval West and East.[10] Such punishments, however, had to be weighed against the considerations of the utility of the person's unscathed body to the early medieval warband, as Daniela Fruscione has recently pointed out.[11]

I have suggested elsewhere that many of the facial injuries described and penalised in the laws should be understood not in terms of actual, *physical* impairment, but as potential starting points for a person to be *socially* disabled, that is, shamed or dishonoured by the fact that their appearance – especially in the region of the head and face – was altered in some way.[12] Damage to ears was a case in point: early medieval law codes make provision for compensation even if the ear is only injured without sensory loss. Even a mutilated, but not missing, ear required explanation. Psychologists Vicky Bruce and Andy Young, discussing how human interactions are shaped largely by face perception, point out that "[e]ars tend to be an unremarkable aspect of human facial appearance *unless they are noticeably unusual in shape*".[13] A late Roman legal maxim preserved in Justinian's *Digest*, relating to the theft of part of something, uses the maxim, "one who touches the ear of a person touches the whole person", neatly conveying the sense that ears are unremarkable if left alone, but noticeable if modified or removed.[14] The concern was mainly with visual impact, and linked to the contemporary practice of cutting off or nicking the ears of traitors and escaped slaves.[15]

[9] W.I. MILLER, *Eye for an Eye* (Cambridge, 2006), pp. 35-36, 109-129.

[10] WHEATLEY, *Stumbling Blocks*; G. BÜHRER-THIERRY, "'Just anger' or 'vengeful anger'? The punishment of blinding in the early medieval West", in: *Anger's Past: The Social Uses of an Emotion in the Middle Ages*, ed. B.H. ROSENWEIN (Ithaca, NY, and London, 1998), pp. 75-91.

[11] D. FRUSCIONE, "Beginnings and legitimation of punishment in early Anglo-Saxon legislation from the seventh to the ninth century", in: *Capital and Corporal Punishment*, pp. 34-47, at p. 37.

[12] SKINNER, *Living with Disfigurement*; EAD., "Visible prowess? Reading men's head and face wounds in early medieval Europe to 1000 CE", in: *Wounds and Wound Repair in Medieval Culture*, ed. K. DEVRIES and L. TRACY (Leiden, 2015), pp. 81-101.

[13] V. BRUCE and A. YOUNG, *Face Perception* (London and New York, 2012), p. 7, my emphasis.

[14] *The Digest of Justinian*, 47.II.21. ed. and tr. A. WATSON, 4 vols. (Philadelphia, 2011), 4, pp. 251-273.

[15] As reported, for example, in Gregory of Tours' sixth-century histories: *Gregorii Episcopi Turoniensis Libri Historiarum X*, V.48, VIII.29, and IX.38, ed. B. KRUSCH and W. LEVISON (Hanover, 1937-1951: *MGH SRM* 1.1), pp. 257-258, 391-393, 458-459.

Other injuries to the ear, however, were clearly envisaged as having rather more serious consequences, including partial or total impairment of hearing: several codes allow for the possibility that removal of the outer ear, leading to the closure of the wound and, presumably, an obstruction to the ear channel, might cause deafness.[16] It is telling that in at least one later author the Latin adjective *surdus* was also used to indicate stupidity rather than deafness.[17] This suggests that being deaf could so severely impair the ability to communicate that the person was considered mentally impaired as well. Luke Demaitre highlights later medieval texts that make this association explicit, underscoring the "auditory nature" of the era.[18] 'Deaf and mute' is a common combination in narrative texts, modelled on Christ's healing miracle in Mark 7:31-37, but the biblical text highlights not muteness, but a speech impediment or stammer. Again we meet the gradations of impairment – inability to speak clearly, it seems, rendered a person 'mute'. In terms of alternative forms of communication, much has been made of the adaptive power of medieval monks, forced by their rules of silence to create and use a sign language, but less is known about similar strategies among lay people.[19]

By far the most important sense was that of sight. Edward Wheatley's work on blindness in the Middle Ages points out that sight impairment does not necessarily imply total sight deprivation, but it is often treated as a monolithic condition, ignoring the spectrum of actual, physical impairments categorised as 'blindness'.[20] Rosemarie Garland-Thomson remarks that the "ocularcentric" modern world actually underestimates "the advantages of blindness, such as being able to navigate without artificial light or engaging fully with other senses such as touch and smell".[21] Whilst I do not fully share her optimistic view, it is certainly the case that medieval life and work often took place in

[16] E.g. the *Laws of King Aethelberht of Kent* (560×616), ed. L. OLIVER (with revised numbering) online at <http://www.earlyenglishlaws.ac.uk/laws/texts/abt/> [accessed 20 May 2015], c. 38; the two recensions of Alemannic law dating to the early eighth century, *Leges Alamannorum*, A., LVII, 9 and *Pactus Legis Alamannorum*, VI.2, ed. K.A. ECKHARDT, *Leges Alamannorum* (Hanover, 1966: *MGH LL Nat. Germ.* 5.1), pp. 118 and 22 respectively.

[17] Orderic Vitalis uses the adjective to refer to the personal physician of King Henry I of France after the king died: *The Ecclesiastical History of Orderic Vitalis*, ed. M. CHIBNALL, 6 vols. (Oxford, 1969-1980), 2, pp. 88-89.

[18] L. DEMAITRE, *Medieval Medicine: The Art of Healing from Head to Toe* (Santa Barbara, CA, 2013), p. 183 (discussing Bernard de Gordon).

[19] S. BRUCE, *Silence and Sign Language in Medieval Monasticism: The Cluniac Tradition, c. 900-1200* (Cambridge, 2007).

[20] WHEATLEY, *Stumbling Blocks*, pp. 23 and 189.

[21] R. GARLAND-THOMSON, *Staring: How We Look* (Oxford, 2009), pp. 25-26.

poorly-lit environments (whether during the day or at night), so that a certain amount of groping around in the dark or half-light was probably commonplace even for the sighted. Moreover, ability to see in poor light deteriorates quite markedly with age, the condition known as presbyopia, which also manifests as a growing inability to see things close by, making reading increasingly difficult. Predictably, those most likely to live into their sixth decade in the medieval past, monks and clergy, often refer to their failing sight as they write. Abbot Guibert of Nogent is a case in point, complaining that his sight had grown dull, but contrasting this with the more important 'internal' sight, a common trope.[22]

Touch and smell, therefore, whilst not featuring heavily in the legal texts or discussions of impairment in chronicles, may have been far more important in the past than might be expected, at least for purposes of moving around. In the words of Piero Camporesi, the sense of smell, in particular, "has now plunged to infamous depths amongst a sensory hierarchy much changed in character ...".[23] Utilising touch does indeed figure in accounts of deliberately blinded men, whether prisoners or political opponents. Gerald of Wales tells the story of a blinded prisoner in the castle of Chateauroux in France who had committed all the passageways and stairs of the castle to memory, and was able to use this knowledge to seize a hostage. Rather sunnier is Anna Komnena's account of the blinded Byzantine aristocrat Nicephorus, who received instruction in geometry, including touching raised figures to understand the shape: her comparison of Nicephorus with the late antique exegete Didymus the Blind, of course, sheds doubt on the veracity of this tale, but it does in passing demonstrate that impairment could be mitigated if a person had the resources to buy assistance.[24]

[22] J. RUBENSTEIN, *Guibert of Nogent: Portrait of a Medieval Mind* (London and New York, 2002), p. 213, points out that Guibert was not *blind* at this point. On outer and inner sight, see also Thietmar of Merseburg and Gerald of Wales: *Thietmar Mersebergensis Episcopi Chronicon*, VII, cc. 55 and 67, ed. R. HOLTZMANN (Berlin, 1935: *MGH SS rer. Germ.*, n.s. 9), pp. 468-469, 481-482; Gerald of Wales, *The Journey through Wales*, I, c. 1, trans. L. THORPE, *Gerald of Wales – The Journey through Wales / The Description of Wales* (Harmondsworth, 1978), pp. 77-78.

[23] P. CAMPORESI, *The Incorruptible Flesh: Body Mutation and Mortification in Religion and Folklore*, trans. T. CROFT-MURRAY and H. ELSOM (Cambridge, 1988), p. 209.

[24] Gerald of Wales, *The Journey through Wales*, I, c.11, pp. 142-143; Anna Comnene, *Alexiade*, IX,10, ed. and trans. B. LEIB, 3 vols. (Paris, 1967), 2, pp. 184-185. On Didymus the Blind (*c.* 313-398) and his reception in Byzantine authors, R.A. LAYTON, *Didymus the Blind and His Circle in Late-Antique Alexandria* (Champaign, IL, 2004).

The spectrum of sight impairment, which we might term the *variability* of sight, is also visible in the early laws.[25] Almost all distinguish, in their tariff lists of illicit injury, between harm to the eye and its total removal, but the *Lex Alamannorum* of the seventh century describes injury resulting in impaired sight, "*ita quod quasi vitro remaneat*" ("as if seeing through glass").[26] Other injuries include damage to the eyelids, so that one could not close the eye or hold its tears. Both could result in damage to sight or, at the very least, repeated eye infections.[27]

It is, however, difficult to place the one-eyed man of the title on this continuum of full, partial or complete loss of sight. Uniquely documented in the seventh-century Edict of King Rothari of the Lombards, the offence of putting out the only eye of a one-eyed, free man is expressed succinctly:

> *Si quis hominem liberum unum oculum habentem ipsum excusserit, duas partes pretii ipsius, quod adpretiatus fuerit si eum occidissit componat. Si autem haldium aut servum alienum unum oculum habentem ipsum excusserit, conponat eum pro mortuo.*[28]

> If someone puts out the eye of a one-eyed freeman, he should pay two-thirds of what would have been given if he had killed him. If he puts out the eye of another's *aldius* or slave, he should pay the compensation as if he had killed him.

Thus rendering an already vulnerable man completely blind was penalised almost as heavily as the penalty that would have been payable on his murder, his *wergeld*. Deprived of his other eye, the victim of such an attack would need to adapt to complete blindness. There are isolated reports in chronicles of attempted blindings going wrong, and some sight being retained, but this is not, I would argue, the scenario being envisaged here. This clause appears late in Rothari's code (it is clause 377 out of 388), separated from the detailed tariff list of head and facial injuries, and it is tempting to think that the law arose from a specific case that was not covered in the rest of the legislation. Taking out an eye (of a freeman, a semi-free *aldius*, and a slave) was certainly covered,

[25] 'Variability' here draws on the work of Chris Mounsey: C. MOUNSEY, "Variability: Beyond sameness and difference", in: *The Idea of Disability in the Eighteenth Century*, ed. C. MOUNSEY (Plymouth, 2014), pp. 1-30.

[26] *Leges Alamannorum*, A, LVII,13, p. 119.

[27] e.g. *Laws of King Aethelberht*, c. 43; *Lex Baiwariorum*, IV, 15, ed. E. VON SCHIND, (Hanover, 1926: *MGH LL nat. Germ.* 5.2), p. 338; *Leges Alamannorum*, A, LVII, 11-12, p. 118.

[28] *Edictus Langobardorum*, c. 377, ed. F. BLUHME, (Hanover, 1868: *MGH LL* 4), pp. 87-88.

each being compensated with half the amount that would have been payable had they been killed.[29] But the specific case of taking out a man's one *remaining* eye, with its implication of total incapacity, clearly had not been thought about, and was compensated for more heavily. By the time Rothari's laws and those of his successors were redacted into a concordance in the early ninth century, this clause found its place just after those relating to single eye removal, expressing the tidying-up of such outliers.[30]

Compensation for injury was calculated not only according to the level of impairment it left, but also weighted, as is made clear, in terms of the social status of the victim: a Lombard freeman so blinded was paid two-thirds of his *wergeld*, whilst the same injury to a semi-free or unfree man was payable in full as if they had been killed. Total sight loss, after all, closed down most forms of economic activity except for begging, and rendered a semi-free peasant or slave virtually useless for most physical tasks, particularly agricultural work or work as a herdsman. At least, this is the tenor of a law that effectively demanded the cost of a replacement. Did the legislators consider a freeman likelier to be able to find a network of support amongst kin and community, whilst the fate of the *aldius* and slave was far more linked to the whim of their masters? Even so, the two-thirds fine expressed the seriousness of his plight. Although the Lombard law was the only one to make this connection of effective social or economic death, its heavy penalty was also designed to ensure that talionic revenge, the biblical 'eye for an eye', was not carried out – the metaphorical death of the blinded man was to be repaid as if he had been killed, but physical violence was not to be reciprocated.[31]

To what extent was the law gendered? Was the "one-eyed man" here meant to stand for any person, male or female, who suffered the same fate? Jinty Nelson and Alice Rio have suggested that early medieval laws did *not*, as a general rule, differentiate by gender, only doing so when the offence committed was specified as being against a woman.[32] Of all the early medieval codes, the Lombard laws, however, seem to have had the clearest sense of demarcation between the sexes when it came to impairment and injury, and Ross Balza-

[29] *Edictus Langobardorum*, cc. 48, 81, and 105, pp. 21, 25, and 27.

[30] *Liber Legis Regum Langobardorum, Concordia Dictus*, Tit. XIII, 7, ed. F. BLUHME (Hanover, 1868: *MGH LL* 4), p. 246.

[31] On talionic punishments and their shifting cultural meanings, see MILLER, *Eye for an Eye*.

[32] J.L. NELSON and A. RIO, "Women and laws in early medieval Europe", in: *The Oxford Handbook of Women and Gender*, ed. J. BENNETT and R. MAZO KARRAS (Oxford, 2013), pp. 103-117, at p. 105.

retti has highlighted the ideological denial of women's capacity to become enmeshed in fights, and the dismissal of any claims to compensation for injuries received if they did so.[33] King Liutprand adds more laws relating to women, such as penalising stealing their clothes whilst they bathed.[34] This was a shaming act, and specific clauses relating to women suggest that most injuries and impairments were coded male in Lombard society. Moreover, Lombard law allowed a prospective groom to break off a betrothal if his future wife became blind (or was found to be blind) in both eyes ("*ambos oculos*").[35] The reverse does not appear to have been allowed for, however, suggesting that marriage might well have been seen as an opportunity to delegate the care of an impaired man to his new wife.[36] A woman without sight, however, was clearly not deemed capable of sustaining the marital home or caring for any children. We shall return to a female perspective later on.

The lack of reciprocal violence in the Lombard laws stands in contrast to contemporary and later Byzantine practice, but the same fear of total sight loss underpins a series of clauses in the Novels of Emperor Leo VI of Byzantium (r. 886-912). Novel 92 punishes the person who blinds someone else, noting that "it is not possible to repair the damage done to a blinded man's eyes". This principle, however, guides Leo's punishment of the perpetrator – whilst it would be tempting to inflict blinding in return, Leo suggests that a better way is to engender remorse in the perpetrator and help the victim of the act. So if one eye has been removed in the attack, the perpetrator should lose one eye, but if the perpetrator has taken *both* eyes, only one eye should be put out in retaliation and, in lieu of losing the hand that did the deed, two-thirds of the perpetrator's goods be confiscated and given to the victim. By restricting the punishment, Leo was ensuring that the perpetrator was suitably shamed, whilst not creating the circumstances for him to evoke pity for his condition. At the same time, this law demonstrates a practical approach to supporting the victim

[33] R. BALZARETTI, "'These are things men do, not women': The social regulation of female violence in Langobard Italy", in: *Violence and Society in the Early Medieval West*, ed. G. HALSALL (Woodbridge, 1998), pp. 175-192.

[34] Bathing: *Edictus Langobardorum*, Liudprand, c. 135, ed. BLUHME (Hanover, 1868: *MGH LL* 4) 135, p. 166; blocking the way: *Edictus Langobardorum*, Rothari, c. 26, p. 17.

[35] *Edictus Langobardorum*, Rothari, c. 180, p. 42; *Liber Legis Regum Langobardorum*, Tit. XXI, 3, ed. BLUHME (Hanover, 1868: *MGH LL* 4), p. 254.

[36] Campaigners against modern forced marriage often find this used as a tactic, although more often in cases of learning disability: <https://www.gov.uk/government/uploads/system/uploads/attachment_data/file/35533/fmdisability-guidelines.pdf> [accessed 22 June 2015].

economically. Only if the perpetrator was already poor and unable to pay is full blinding ordered.[37]

Whilst the sole extant first-person narrative of the aftermath of a deliberate blinding, by the priest Wipert, might make much of the spiritual benefits his condition of sightlessness brought him and those who helped him (he was, after all, on a mission to the Rus at the time), his account is shaped by the clerical distinction between physical and spiritual or moral sight.[38] Being blind may have made him a better person, but his economic and social vulnerability, wandering as a humble pilgrim across Europe and begging to sustain himself, is apparent. Hagiography from England in fact includes stories of deliberately-blinded men having their eyes and sight restored by the saints. The most famous is the case of Ailward of Westoning, cured by St Thomas Becket,[39] but of equal or possibly greater interest is the account of St William of York helping a certain Ralph. Beaten in judicial combat, Ralph suffered the loss of one eye at the hands of his opponent, Besing; *because* he had lost his appeal, he was then handed over to the justices and deprived of his *other* eye. A servant retrieved both eyes, a gruesome detail that presumably heightens the horror of the reader, before William intervened and restored the man's eyes and his sight.[40] Whilst such tales primarily depict their protagonists as restorers of justice (morally, if not always legally), they also acknowledge the difficulties of living as a blinded man in twelfth-century England.

But what about living as a one-eyed man? Here we have evidence of a form of sensory deprivation that has eluded the attention of disability historians, perhaps because the person concerned could still see. It is doubtful whether the one-eyed person would even have been considered impaired, although their condition was not entirely without impact on their lives. Many people today live with monocular vision, whether from birth or through accident, injury, or illness, but acquired monocular vision comes with considerable drawbacks: a

[37] *Les Novelles de Léon VI Le Sage*, ed. and trans. P. NOAILLES and A. DAIN (Paris, 1944), pp. 300-305.

[38] Wipert's eleventh-century account is reproduced in the preliminary matter to the *Vita S. Adalberti Episcopi*, ed. G.H. PERTZ (Hanover, 1841: *MGH SS* 4), pp. 579-580.

[39] The *Miracula of Benedict of Peterborough*, reproduced in: *English Lawsuits from William I to Richard I, 2, Henry II and Richard I*, ed. R.C. VAN CAENEGEM (London, 1991), No. 471B, pp. 509-514.

[40] *English Lawsuits*, 2, ed. R.C. VAN CAENEGEM, No. 505, p. 558.

loss of depth perception and up to 25% decrease in the field of view, particularly peripheral vision.[41]

For a layman in medieval Europe, the threat of losing an eye and living a monocular life might have had fatal consequences in a society where elite masculinity, at least, was expressed through physical completeness and participation in warfare, weapons practice and hunting. Judith Butler's framing of gender identity as one that needs constant performance has been influential in discussions of masculinity, but more recent work has criticised her for ignoring those who were physically unable to perform.[42] Paul McIlvenny asks, "[w]hat happens to the theory [of performativity] when the cultural inscription of disability is one of failure or the inability to act or perform – does the theory omit the disabled body from its purview?"[43] This is a key question to consider when exploring an acquired, as opposed to congenital, sensory impairment, because its acquisition could reduce or completely curtail a man's ability to maintain his status through his martial prowess. Practice and mock combat, in particular, could end with accidental and quite severe head injuries, such as that suffered by Charles the Bald's eponymous son in 864. It is not commented whether he lost an eye from the sword stroke that cut from his left temple to the right part of his jaw, but he was clearly incapacitated in the subsequent two years before his death.[44]

Lacking an eye did not pass without comment, it seems, particularly among highly visible elites. The chronicler Orderic Vitalis reports that Robert of Courcy was wounded in battle, losing his right eye, and such cases of survivable head injury seem to have been quite frequent. Arrow strikes, in particular,

[41] T. POLITZER, "Implications of acquired monocular vision (loss of one eye)", at the Neuro-Optometric Rehabilitation Association website: <https://nora.cc/for-patientsmainmenu-34/loss-of-one-eye-mainmenu-70.html> [accessed 29 May 2015].

[42] J. BUTLER, "Performative acts and gender constitution: An essay in phenomenology and feminist theory", *Theatre Journal* 40 (1988), pp. 519-531, especially p. 528: "That gender reality is created through sustained social performances means that the very notions of an essential sex, a true or abiding masculinity or femininity, are also constituted as part of the strategy by which the performative aspect of gender is concealed".

[43] His answer, speaking as someone with spina bifida, was 'yes', but his response is to perform his masculinity through drawing an autobiographical comic book: P. MCILVENNY, "The disabled male body 'writes / draws back': Graphic fictions of masculinity and the body in the autobiographical comic *The Spiral Cage*", in: *Revealing Male Bodies*, ed. N. TUANA, W. COWLING, M. HARRINGTON, G. JOHNSON and T. MACMULLAN (Bloomington, IN, 2002), pp. 100-124, at p. 101.

[44] *Annales Bertiniani*, ed. G. WAITZ (Hanover, 1883: *MGH SS rer. Germ. in usu scholarum* 5), *s.a.* 864.

could do plenty of damage without actually penetrating the eye socket.[45] Literally having a 'blind side' opened one up to unseen attack, but the need to turn the head in the direction of the blinded or missing eye, ironically, left the sighted side just as vulnerable. The loss of an eye in battle does not appear to have been a mark of honour, if the tenth-century Saxon chronicler Widukind's account of Count Ecgbert is any indicator. According to Widukind, Ecgbert nursed a grudge against Otto I for the "reckless battle" in which he had lost his eye (and subsequent German chroniclers, for example Thietmar of Merseburg, add the epithet "*monoculus*" to Ecgbert's name).[46] Later on, William of Auvergne would comment that "a man with only one eye is physically displeasing".[47] So frequent were such injuries, however, that Gerald of Wales was able to suggest in the twelfth century that King Harold was only injured in his left eye at Hastings, and survived to become a fugitive on the Welsh border before his death and burial at Chester.[48]

For other one-eyed men documented in the early medieval sources, the disadvantages of their situation may have been mitigated by their occupation: the Byzantine chronicler Theophanes (writing in the late eighth / early ninth century) mentions Maximus, who became patriarch of Jerusalem in the early fourth century despite lacking an eye. Theophanes explains that Maximus had "endured many tortures", implying that he had lost his eye during the last great persecutions of Christians before toleration was decreed by Constantine, and thus could be presented as a hero for his faith. His impairment, whilst technically disbarring him from serving as a bishop according to the principles set out in Leviticus, was overwritten by his heroism and the fact that he had acquired his injury *after* he had entered holy orders. And as a cleric his possibly impaired motor skills (a direct result of loss of depth perception) would probably not have had much impact on his daily life.[49] (This assumes, of course, that

[45] J. BRADBURY, *The Medieval Archer* (Woodbridge, 1985), *passim*, features many examples.

[46] *Die Sachsengeschichte des Widukind von Korvei*, III, c. 19, ed. P. HIRSCH and H.E. LOHMANN and P. HIRSCH (Hanover, 1935: *MGH SS rer. Germ. in usu scholarum* 60), p. 114; *Die Chronik des Bischofs Thietmar von Merseburg*, IV, c.1, pp. 131-132.

[47] William of Auvergne, *Tractatus de Bono et Malo*, cited in U. ECO, *On Beauty* (London, 2004), p. 132.

[48] *The Ecclesiastical History of Orderic Vitalis*, ed. CHIBNALL, 5, Book X.7.IV.33, pp. 226-227; Gerald of Wales, *The Journey through Wales*, II, c. 11, pp. 198-199.

[49] *Chronicle of Theophanes*, AM 5817 (324/5 CE), trans. C. MANGO and R. SCOTT, *The Chronicle of Theophanes Confessor: Byzantine and Near Eastern History AD 284-813* (Oxford, 1997), p. 42; Greek: ed. C. DE BOOR, 2 vols. (Leipzig, 1883-1885), 1, p. 27.

he was not a martial bishop: Thietmar of Merseburg's account of Bishop Michael of Regensburg losing an ear fighting the pagan Hungarians, "to his greater honour", suggests that we should not draw too hard and fast a distinction between elite laymen and their clerical peers.[50])

Clergy and women are all too often lumped together as excluded from the concerns of elite lay masculinity, and certainly cases of women suffering deliberate blinding or attacks to their eyes are few and far between – even the notorious condemnation to blinding of Alice Crithecreche as an accessory to theft and murder in Shropshire in 1203 does not indicate whether the sentence was carried out.[51] What is striking in this context, however, is a later compilation of the Lombard laws made and glossed at Pavia in the eleventh century, revisiting the question of the betrothed woman found to be blind in both eyes and thus considered unmarriageable. What exercised the scholarly compiler was precisely the spectrum of blindness that we have already met elsewhere. Was a one-eyed bride who subsequently lost her other eye included in the original provision issued by Rothari?[52] The Pavian scholar thought hard about this:

> *In hoc quod dicit "aut de ambobus oculis excecata apparuerit" dicebant antiqui, quodsi quis sponseret aliquam monoculam, et postea ex ipso oculo excecata appareret, quod cogendus esset accipere: quia hec lex aliam non facit relinqui, nisi eam que ex utrisque oculis postea excecata apparuerit. Sed male dicebant: quia hec lex non ideo dixit "de ambobus oculis" quia illa, que tantum ex uno excecata postea apparuerit, non possit relinqui, sed ideo dixit ut illa, que, postquam sponsata fuerit, monocula apparuerit, relinquatur.*

> In this law that said "or will appear to be blind in both eyes" the ancients said, that if someone should become engaged to a one-eyed woman, and afterwards she should appear blind in this one eye, it should be inferred that he accept her: because this law allows none other than a woman found to be blind in both eyes afterwards to be left. But they spoke wrongly: because this law does not say "in both eyes" so that she, who will appear just as a blind woman, cannot be left, but so that she, who after the betrothal appears one-eyed, can be left.

[50] Thietmar, *Chronicon*, II, c. 27, p. 72: "... *ad honorem magis*".

[51] *Select Pleas of the Crown*, 1, *AD 1200-1225*, ed. F.W. MAITLAND (London, 1888), pp. 33-34.

[52] *Liber Legis Langobardorum Papiensis Dictus*, ed. A. BORETIUS (Hanover, 1868: *MGH LL* 4), p. 332.

The gist of the argument is that being blind "in both eyes" should also apply to a blind woman even if she only had one eye, and to exclude a one-eyed woman from the ruling was an inadmissible technicality. However, the last sentence does appear to open up – theoretically at least – the possibility that a monocular, but still sighted, girl might also be rejected. This would represent a significant hardening of the original law's provision, and whilst some eleventh-century charter evidence from northern and southern Italy does sometimes cite Lombard law (particularly around the protection of and the rights of women over their property), it is doubtful whether this legalistic glossing had much effect on the practical matters of betrothals.

The legal semantics visible in this extract highlight the major problem of using law codes to examine the reality of life as an impaired person in medieval Europe. Whilst they might provide for a number of disabling injuries, and look to keep the peace by outlawing reciprocal violence and establishing compensation tariffs and fines, ultimately these provisions were works of hypothesis, envisaging situations that might or might not occur. I have suggested that the clause about the one-eyed man in Rothari represented a response to an actual case, largely due to its isolation in the Edict from other clauses dealing with eye injuries and lack of parallels in other early medieval codes. Yet it might equally have been the product of an imaginative legislator, eager to ensure that no possible injury was overlooked in this comprehensive document claiming and expressing royal authority, and recognising that completely blinding a one-eyed man represented a plausible scenario in a world where warfare was endemic and men with one eye not uncommon. We return to the vulnerability of such men: in a fight, their peripheral vision would already be impaired, and so the likelihood of serious injury was increased. The apparent anger felt by Count Ecgbert, particularly if he acquired his nickname *Monoculus* in his lifetime, may have related not only to his impaired appearance, but to the weakening of his capacity to perform his role as an elite warrior. Since verbal injury was also recognised in most medieval law codes, simply the insult of being called One-Eyed may have been enough to start a brawl. Ultimately, the sensory impairment was physical, but the disability was social, and could be devastating.

Dis-embodied Cognition and Sensory Perception in *Sólarljóð*

PETE SANDBERG

> We paint, sculpt, compose, and write with sensations. We paint, sculpt, compose, and write sensations (Gilles Deleuze and Félix Guattari, *What Is Philosophy?*).[1]

How does the poet's body affect the poem? This seems like an interesting enough question, but before attempting to answer it one might do well to reconsider the causal relationship between body and language that the question implies. For the body to *a*ffect the poem, it is necessary for language to have some sort of existence anterior to and separate from the body. But as language is ultimately a product of the body, this cannot straightforwardly be the case, and this observation has influenced the development of a concept of 'embodied cognition'. The *Stanford Encyclopedia of Philosophy* entry on this term points out that "sometimes the nature of the dependence of

[1] G. DELEUZE and F. GUATTARI, (1994): *What is Philosophy?*, trans. H. TOMLINSON (London, 1994), p. 166.

Sensory Perception in the Medieval West, ed. Simon C. THOMSON and Michael D.J. BINTLEY, *Utrecht Studies in Medieval Literacy*, 34 (Turnhout: Brepols, 2016), pp. 195-206.

BREPOLS PUBLISHERS DOI 10.1484/M.USML-EB.5.109511

cognition on the body is quite unexpected", and further highlights the tendency of an embodied-cognitivist approach to manifest as a critique of "traditional approaches to cognition and cognitive processing".[2] Lawrence Shapiro delineates three broad categories of embodied-cognitivist inquiry, one of which is "[c]onceptualization", which "aims to reveal the extent to which the body shapes or constrains the concepts an organism comes to possess or, more generally, how organisms think".[3] Shapiro dubs this school of thought "body determinism" (comparing it to the similar concept of *linguistic* determinism) and concludes that, while compelling, the evidence for it is ambiguous and difficult to test.[4]

The difficulty in empirically verifying causal connections is one that plagues the historical debate around the nature of the mind and its relationship to the body going back at least as far as Descartes; and yet the fundamental premise of, and insights provided by, the embodied-cognitivist approach are difficult to dismiss. Being fundamentally unable to escape our bodies, how can we say definitively that the conceptual tools we use are not shaped by the peculiarities of the human organism? What would it be like to be *dis*embodied? Can we imagine such a thing without resorting to embodied concepts? The importance of sensory information to linguistic description is so great that it is difficult, perhaps even impossible, to imagine how one might describe any sort of conceivable experience without appeal to it. Indeed, it is one of the general observations of cognitive poetics that conceptual metaphors (to use the term coined by George Lakoff and Mark Johnson)[5] tend to rely on 'biophysical' schemata.[6]

So to revisit our initial question, in the particular case of the thirteenth-century Icelandic poem *Sólarljóð* (*Song of The Sun*),[7] the question one might

[2] R.A. WILSON and L. FOGLIA, "Embodied cognition", in: *The Stanford Encyclopedia of Philosophy* (Fall 2011 Edition), ed. E.N. ZALTA, <http://plato.stanford.edu/archives/fall2011/entries/embodied-cognition>.

[3] L. SHAPIRO, "Embodied cognition: Lessons from linguistic determinism", *Philosophical Topics* 39 (2011), pp. 121-140, at p. 122.

[4] SHAPIRO, "Embodied cognition", p. 139.

[5] G. LAKOFF and M. JOHNSON, *Metaphors We Live By* (Chicago, 1981).

[6] O. JÄKEL, "Hypotheses revisited: The cognitive theory of metaphor applied to religious texts", *Metaphorik* 2 (2002), pp. 20-42, at p. 22.

[7] On the dating of this text, which is only preserved in manuscripts going back to the seventeenth century, see H. FALK, *Sólarljóð* (Oslo, 1914: *Videnskapsselskapets skrifter* II, *Hist-Filos. Kl.* 7 (Oslo, 1914); B.M. ÓLSEN, *Sólarljóð – Gefin út með skíringum og athugasemdum* (Reykjavik, 1915); F. JÓNSSON, *Den oldnorske og oldislandske litteratturs historie* (Copenhagen, 1920-1924); B. FIDJESTØL, *Sólarljóð: Tyding og tolkingsgrunnlag* (Bergen, 1979).

rather ask is, "How does the poet's body *e*ffect the portrayal of a *dis*embodied voice?" Here we have changed the emphasis from a question of influence (*a*ffecting the poem) to a question of how the poem is made possible at all (*e*ffecting the poem): as I hope to demonstrate here, the idea or schema of the body is not merely decorative in *Sólarljóð,* but actually constitutes the means of constructing the poem's central scene. In this volume we are trying to make some sense of the medieval mind in its interaction with the physical world, embedded in its environment. This particular text displays an implicit belief in the clear distinction between the soul and the body, or perhaps rather the independence of the soul from the body; that the soul can have a disembodied existence. As the wide circulation of later body-and-soul debate literature based on the *Visio Philiberti* shows,[8] this concept of the distinction between body and soul was highly prevalent in medieval Christian thought. However, as we shall see in the case of *Sólarljóð,* a certain paradox arises when one attempts to conceptualise a disembodied soul, let alone the experience of *being* a disembodied soul: the narrator must necessarily appeal to the faculty of the physical senses in order to construct a scene.

Sólarljóð is unusual among Old Norse poetry. It recycles and recombines elements from various earlier poems of what we now call the 'Eddic' genre, it uses the Eddic *ljóðaháttr* metre and, like other Eddic poems, it is anonymous, not attributed to a particular poet. This genre of Old Norse poetry is strongly associated with legendary or mythological narratives,[9] and often uses the first-person voices of mythological characters, either as dialogue (such as in *Grímnismál*, *Vafþrúðnismál*, *Lokasenna*) or as a first-person narrative voice (such as in *Hávamál*, *Vǫluspá*). The most immediately striking thematic aspect of *Sólarljóð* is its deployment of pre-Christian mythological motifs in what is otherwise an overtly Christian context, and this aspect has inspired much of the existing scholarship on the poem. Bjarne Fidjestøl points out most succinctly that the poet seems to deliberately use archaic, pre-Christian terms ("*heidne religiøse ord*") in a Christian context, and argues further that the poet uses pre-Christian motifs to describe specific Christian concepts.[10] However, as Carolyne Larrington also notes,[11] this does not seem to reflect an actual religious syncretism;

[8] M-A. BOSSY, "Medieval debates of body and soul", *Comparative Literature* 28 (1976), pp. 144-163.

[9] M. CLUNIES ROSS, *A History of Old Norse Poetry and Poetics* (Cambridge, 2005), pp. 10-12.

[10] FIDJESTØL, *Sólarljóð*, p. 42.

[11] C. LARRINGTON, "Freyja and the organ-stool: Neo-paganism in *Sólarljóð*", in: *Germani-*

rather, it appears to be a highly original poetic or rhetorical device, reflecting the same association in the Old Norse cultural mind between archaic pre-Christian mythology and poetry which motivated Snorri Sturluson to compose *Snorra Edda*, intended to be both a compendium of mythology and a handbook for composers and consumers of poetry.

Sólarljóð is ordered into distinct sections, beginning with a series of short *exemplum*-like tales followed by a list of counsels reminiscent of the advice section of the Eddic poem *Hávamál* (which is apparently narrated by the god Óðinn) as well as *Hugsvinnsmál* (an Old Norse translation of the Latin *Disticha Catonis*). The tales in the first section focus primarily on the treachery of worldly things (in particular wealth, power, and women) and the various downfalls of sinful men, while the counsels that follow are concerned with the necessity of avoiding sin and trusting in God. After this (from approximately stanza 33), the content changes significantly, becoming more immediate and personal rather than abstract and general. Yet at the same time the language becomes more cryptic, both in the sense that little context is given for the scene and in the sense that the mystical and the worldly blend into one another, as we shall see below. There is a shift from stories narrated in the third person and general advice delivered to a second person to a first-hand account by the narrator, in which first-person pronouns are used prominently. Here we are dealing with the central portion of the poem, that which gives it its name: this section culminates in seven stanzas (39-45) beginning with the refrain "*Sól ek sá*" ("I saw the sun").[12] Thus we have seven stanzas where not only is the first person distinctly emphasised, but also the sensory aspect of the scene is brought to the foreground. This section narrates the mystical process of the narrator's death and the departure of his soul from his body. The nature of the events being described is unclear, and so it seems possible that we should interpret this narrative allegorically. However, unlike other parts of the poem, in which fixed abstract or cultural concepts are juxtaposed in order to produce meaning (such as in the aforementioned distinctive juxtaposition of Christian and pre-Christian motifs), this series of visions is constructed entirely from sensory phenomena; in spite of its mysticism, its components are almost entirely material.

sches Altertum und christliches Mittelalter: Festschrift für Heinz Klingenberg, ed. B. BROGANYI (Hamburg, 2002), pp. 177-196, at p. 192.

[12] All references to the primary text are to F. JÓNSSON, *Den Norsk-Islandske Skjaldedikting*, 4 vols. (Copenhagen, 1912-15), 1, pp. 635-648.

This materiality is, to a certain extent, inherent in the term *vision.* The faculty of vision has primacy over other senses throughout this poem, just as the Revelation to St John (and medieval dream-vision literature stemming from it) is ordered primarily as a series of *visions,* as if the narrator is a sort of camera: the scene focusses outward from the narrator in much the same way that one's own vision is focussed outward from the body. With this outward visual focus, the role of the viewing narrator becomes more assumed than shown. Though (to a modern reader, at least) a body would seem necessary for vision to occur, this narrative strategy also has the effect of emptying the text of the narrative presence (much as the camera often seeks to do), appealing to the reader's or listener's senses to construct the image in their minds while to some extent burying or obscuring the presence of the viewing narrator. In this case the narrator reinstates himself in the text with the constant repetition of the first-person pronoun (especially in the distinctive refrain of the seven "Sun" verses), as well as adding his own abstract interpretations of some of the things he experiences. However, in spite of this assertion of his personality in the scene he is describing, his descriptions tell us less about him than about the sights and sounds that make up his experience.

Each of the seven visions in these seven stanzas are visions of the sun, and therefore primarily visions purely of *light* rather than visions of objects, perhaps more properly *sensations.* In fact, the narrator barely describes the sun itself at all, but juxtaposes his vision of it, and the sensuous details of that vision, with other sensory information or with intangible states, as we shall see below. The most conspicuous opposition to the pure light of the sun is the sensation of *sound.* Here the narrator sets up an association of sound with death, mortality, and hell that persists for the rest of the text. Twice the narrator hears a loud, cacophonic sort of sound, and in both of these instances the sound is portrayed as coming from "*annan veg*" (39:5, 42:5), from the "other side" or the "other direction" from the light. The first sound is said specifically to be the creaking of the gate of hell, *"en heljar grind / heyrða ek annan veg / þjóta þungliga"* ("and hell's gate / I heard from the other direction / howl heavily", 39:4-6), and the second sound is caused by currents of water mixed with blood, *"en gylfar straumar / grennjuðu annan veg / blandnir mjǫk við blóð"* ("and the seas' currents / roared from the other direction / mixed greatly with blood", 42:4-6). The obvious syntactic similarity of the sentences describing these two sounds provides an additional link between them, showing their thematic affinity and uniting them as experiences opposed to that of viewing the sun. Water also plays a role in the ending of this section, closing over the narrator and ending his vision, presumably signalling his final descent into death, but most importantly obscuring his vision of the sun.

In addition to these aural experiences, the narrator also juxtaposes the vision of the sun with two expressions of his own emotional state described as physical bodily conditions, one with a particularly tactile image. The first of these is the image of the narrator's heart shattered into pieces: "*Sól ek sá / á sjónum skjálfandi / hræzlufullr ok hnipinn, / þvít hjarta mitt / var harðla mjök / runnit sundr í sega*" ("I saw the sun / with shaking vision, / fearful and despondent, / because my heart / had been very greatly / torn to shreds", 43). The second image is that of the narrator's tongue turned cold and wooden: "*tunga mín / var til trés metin / ok kólnat fyrir útan*" ("My tongue / had become like wood / and chilled on the outside", 44:46). These images illustrate the narrator's more abstract description of his emotional state as being fearful, afflicted, and distressed, most likely due to the trauma of death. But by putting them in specifically bodily terms, he creates an equivalence between sensory and emotional feeling, and also demonstrates his dependence on biophysical categories in his language. The corporeal and the abstract are both united and implicitly contrasted in these images, though perhaps this is more the case in the first image, in which the "heart" is acting primarily in its role as the container of the soul and therefore its tearing to pieces is to be understood in a partly metaphorical sense, than in the second, which more clearly describes the actual physical condition of a dry, cold mouth that might be caused by a traumatic experience. However, in these images both the heart and the tongue are given a materiality that exceeds the corporeal, being compared to *wood.* In the case of the heart, this seems to illustrate the heart's metaphorical nature in this image (presumably the narrator's heart is not actually being damaged here, but rather stands for his intangible emotions); while in the case of the tongue it is more clearly a tactile comparison that illustrates the physical sensation being described. Additionally, the visceral and aversive mental states being described are contrasted with the pure, disorienting light of the sun in much the same way as the hellish noises were.

Throughout this scene we have no way of orienting ourselves except by this particular set of sensory information. We do not know where we are, where the narrator is. We only know that the light of the sun is shining from one direction, and the sounds of hell are emanating from another. The sun is indeed described as disorienting the narrator, causing his vision to shake, making him feel as if he "knows nothing": "*Sól ek sá / svá hon geislaði / at ek þóttumz vætki vitta*" ("I saw the sun / she shone so / that it seemed to me that I knew nothing", 42:1-3). The effect is heightened by the confusion of the abstractly emotional with the bodily and the tactile. This is, presumably, the confusion and distress of being between life and death. The narrative is physical and embodied, but the state being described is one of partial disembodiment, where otherworldly influences can play a material part. And although the narrator offers a tentative interpretation of the vision to him, the use of "*þótti mér*" ("it seemed") that he was looking upon God (41:1-3), implies that the sun is *not* God. The idea of a theological interpretation is suggested, but the sun is not transformed into a pure metaphor and remains material. This seems to be affirmed in the closing stanza of this section, in which the narrator states that "*Sól ek sá / síðan aldri / eptir þann dapra dag*" ("I saw the sun / never again / after that gloomy day"). As the journey of the narrator's soul eventually takes him to heaven, this stanza strongly implies that the light of the sun seen in these visions is the sunlight solely of the material, mortal world.

After this section, the narrator's (now entirely disembodied) soul goes on a Dantean tour of hell and heaven. Vision again takes primacy as the most important means of structuring the narrative, but other sensory information continues to play a role even after the complete abandonment of the body, and indeed the narrator's fixation on bodies comes to the fore in his visions of hell. Here the "*Sól ek sá*" formula changes to "*menn sá ek þá*" ("I saw men then", 61-67, 69-72). From a more abstract point of view, each vision of a torment in hell conveys its particular moral message without much subtlety: groups of souls are punished in specific ways for specific sins. In material or biophysical terms, the treatment of bodies (and again we must bear in mind here that these are in fact *souls,* merely rhetorically constructed from bodily terms) amounts to scenes of body *horror.* It is primarily the violation of the boundaries and integrity of human bodies that functions as a means of torture here; the horrifying problematisation of the body. The body in this vision of hell is (again, somewhat paradoxically) the site upon which the soul receives its punishment. Faithless women's hearts hang *outside* their breasts (57-58); poison-dragons run *through* the breasts of thieves and murderers (64); hell's ravens tear the eyes *out of* the heads of slanderers (67). Heaven's rewards, by contrast, are largely incorporeal: angels bow to (71) and read heavenly texts to (70) the souls of the faithful, who travel on paths to God (74). It hardly seems an appropriate counter-balance for the far more evocative torments of hell, but the contrast between the punishments of hell and the rewards of heaven also seems to be a contrast between the material or bodily on the one hand, and the abstract or intellectual on the other.

The majority of the poem, as we have seen, deals with the disembodied person of the narrator, and at the end it is confirmed that he is delivering this narrative from a state of disembodiment after death (82-83). But we have also seen how the narrator must necessarily rely on biophysical schemata to construct images of otherworldly scenes: sensory information and images of bodies make up much of the poem's content. How, then, are these images to be interpreted? Again, it is possible that the visionary content of the poem is entirely (or partly) metaphorical or allegorical, but this is not made explicit by the narrator. Furthermore, the sections of sensory information and bodily images stand in contrast to more obviously symbolic visions such as that of the "*sólar hjǫrt*" ("hart of the sun", 55), possibly representing Christ,[13] or the far more obscure allusions to pre-Christian mythology that crop up at the end of the poem in a style that evokes the cryptically allusive tone of earlier Eddic mythological poetry. In these sections the narrator signals an allusion relatively clearly by exploiting the conventions of his poetic genre. For example, various fragments of mythology that have not survived in any other existing source seem to be alluded to in stanzas 76-80, such as *"þær rúnir, / sem ristit hafa / Njarðar dœtr níu*" ("those runes which / have been carved by / the nine daughters of Njǫrðr", 79:1-3), and in a way that displays the narrator's knowledge while remaining cryptic, comparable to the tone used by the narrator of *Vǫluspá*. The focus of these allusions is mythological, referring primarily to pre-Christian gods and the supernatural, and adds a characteristically Eddic flourish to the tone of the poem, though without access to the relevant mythological material it is unfortunately impossible for the modern reader to know what purpose these allusions might serve. But in the seven sun-visions (and, to a somewhat lesser extent, in the visions of heaven and hell), by contrast, the poet creates images not primarily by juxtaposing abstract symbols but rather by constructing fresh sensory scenes from the most basic of elements.

But the subject of these images is a world that, though perhaps very real in the poet's mind, is somehow beyond the material and the embodied. It is particularly striking, then, that the poet uses such strictly (albeit creatively) biophysical language to construct disembodiment and the incorporeal afterlife. The

[13] N.P. NJARÐVÍK, *Sólarljóð* (Reykjavik, 1991), p. 84; FALK, *Sólarljóð*, p. 35; F. PAASCHE, *Hedenskap og kristendom: Studier i norrøn middelalder* (Oslo, 1948), pp. 149-150.

basic inability of the poet to speak of an incorporeal world in anything other than corporeal terms highlights the dependence of language and cognition on the body, of the linguistic imagination on sensory experience. The poet has to use the tools that he has – real and material sensations such as the blinding light of the sun, the sound of rushing water, or the groaning of a gate. These images do not, however, add up to an objectively descriptive or mimetic poem, rather, they are creatively and non-realistically applied to an abstract idea of what the afterlife, heaven and hell, and the experience of becoming disembodied, might be like. Indeed, the descriptions of the sun-visions are constructed from known or knowable sensory experiences, but the way these sensations fit together corresponds to nothing in the everyday material world.

By way of highlighting the distinctively sensory and corporeal language of *Sólarljóð,* one might productively compare it to another major Old Norse poem written in an overtly Christian context, the twelfth-century *Geisli.* From their titles alone, *Geisli* (*Beam*, i.e. of light) and *Sólarljóð* would seem to have an affinity with one another. The titular 'beam' of *Geisli* refers to St Óláfr, who is referred to in the poem through the kenning "*gǫfgan geisla guðs hallar*" ("the splendid [light] beam of God's hall", 7:1-2).[14] Unlike *Sólarljóð, Geisli* uses the quintessentially skaldic *dróttkvætt* metre.[15] Throughout the poem, its composer Einarr Skúlason uses elaborate kennings to refer primarily to his subject St Óláfr, as well as to God and Christ. Though Einarr wields kennings with a virtuosic hand, he is restricted in his construction of kenning-images by the formal constraints of that particular poetic device, which tends to rely on a conventional set of poetic associations (as Snorri Sturluson sought to map out in *Skáldskaparmál*), and which adheres to a general grammatical schema requiring two groups of nouns of which one is a determinant of the other.[16] The terms Einarr uses to denote God in particular show a trend of using less material and more abstract associations, cultural symbols rather than descriptions based on raw sensory information such as the *Sólarljóð* poet creates. God, Christ and St Óláfr are all associated with the sky, but only insofar as the sky is associated with or the site of heaven. God is referred to as "*vísi veðrhallar*" ("lord of the weather hall", 2:3-4), "*jǫfurr hreggsalar*" ("king of the storm hall", 64:5-6), and "*salkonungr himna*" ("hall king of the heavens", 66:6). In

[14] *Einarr Skúlason's Geisli: A Critical Edition*, ed. M. CHASE (Toronto, 2005).

[15] On this generic distinction, see CLUNIES ROSS, *A History of Old Norse Poetry*, pp. 21-28.

[16] On which see for example F. AMORY, "Kennings", in: *Medieval Scandinavia: An Encyclopedia*, ed. P. PULSIANO and K. WOLF (New York and London, 1993), pp. 351-352.

these kennings in particular, the sky is, rather strikingly, domesticated by being combined with the social concepts of hall and ruler in order to produce the meaning 'heaven'. We also see in these kennings a pervasive tendency in *Geisli* toward comparing God to an earthly ruler or king, with Óláfr himself providing a bridge between earthly and heavenly kingship. There even seems to be a sort of social hierarchy being created in Einarr's system of kennings, with Óláfr designated as "*guðs ríðari*" ("God's knight", 18:6). The reliance here on abstract concepts that themselves rely on socially symbolic connotations to create and connect meanings is quite at odds with the starkly sensuous visions of the *Sólarljóð* poet that we have examined above. During the sun-vision episode, the sensory information related by the narrator presents the image of clear, blinding light that confounds his own attempts to make any sort of meaning out of it; and though this is contrasted to the "*dynheimar*" ("noise-world", 39:3) of mortal life, we have seen that the sun described in these visions does not rhetorically stand for God or Christ or anything else; it is simply the sun itself.

Throughout *Sólarljóð*, the narrator retains identity, selfhood, subjectivity, even after his body is no more. In spite of his own rather grimly materialistic proclamation earlier in the poem that "*ýta synir / verða nauðgir at náum*" ("the sons of men / necessarily become corpses", 33: 5-6), he continues to be a narrative agent after death without being substantially transformed, retaining his identity. The creative and often striking use of voice that we noted above as a characteristic of Eddic poetry has here been taken to a certain extreme: this is a voice without any body at all, a voice that cannot be. Carolyne Larrington has called the use of pre-Christian symbols in the poem a "late pastiche of paganism"[17] rather than a representation of truly syncretic beliefs, and the way in which the *Sólarljóð* poet seems to knowingly re-purpose the Eddic style ("self-consciously archaising and imitative of ... Eddic poems", as Margaret Clunies Ross puts it[18]) arguably corroborates this view. Other Eddic poems that were sufficiently widely circulated so that they have survived for modern audiences tend to use the voices of characters who are clearly fictional or often in some way non-human, such as giants, gods, and seeresses. In *Sólarljóð* this generically Eddic use of the fictional voice has been put to a novel purpose, with the use of the disembodied voice of a soul speaking from beyond the grave as the narrative voice. But with the intrusion of the sensuous and bodily into the

[17] LARRINGTON, "Freyja and the organ-stool", p. 192.

[18] CLUNIES ROSS, *A History of Old Norse Poetry*, p. 216.

poem, with the poet's inability to construct an image without appealing to the senses, the body seems to have had its revenge. In its extensive and creative use of sensory information in its language, *Sólarljóð* actually indicates the absurdity inherent in its own agenda, the portrayal of the incorporeal.

In these terms, the persistence of the corporeal and sensuous in the language of *Sólarljóð* may sound like a conceptual or stylistic failure on the part of the poet, but we have also seen that the ways in which sensory details are employed in the poem are striking and highly creative. I began this essay with an epigraph taken from the seventh chapter of French philosophers Gilles Deleuze and Félix Guattari's final collaboration, *What Is Philosophy?* This chapter, entitled "Percept, affect, and concept", deals very broadly with the idea of the work of art.[19] Deleuze and Guattari hold up the idea of the work of art as "percept", or a group of "percepts" or "a bloc of sensations", "a compound of percepts and affects".[20] Like the montage of sensory information we have examined in the sun-vision section of *Sólarljóð* above, Deleuze and Guattari's percepts "are not perceptions referring to an object (reference): if they resemble something it is with a resemblance produced with their own methods".[21] The sensory perceptions of everyday life provide a sort of raw material for the work of art, but their composition as percepts amounts to more than mere mimesis (even in the case that the work of art is conceptualised, by its creator or by its consumers, as mimetic). In the central section of *Sólarljóð* we have seen the conceptual paradox faced by the poet of attempting to resemble something that cannot be experienced by the living, and we have also seen how the poet creatively juxtaposes perceptual images, "blocs of sensation", to realise this objective. For Deleuze and Guattari

> the aim of art is to wrest the percept from perceptions of objects and the states of a perceiving subject, to wrest the affect from affections as the transition from one state to another: to extract a bloc of sensations, a pure being of sensations.[22]

Sólarljóð is framed by its social and cultural Christian agenda, beginning with its *exempla* and gnomic advice sections and concluding with visions of heaven and hell that serve primarily to reinforce Christian concepts. But the central section of the seven sun-visions exceeds or transcends these concerns

[19] DELEUZE and GUATTARI, *What is Philosophy?*, pp. 163-199.
[20] DELEUZE and GUATTARI, *What is Philosophy?*, p. 164.
[21] DELEUZE and GUATTARI, *What is Philosophy?*, p. 166.
[22] DELEUZE and GUATTARI, *What is Philosophy?*, p. 167.

just as the sensory percepts used by the poet exceed the sensory memories recalled in order to create them. They are re-purposed for the creation of the poem, just as the poet has re-purposed an archaic art form, archaic poetic language, and archaic mythological figures. The narrator in the central section of *Sólarljóð* is between states of life and death, "*mjǫk ... ór heimi hallr*" ("greatly declining out of this world", 40:3, 44:3), experiencing otherworldly perceptions, but still experiencing them corporeally. The visions and sensations he experiences are "not independent" of his "supposed perceptions", "and, through them, of the author's perceptions and memories",[23] but for Deleuze and Guattari, "[c]haracters can only exist, and the author can only create them, because they do not perceive but have passed into the landscape and are themselves part of the compound of sensations".[24] The narrator of *Sólarljóð* is at least halfway into the state of disembodiment in the poem's central section. In spite of his attempts to empty the text of himself by focussing the narration on vision, he has himself become a part of the perceptual composition. In the end, perhaps the investigation of this section of the poem has not been a phenomenology of the proper "material" with which the poet works, that is, language itself, but rather a phenomenology of the sensory percepts conveyed (via the problematic relationship between linguistic concepts and sensory, bodily phenomena highlighted by the embodied-cognitivist approach) in that material. In spite of its jarring distinctiveness from the other sections of the poem, it seems fitting that the sun-vision section, in which sensory percepts conveyed through language exceed the status of sensory memories or mimetic devices, should give *Sólarljóð* its name.

[23] DELEUZE and GUATTARI, *What is Philosophy?*, p. 169.

[24] DELEUZE and GUATTARI, *What is Philosophy?*, p. 169.

(Re-) Viewing "*Iuxta Morem Romanorum*": Considering Perception, Phenomenology, and Anglo-Saxon Ecclesiastical Art and Architecture

MEG BOULTON

The foundational scholarship concerning the identification of Anglo-Saxon Architecture as a discrete style (scholarship that prioritised the recognition, cataloguing, classification and description of the extant architecture) came from a predominantly antiquarian milieu, as I have discussed at length elsewhere.[1] Since this initial antiquarian interest there has

[1] See M. BOULTON and J. HAWKES, "The early churches of Kent: Rome and Jerusalem in Anglo-Saxon England", in: *The Church in Kent*, ed. P. BIDWELL and S. BROWN (Oxford, 2015), pp. 92-118. For further reading providing a brief history of the scholarly engagement with Anglo-Saxon architecture see T. RICKMAN, *An Attempt to Discriminate the Styles of English Architecture from the Conquest to the Reformation* (London, 1817); see e.g. J.T. MICKLETHWAITE, "Description and history of the church of St Pancras", *Archaeological Journal* 55 (1896), pp. 343-344; G. BALDWIN BROWN, *The Arts in Early England*, 2, *Anglo-Saxon Architecture* (London, 1925); A.W. CLAPHAM, *English Romanesque Architecture Before the Conquest* (Oxford, 1930); E.A. FISHER, *An Introduction to Anglo-Saxon Architecture and Sculpture* (London, 1962); E.C. FERNIE, *The Architecture of the Anglo-Saxons* (London, 1983); H.M. TAYLOR and J. TAYLOR, *Anglo-Saxon Architecture*, 3 vols. (Cambridge, 1965-1972); R. MORRIS, *The Church in British Archaeology* (London, 1983); C.B. MCCLENDON, *The Origins of Medieval Architecture: Building in Europe A.D. 600-900* (London and New Haven, CT, 2005).

Sensory Perception in the Medieval West, ed. Simon C. THOMSON and Michael D.J. BINTLEY, *Utrecht Studies in Medieval Literacy*, 34 (Turnhout: Brepols, 2016), pp. 207-226.

BREPOLS PUBLISHERS DOI 10.1484/M.USML-EB.5.109512

been considerable scholarly discussion of the subject, resulting in a multiplicity of publications devoted to the classification and description of architecture from this period. These range from Rickman's foundational *Attempt to Discriminate the Styles of English Architecture* in 1817,[2] to the comprehensive catalogue produced by Taylor and Taylor in the 1960s, to recent work addressing the importance and significance of architecture in a more synthetic manner, such as Helen Gittos' recent publication on *Liturgy, Architecture, and Sacred Places in Anglo-Saxon England*,[3] and Charles McClendon's impressive work *The Origins of Medieval Architecture: Building in Europe A.D. 600-900*.[4]

The churches of Anglo-Saxon England, built by Augustine and his successors, of stone, brick and glass "in the Roman manner",[5] are remarkable structures.[6] Besides offering insight into the architectural, intellectual and ecclesiastical climate of the now much fragmented milieu of Anglo-Saxon England for the modern viewer seeking to reconstruct this landscape, they may also be understood as monumental archetypes that represent concepts of place and identity. In such an archetypal model these structures recall, establish and actualise the architectural vocabulary of disparate places such as Rome, or Jerusalem within Anglo-Saxon England, while providing multivalent experiential encounters with sacred spaces beyond the earth.[7] This contribution builds on such understandings of these monumental structures, sculptures and spaces, to address how the art and architecture of this period may be conceptualised by those engaging with it, in addition to the widely recognised ability of these buildings to recall and actualise far-off spaces and places through their associations with Rome or Jerusalem and their embedded *romanitas*, or other such connotations.[8] Taking such established understandings further, it argues that by

[2] RICKMAN, *Styles of English Architecture*.

[3] H. GITTOS, *Liturgy, Architecture, and Sacred Places in Anglo-Saxon England* (Oxford, 2013).

[4] MCCLENDON, *Origins*. For an analogous approach to medieval architecture that is challenging and holistic in its treatment of the subject, although addressing a slightly later period, see E.C. FERNIE, *Romanesque Architecture* (New Haven, CT, 2014).

[5] See Bede, *Historia Ecclesiastica gentis Anglorum* (hereafter *HE*), I, 22-27, ed. B. COLGRAVE and R.A.B. MYNORS, *Bede, Ecclesiastical History of the English People* (Oxford, 1969), pp. 68-79.

[6] J. HAWKES, "*Iuxta morem Romanorum:* Stone and sculpture in Anglo-Saxon England", in: *Anglo-Saxon Styles*, ed. C. KARKOV and G. HARDIN BROWN (Albany, 2003), pp. 66-99.

[7] For further discussion see M. BOULTON, *The Conceptualisation of Sacred Space in Anglo-Saxon Northumbria in the Sixth to Ninth Centuries*, 2 vols. (unpublished doctoral thesis, University of York, 2013).

[8] For selected readings on phenomenology see E. HUSSERL, *Logical Investigations*, trans.

employing phenomenological and performative methods of 'looking' we may, as modern viewers, gain further appreciation of their potential sophistries as architectural structures and representations, which may seem alien when perceived by our (largely secular) modern gaze. Both phenomenology and performativity are established methods of viewing within wider art historical discourse, which engage with and act on the body and psychology of the viewer by placing them, as body, in direct relationship with the work in question, which, from a phenomenological perspective, also performs as body. In the discussion of methodologies of viewing presented here, it is suggested that a quasi-phenomenological encounter with medieval imagery – whereby the image is allowed to 'speak' to its viewer / reader on a fundamental level, outside the constraints of period, chronology or animation – should be set alongside the period-specific exegetical understanding of the image (understood to be common to the medieval milieu). It is suggested that the acknowledgement of such trans-historical epistemological awarenesses when embedded in deliberate, anachronic modes of viewing (whereby objects – and the scholarly methods used to interrogate them – are understood to perform across and outside expectations and methodologies dictated by time and period),[9] might further the discussion of the medieval from the vantage of the modern. In employing such a methodology this discussion seeks to question what we know, how we know, and the experience of knowing as we look at medieval material as modern scholars. In so doing it is to be hoped that the resulting relational impressions of image, object, and viewer may go beyond the architectural classifications and spatial discussions that have been confined to the surface of the images, objects, and structures that have formed the backbone of scholarship thus far.[10]

J.N. Findlay and K. Paul, 2 vols. (London, 1970); F. Brentano, *Psychology from an Empirical Standpoint*, trans. A.C. Rancurello, D.B. Terrell and L.L. McAlister (London and New York, 1995); M. Heidegger, *The Basic Problems of Phenomenology*, trans. A. Hofstadter (Bloomington, IN, 1982); D. Moran, *Introduction to Phenomenology* (Abingdon, 2000); M. Merleau-Ponty, *Phenomenology of Perception*, trans. D.A. Landes (London and New York, 2012); D. Zahavi, *The Oxford Handbook of Contemporary Phenomenology* (Oxford and New York, 2012) and D.W. Smith, *Husserl* (London and New York, 2013). See also S. Ahmed, *Queer Phenomenology: Orientations, Objects, Others* (Durham, NC, 2006). For ideas of phenomenology relating to the arts see *Art and Phenomenology*, ed. J.D. Parry (Abingdon, 2011).

[9] For reading around anachronic viewing see G. Didi-Huberman, "Before the image, before time: The sovereignty of anachronism", in: *Compelling Visuality: the Work of Art in and out of History*, ed. C. Farago and R. Zwijnenberg (Minneapolis, MN, 2003), pp. 31-44; A. Nagel and C.S. Wood, *Anachronic Renaissance* (New York, 2010); and A. Nagel, *Medieval Modern Art Out of Time* (London, 2012).

[10] For discussion of various types of 'viewing' in relation to art see J. Berger, *Ways of*

As stated, the historiographic and iconographic scholarship on the places, structures and objects of Anglo-Saxon England is well established, and the view of medieval art (and architecture) as 'barbaric' or the work of 'blind copyists' espoused by some early scholars is (thankfully) a thing of the past.[11] Despite this, the perceived gap between medieval and modern ways of understanding, articulating and viewing medieval images, objects, and structures is consistently highlighted within the scholarship, particularly in terms of differing perceptions of space, plane and surface,[12] while the fragmented architectural spaces that remain give little immediate impression of the grandeur and intellectual sophistication of the original building schemes. This spatial dislocation – seen consistently across discussion of medieval image and surface – does not arise solely from perceived fragmentation, resulting from anachronistic viewing of unfamiliar objects, but also from the scholarly precept of a fundamental difference in the way space is conceived across centuries. Contemporary art historians tend to perpetuate this difference somewhat, frequently relying on vocabularies of depth, perspective, quantifiable and (moreover) *complete* space to draw conclusions about the studied object; judging pre-Renaissance space and surface by standards developed to discuss Renaissance and post-Renaissance imagery, as we look back to the flat, seemingly surface-bound images and fragmented structures of medieval art and architecture. In other words, medieval images and structures are defined in terms of what they are *not* as much as what they *are* – judged against later standard forms and discussed in anachronistic terms. The formalised consideration of space and

Seeing (London, 1972); *Reading Medieval Images: The Art Historian and the Object*, ed. E. SEARS and T.K. THOMAS (Ann Arbor, MI, 2002); *The Four Modes of Seeing: Approaches to Medieval Imagery in Honor of Madeline Harrison Caviness*, ed. E. STAUDINGER LANE *et al.* (Aldershot, 2009).

[11] See CLAPHAM, *English Romanesque Architecture*; T.D. KENDRICK, *Anglo-Saxon Art to A.D. 900* (London, 1938); F. SAXL and R. WITTKOWER, *British Art and the Mediterranean* (Oxford, 1948) for numerous references to so-called 'barbarous' art in Britain.

[12] For discussion of this see BOULTON, "The conceptualisation of sacred space"; M. BOULTON, "'The end of the world as we know it': The eschatology of symbolic space/s in insular art", in: *Making Histories: Proceedings from the Sixth International Insular Arts Conference*, ed. J. HAWKES (Donnington, 2013), pp. 279-290. For other art historical engagements with space, historic images and ways of viewing, see E. PANOFSKY, *Perspective as Symbolic Form* (New York, 1927); BERGER, *Ways of Seeing*; M. BAXANDALL, *Painting and Experience in Fifteenth-Century Italy: A Primer in the Social History of Pictorial Style* (Oxford, 1988); DIDI-HUBERMAN, "Before the image, before time", pp. 31-44; D. SUMMERS, *Real Spaces: World Art History and the Rise of Western Modernism* (London and New York, 2003).

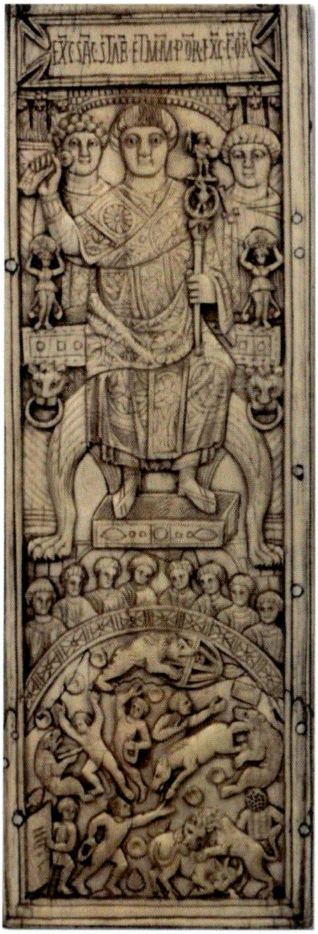

Fig. 12.1 Consular Diptych of Areobindus. Paris, Musée de Cluny – Musée du Moyen Âge, inv. no. Cl. 13135.

surface has been a prevalent facet of art historical research; ushered into the canon of visual analysis with the advent of perspective and the consistent centrality of the classicising gaze, which has resulted in the concomitant, pervasive and erroneous tendency to confuse a proficient use of perspective with a sophisticated understanding of space. This has, in turn, restricted the attention paid to the complex relationalities of space and surface, viewer and viewed object within this period, which has only recently begun to be readdressed.[13]

Underlying this pervasive model is the presupposition that, because the Anglo-Saxon method of depicting space and adorning surfaces is planar rather than perspectival, seemingly confined to two dimensions on the surface of the image / object, the method of conceptualising space is also two-dimensional. This is clearly not the case in the late antique and early medieval periods, as examination of the spatial complexities of images such as that of the Consular Diptych of Areobindus (*c.* 506) (Fig. 12.1),[14] or the so-called

[13] Boulton, "The conceptualisation of sacred space", and Boulton, "'The end of the world'", pp. 279-290. For scholarship revisiting these ideas see J. O'Reilly, "Introduction", in: Bede, *De Templo*, trans. S. Connolly, *On the Temple* (Liverpool, 1995), pp xvii-lv; M. Carruthers, *The Book of Memory: A Study of Memory in Medieval Culture* (Cambridge and New York, 1990) and ead., *The Craft of Thought: Meditation, Rhetoric, and the Making of Images, 400-1200* (Cambridge, 1998); J. Hawkes, "Stones of the north: Sculpture in Northumbria in the 'Age of Bede'", in: *Newcastle and Northumberland, Roman and Medieval Architecture and Art*, ed. J. Ashbee and J. Luxford (Wakefield, 2013), pp. 34-53; and J. Hawkes, "A sculptural legacy: Stones of the north from the 'Age of Wilfrid'", in: *Wilfrid: Abbot, Bishop, Saint: Papers from the 1300th Anniversary Conference*, ed. N. Higham (Donnington, 2013), pp. 124-135.

[14] Consular Diptych of Areobindus, Musée National du Moyen Âge –Thermes et Hôtel de Cluny, Paris, *c.* 506 a.d., *Classement*: 13135. Ivory, 39 × 13 cm. For scholarly discussion see

Temptation page in the *Book of Kells* demonstrates (Fig. 12.2);[15] but it may require a greater flexibility on the part of modern viewers to fully recognise the complexities at play in this type of imagery.[16] With this in mind, a phenomenological approach may be of use when reconsidering our modern perceptions of these spaces and structures in order to shift our gaze (as modern viewers) away from a practice of looking that relies on a verbal, formally intellectual and intellectualising engagement with medieval images, objects and spaces – often derived from anachronistic art historical vocabularies – toward something more instinctive, existing between self and object, between consciousness and sensory experience which may be provided by a phenomenological method of viewing. Such a phenomenological encounter is produced here by an intentional, embodied experiential encounter with medieval surface/s and structures on the part of the modern viewer, in combination with the exegetical manner of reading and looking understood to exist among medieval ecclesiastical viewers and scholars, in order to encounter these images, spaces and surfaces both as they appear, and also as they may be actualised in the imagination, then and now. Thus the surface-spaces and structures discussed here are encountered somewhere between experience, (actualised) existence, and imagination – pulling them into sharper focus in the mind of the modern viewer, in a process of looking that entails (re-) making/s and (re-) newed meaning/s for viewer and viewed object alike.

Rom und die Barbaren: Europa zur Zeit der Völkerwanderung: 22. August bis 7. Dezember 2008 in der Kunst- und Ausstellungshalle der Bundesrepublik Deutschland, Bonn, ed. J. FRINGS, H. WILLINGHÖFER, and J. AILLAGON (Munich, 2008), p. 211, no.16, Pl. II; see also J. NATANSON, *Early Christian Ivories* (London, 1953).

[15] Book of Kells, MS Dublin, Trinity College Library, MS A. I. (58), f. 202v (*c.* 800). For discussion see B. MEEHAN, *The Book of Kells* (New York, 1995); ID., "Looking the devil in the eye: The figure of satan in the Book of Kells", in: *Making and Meaning in Insular Art: 5th International Conference on Insular Art, 25-28 August 2005*, ed. R. MOSS (Dublin, 2007), pp. 268-274, and ID., *The Book of Kells* (London, 2012); see also F. HENRY, *The Book of Kells* (New York, 1974); G. HENDERSON, *From Durrow to Kells: the Insular Gospel-books, 650-800* (London, 1987), pp. 168-174; C. FARR, *The Book of Kells: Its Function and Audience* (London, 1997); C. BOURKE, "The Book of Kells: New light on the Temptation scene", in: *From Ireland Coming: Irish Art from the Early Christian to the Late Gothic Period and its European Context*, ed. C. HOURIHANE (Princeton, NJ, 2001), pp. 49-60. For discussion of the Temptation miniature, see further J. O'REILLY, "Exegesis and the Book of Kells: The Lucan Genealogy", in *The Book of Kells: Proceedings of a Conference at Trinity College Dublin 6-9 September 1992*, ed. F. O'MAHONEY (Dublin, 1994), pp. 370-397; and H. PULLIAM, *Word and Image in the Book of Kells* (Dublin, 2006).

[16] For discussion of the manner in which these spaces may function 'dimensionally' in the mind of a viewer see BOULTON "'The End of the World'", pp. 279-290.

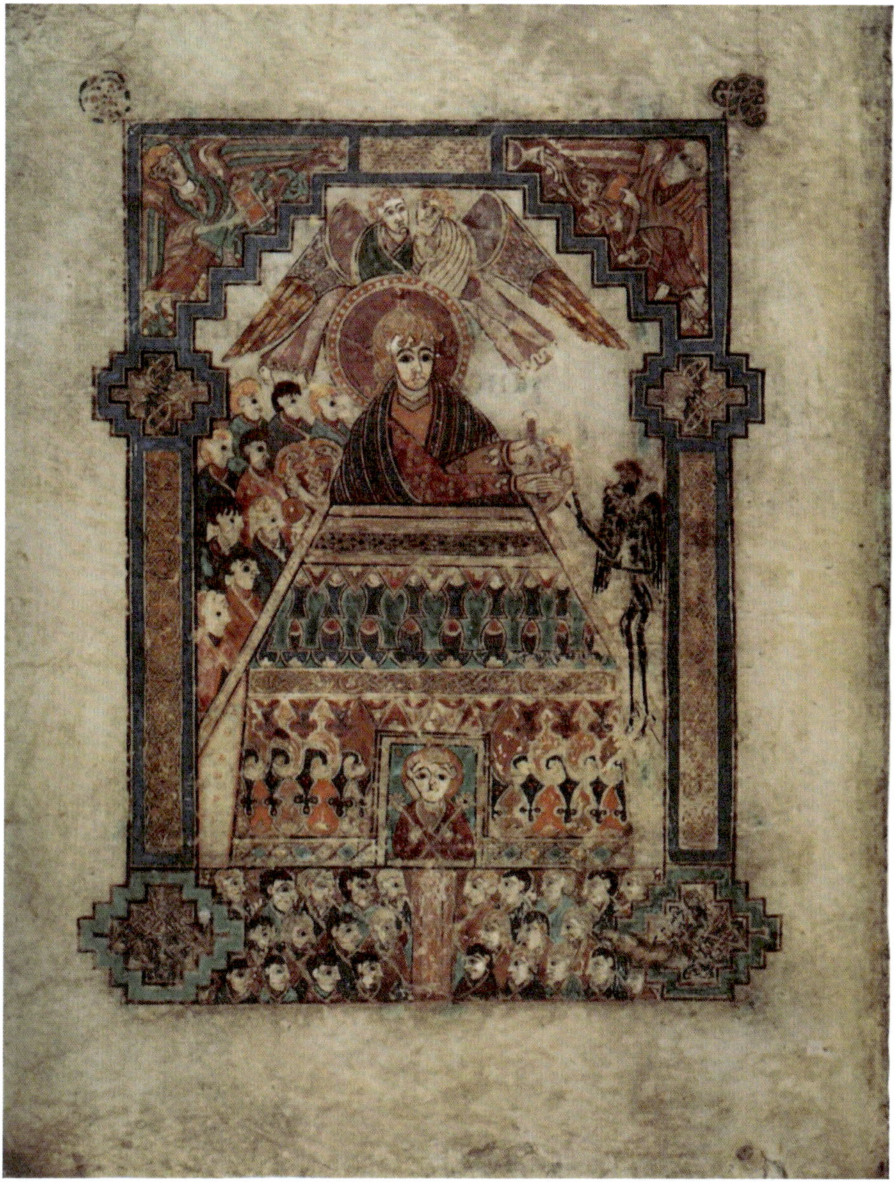

Fig. 12.2 Temptation page from the *Book of Kells*. MS Dublin, Trinity College, A.I.6, f. 202v. By permission of Dublin, The Board of Trinity College Dublin.

Two-dimensional depicted space as visualised by the modern is not necessarily the same as depicted space in the early medieval, either in the way it is constructed, or in the way it is understood. Yet, despite the differences in perceptions and understandings of space across periods, intellectual frameworks, and epistemological vocabularies, which *are* real, if not as all-important as they are sometimes perceived to be, by reconsidering our approach to these surfaces and structures as cognate, embodied viewers, they may be (re-) negotiated. Such a shift has the potential to bring the instinctive viewing practices of the modern closer to those of the medieval, facilitating a fuller exploration *of* the visual – and thus of the conceptual potential exhibited by such pre-perspectival imager and monumental structures as those produced in Anglo-Saxon England.

In terms of appropriating a 'phenomenological' methodology, I am largely drawing on Sara Ahmed's seminal work *Queer Phenomenology: Orientations, Objects, Others*,[17] which presents a way of thinking, looking and experiencing that has extremely useful things to offer in terms of locating ourselves as modern viewers looking at the Anglo-Saxon (although this is far from the subject of her work), but that may nonetheless usefully frame an examination of the types of sensory perceptions such encounters may produce. Ahmed begins her discussion by asking "what it means to be oriented?" going on to state:

> If we know where we are when we turn this way or that way, then we are orientated [...] To be orientated is also to be turned toward certain objects, those that help us to find our way. These are the objects we recognize, so that when we face them we know which way we are facing. They might be landmarks or other familiar signs that give us our anchoring points. They gather on the ground, and they create a ground upon which we can gather.[18]

This passage – although developed in a context that is entirely 'other' to that discussed here – nevertheless struck me as both interesting and useful when considered alongside the manner in which we, as modern viewers, locate ourselves in relation to the medieval. This siting of self and object described by Ahmed is a locative act that is integral to our/a/ny encounter with art, medieval or otherwise – in that we, as viewer and as body, make a constantly modified series of deliberate and shifting choices, associations and assumptions in viewing art, relating to surface, structure, space, and body/ies; enacting a fluid series of interrelations between us and the object. These interrelations surround-

[17] AHMED, *Queer Phenomenology,* p. 1.
[18] AHMED, *Queer Phenomenology*, p. 1.

ing viewing practice – of body, object / image and space / place – are complex and particularising, involving serried and nuanced negotiations between where we are, where it is, what we want, what it wants etc.[19] Moreover, particularly when engaging with objects from past periods, all of these nuanced and unfolding reactions between viewer and art, body and thing, must also be considered in terms of how we perceive the lasting spaces and structures produced across disparate times and socio-cultural norms, in wildly different contexts to our own. Given the perceived dislocation between the medieval and the modern perceptions of space and surface outlined above, encountering the Anglo-Saxon often results in modern perception/s being continually disrupted and disorientated by the less familiar practice of viewing required by medieval material. Here, like Ahmed, we may be said to be involved with a queer(ed) phenomenology of viewing.

As she states of her own project, "[p]henomomeology can offer a resource insofar as it emphasises the importance of lived experience, the intentionality of consciousness".[20] An analogous intentionality may be understood to surround art historians engaging with the medieval,[21] as we must consciously engage as a fragmented body (dislocated or disorientated from traditional methodologies of looking), with fragmented things encountered outside their original (lived) contexts in order to encounter / perceive the medieval.

I have argued elsewhere for the importance of a performative gaze when viewing the medieval.[22] To this, I would add the importance of recognising the specificity of the embodied gaze and the necessity of recognising ourselves as embodied viewers, grounded in the modern, looking at the medieval, alongside the resultant sensory perceptions that arise as we reorient ourselves in an aesthetic sensibility which is 'other'. This emphasis on the importance of 'vision' and viewing, here understood to be acts that are both conscious and embodied for the modern viewer, yet simultaneously understood as appropriate terms for

[19] W.J.T. MITCHELL, *What Do Pictures Want? The Lives and Loves of Images* (Chicago, 2005), esp. pp. 5-56.

[20] AHMED, *Queer Phenomenology*, p. 2.

[21] As indeed is the case when engaging with art more widely, but this is arguably heightened when encountering artworks that disrupt the assumed chronology of pictorial space and defy expectations of planar behaviour of surface and actuality, as do medieval images and objects.

[22] BOULTON, "'The end of the world'", pp. 279-290. For a brief introductory to the performative see J.L. AUSTIN, *How to Do Things with Words* (Oxford, 1962); J. BUTLER, *Gender Trouble: Feminism and the Subversion of Identity* (New York, 1990); and A. PARKER and E. KOSOFSKY SEDGWICK, 'Introduction', in: *Performativity and Performance*, ed. A. PARKER and E. KOSOFSKY SEDGEWICK (London and New York, 1995), pp. 1-19.

the manner in which viewers in the medieval world engaged with images / objects, has been recently addressed by Heather Pulliam in her work on the Lindisfarne Gospels.[23] Drawing on Isidore of Seville's statement that

> [e]yes are called *oculi* [...] because they have a hidden, *occultus*, light, that is one placed secretly or within. These, among all the senses, are very close to the soul [*animae*]. In the eyes is every disclosure of the mind [*mentis*]...,[24]

Pulliam states that:

> the mind focuses and wills rays of light from the eyes to the object, touching the object and bringing some aspect of it – its form or image – back into the viewer's body. In so doing, the viewer takes on some characteristics of what s/he has seen, and the object is imprinted onto the viewer.[25]

While not *entirely* analogous with a performative practice of viewing (relying on the transformative properties of light to affect a relationship between viewer and viewed object, rather than an intentional embodied cognisance as would be sought in a phenomenological encounter with an image or the actualised understandings called into being by a performative relationship with art), these statements are, nevertheless, indicative that there was, and *is*, a theorised manner of viewing in and of the medieval which remains to be fully recognised in the scholarship to date. Viewing, as discussed by Isidore, was an act which engaged and *altered* the body, as is recognised by Pulliam in her discussion of the

[23] Lindisfarne Gospels, MS London, British Library, Cotton Nero D. IV. For selected reading around this MS see J. BACKHOUSE, *The Lindisfarne Gospels* (London, 1981); R. GAMESON, "Why did Eadfrith write the Lindisfarne Gospels?", in: *Belief and Culture in the Middle Ages: Studies Presented to Henry Mayr-Harting*, ed. R. GAMESON and H. LEYSER (Oxford, 2001), pp. 45-58; M. BROWN, *The Lindisfarne Gospels: Society, Spirituality and the Scribe* (London, 2003); and H. PULLIAM, "Eyes of light: Colour in the Lindisfarne Gospels", in: *Newcastle and Northumberland*, pp. 54-72.

[24] *The Complete English Translation of Isidori Hispalensis Episcopi Etymologiarum sive Originum Libri XX*, trans. P. THROOP, 2 vols. (Charlotte, VT, 2005), 2. Isidore of Seville, *Etymologies*, XI.I.36, ed. W.M. LINDSAY, *Isidori Hispalensis episcopi Etymologiarum sive Originum libri XX*, 2 vols. (Oxford, 1911), 2 [without pagination]: "*Oculi vocati [...] quia occultum lumen habent, id est secretum, vel intus positum. Hi inter omnes sensus viciniores animae existunt. In oculis enim omne mentis indicium est, unde et animi perturbatio vel hilaritas in oculis apparet. Oculi autem idem et lumina. Et dicta lumina, quod ex eis lumen manat, vel quod ex initio sui clausam teneant lucem, aut extrinsecus acceptam visui proponendo refundant*" (cited after *PL* in PULLIAM, "Eyes of light", pp. 60-62, n. 31).

[25] PULLIAM, "Eyes of light", pp. 60-62.

symbolic significance of colour in the Gospels. The act of viewing in the medieval period is thus understood to be a transformative process that involved an exchange between eyes, mind and soul – a complex exchange between object and viewer often involving embedded cultural associations such as the link between stone and Rome in Anglo-Saxon England. While our modern 'looking' may not involve a spiritual transformation *per se*, it nonetheless requires a transformative engagement, as we must consciously alter our prescriptive expectations of what planar space can or cannot do, and in so doing perceive a fuller range of sensory encounters and exchange generated by medieval images as we view them today, which may be in and of themselves transformative.

Throughout the early Church in the Christian West there was a clear understanding that the decorated, highly ornate spaces of churches were deeply symbolic, both in terms of their architectonic symbolism and the intricate iconographies of the decorative programmes frequently preserved within their interiors – most typically existing in a symbolic symbiosis with the space of the heavenly Jerusalem, recalling and actualising the heavenly city for those on earth. This relationship has been consistently demonstrated textually, architecturally and visually throughout surviving source material in its various forms. Moving away from the images and objects produced in the Anglo-Saxon milieu to the wider symbolic spaces of the early Christian world, some of the most direct and complete examples of this type of symbolic architectural adornment are found in the monumental mosaic programmes of the churches of Rome and Ravenna, particularly in the jewelled borders which surround the wider iconographic programmes of these churches.[26] One clear example of the type of dualistic, performative viewing required by these borders may be found in the church of Sant'Apollinare in Classe outside Ravenna (consecrated in 549).[27] Here, as I have discussed elsewhere, the jewelled borders serve to split and

[26] For specific discussion of the role of these jewelled borders in the iconographic programmes of early Christian churches see M. BOULTON, "Bejewelling Jerusalem: Architectural adornment and symbolic significance in the early Church in the Christian West", in: *Islands in a Global Context: Proceedings from the Sixth International Insular Arts Conference*, ed. C. NEWMAN *et al.* (forthcoming 2016). For discussion of the symbolism of jewels and heaven in this period see D. JANES, *God and Gold in Late Antiquity* (Cambridge, 1998), pp. 80-96, 105, 128-129.

[27] See e.g. R. LANE FOX, "Art and the beholder: The apse mosaic of S. Apollinare in Classe", *Byzantinische Forschungen* 21 (1995), pp. 247-251.

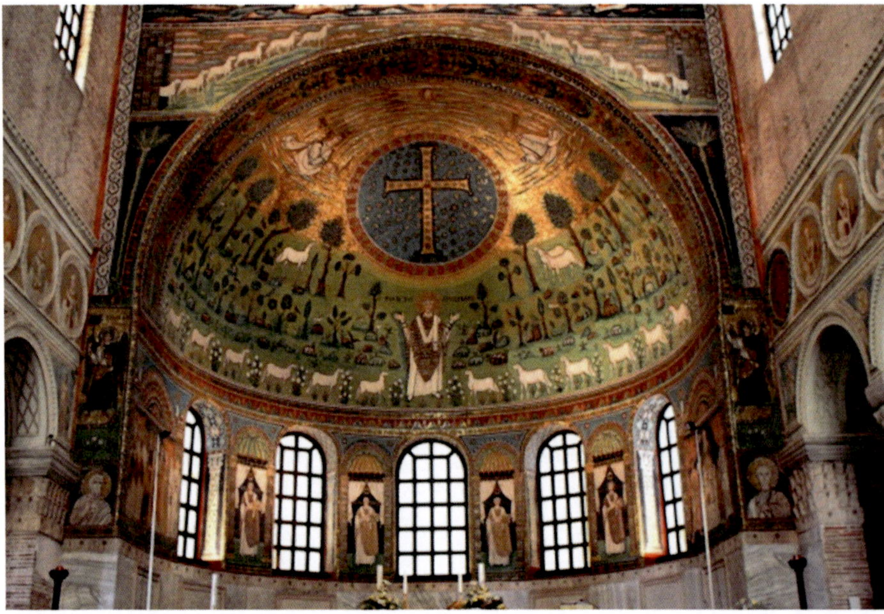

Fig. 12.3 Apse mosaic of Sant'Apollinare in Classe. Photo Meg Boulton.

emphasise the architectural features of the church, wrapping around the physical building, transforming the earthly into the heavenly.[28]

This shifting actualisation of space, surface and structure is articulated in several ways within the overall iconography of the mosaic programme at Classe, which presents a unique take on the iconography of the Transfiguration,[29] wherein the local sacred figure of St Apollinaris (the first bishop of Ravenna and Classe) is presented as a centralised witness to the Transfiguration scene displayed in the apse mosaic. Above the bishop, a large circular bejewelled form encloses a starry sky, with a great jewelled cross set against this cosmological background. The face of Christ (the subject of the transfiguration narrative as it is given in Scripture) is set in the centre of the *Crux gemmata*, while, flanking the gigantic central disc are the figures of Elijah and Moses. Below, in a verdant, paradisial landscape (which is echoic of the local landscape) teeming with flora and fauna, are three lambs symbolising the apostles

[28] BOULTON, "Bejewelling Jerusalem".

[29] Compared to the more traditional representation of the iconography of the Transfiguration seen in the apse mosaic of St Catherine's Monastery, Sinai, *c.* 565-566, which preserves the earliest extant version of the Eastern iconography of the scene.

Peter, James and John (here seen in sheep form); the whole forming an iconographic allusion to the narrative of the Transfiguration of Jesus on Mount Tabor,[30] but portrayed in a very local and distinct decorative vocabulary within the basilica at Classe. The subtleties of the spatial relationships presented within this iconography are manifold, not least that which arguably transforms the floating cosmological roundel occupying the space of the apse into an apparently unique *oculus* 'created' by the decorative programme, as first recognised by Rebecca Sanchez in unpublished work (Fig. 12.3).[31] This transformation, carried out in part through exegetical significance and the illusory cohesion of architectural and decorative forms, is heavily reliant on the use of the jewelled borders within the mosaic. These borders, all too often overlooked within the dynamic iconographies of the wider programme, are far from being a passive or decorative element of the overall design. Rather, if they are considered exegetically and iconographically in light of the text of Revelation 21:19-21 – which describes the walls of heaven as "adorned with all manner of precious stones" – the borders which outline the architectural features of the building can be considered as literally bejewelling the walls of the church. Thus the motif may be understood to actively transform the earthly architecture into its heavenly counterpart – turning the apse into the gate of heaven itself, through a performative process of conscious looking, symbolic surface, exegetical interpretation and actualised space. This process transforms space and structure, viewer and viewed object, calling forth actualised spaces in the mind's eye that go far beyond the limits of surface and representation. The event of the Transfiguration is understood to be a pivotal moment in the Christological narrative through the recognition of Christ's divine nature, and the geographical setting of the event (which takes place on a mountain) is similarly presented as a liminal point where human nature met the divine and where the temporal met the eternal, bridging heaven and earth through the recognition of

[30] Matthew 17:1-9, Mark 9:2-8, Luke 9:28-36.

[31] I am grateful to Rebecca Sanchez for allowing me to build on the idea of the red jewelled circle surrounding the jewelled cross of the Transfiguration being 'read' as a functioning *oculus* within the apse of the church, thus providing a more direct 'view' of the heavenly produced through the earthly architecture and its attendant decorative scheme. Unpublished research.

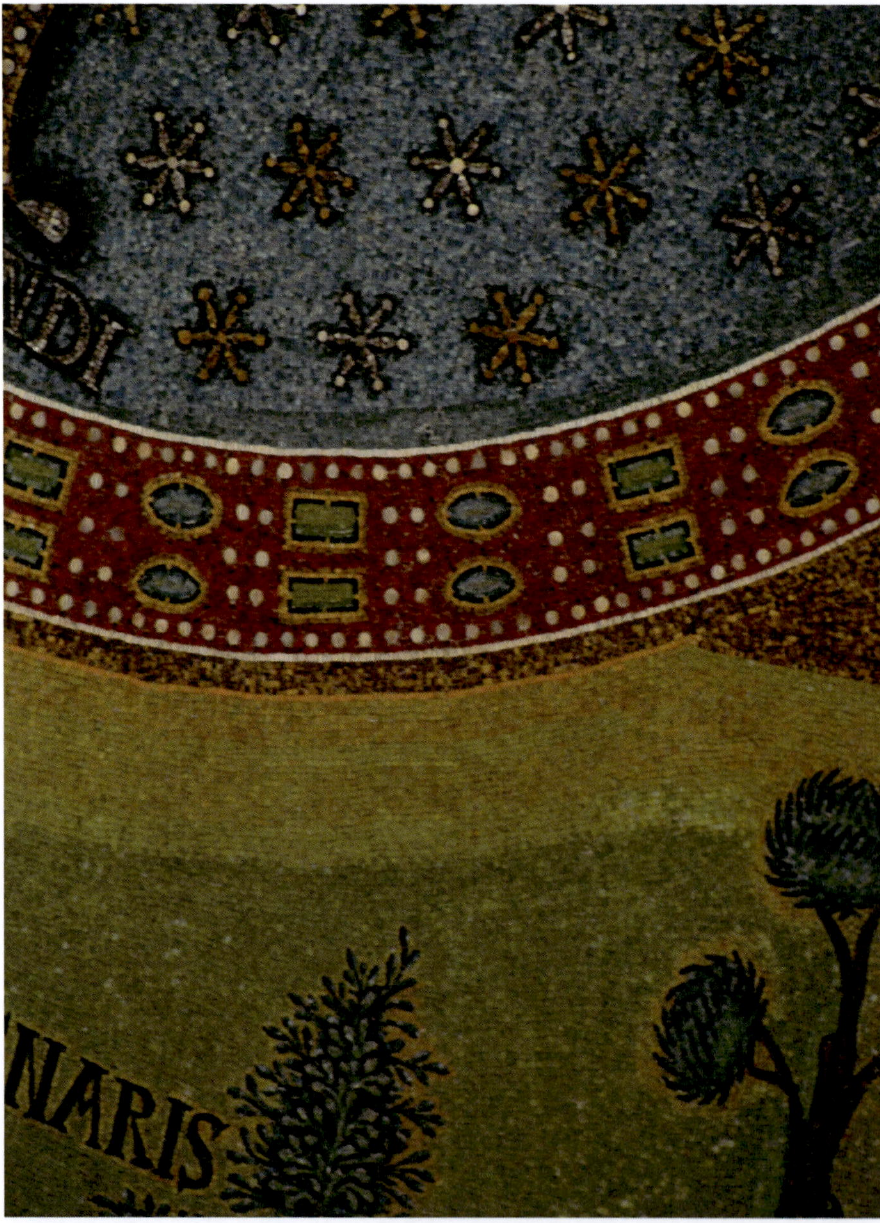

Fig. 12.4 Detail of jewelled border in Sant'Apollinare in Classe. Photo Meg Boulton.

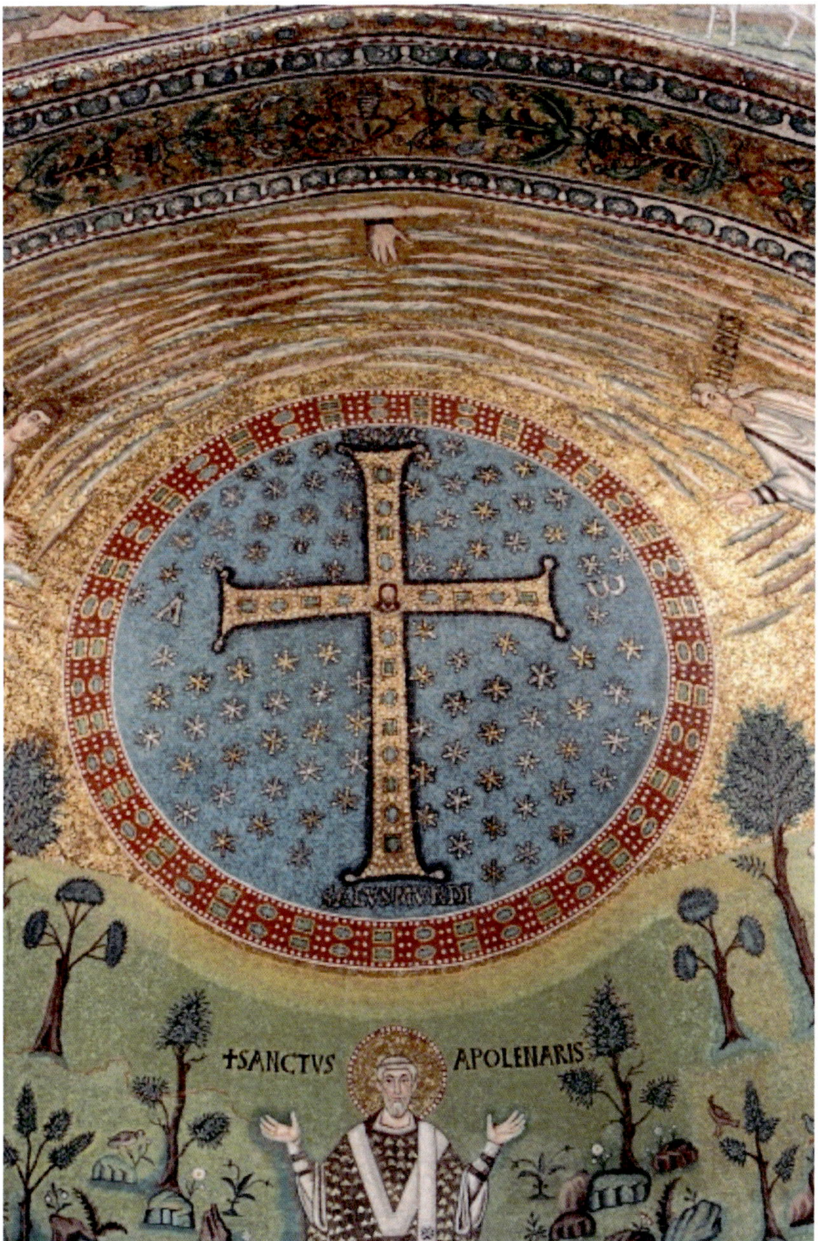

Fig. 12.5 Detail of central roundel in Sant'Apollinare in Classe. Photo Meg Boulton.

the divine body of Christ.[32] In the iconography of the Classe apse mosaic, the ecclesiastical architecture, and the jewelled borders in particular, could be said to enact a similar type of liminal performative transformation for the viewer, transforming the earthly architecture into the timeless expanse of the heavens far beyond the confines of the built structure of the church.

Turning to analogous examples of performative viewing in Anglo-Saxon England, it must be stated from the outset that the jewelled borders which perform such a pivotal function in creating spatial significance and symbolism within the Continental churches do not translate directly into Anglo-Saxon England, in that there is no material evidence for the use of mosaics within Anglo-Saxon ecclesiastical architecture. However, what survives in the contemporary textual accounts and the material record presents strong evidence for an interest *in*, and a marked preference *for*, jewel-toned chromatic adornment, and the practice of decorating the structures and objects of the church with precious stones and shining metal, as well as for a sophisticated interrelation of surface, object and subject which may powerfully act on our contemporary gazes.[33]

Arguably, these 'heavenly materials' were understood to equate heavenly space with earthly place via an association of preciousness in a similar manner to that described for the mosaics of Classe, which present a spatial model symptomatic of that which may be seen across the iconographic programmes of the early Christian churches of the Continent. Consequently, these precious materials can be regarded as denoting the spiritual value of heaven within the medieval Anglo-Saxon Christian community, and as doing so publicly through display and ornamentation. Given the apparently frequent use of gems in the adornment of churches, this public display also served to reinforce the inherent value of the materials as forming an abbreviated iconography of the heavenly Jerusalem.

Additionally, the performative gaze may act on other surfaces and substances of the Anglo-Saxon world, both in terms of their original viewers and

[32] D. LEE, *Transfiguration* (London and New York, 2005). For further discussion of mountains as significant places see also the forthcoming volume based on the conference and exhibition, 'Moving Mountains: Studies in Place, Society and Cultural Representations' held at the University of Edinburgh in June 2014, edited by Emily Goetsch.

[33] The Anglo-Saxon attitude to colour, and more importantly to shining or brightness, as understood in relation to their Latin counterparts is thoroughly discussed by Carin Ruff. See C. RUFF, "Aldhelm's jewel tones: Latin colors through Anglo-Saxon eyes", in: *Anglo-Saxon Styles*, ed. C.E. KARKOV and G. HARDIN BROWN (New York, 2003), pp. 223-238.

in terms of their perception today. Nick Baker, for instance, has discussed contemplation and compunction in relation to insular imagery in a manuscript context, whereby, through an emotive, immersive encounter (alongside a contemplative manner of viewing), viewers may transcend planar space, going beyond the surface of the page in the mind.[34] Similarly, Jane Hawkes, employing the methodologies of performative viewing and engaged planar space, has recently discussed polychrome, mixed-media Anglo-Saxon stone sculpture (often inset with metal and paste glass), as being icons in stone.[35] Such examples of seventh- and eighth-century relief sculptures offer transgressive compositions which break the bounds of their stone surrounds, playing with frame, surface and scene (as discussed in terms of the jewelled decorative borders of the Continental churches), via a systemic "deliberate visual manipulation" as described by Hawkes.[36] The monumental stone sculptures of Anglo-Saxon England frequently show figures breaking the frames of their carved panels, crossing their carved stone surrounds, such as Christ's deeply carved halo on the cross head on the monument at Rothbury and Christ's similar halo in the *majestas* panel on Ruthwell. Both employ the device of high relief carving which quite literally breaks its sculpted frame, protruding from the surface of the cross, into the space of the viewer.[37] These instances of spatial transgression produce a visceral dislocation of surface and subject, producing a tangible 'beginning' for an active process of viewing which goes beyond the frame and the perceived limits of this largely aulic art, which relies on hierarchical scale and symbolic forms to produce meaning, depending on placement and arrangement rather than spatial manipulation to produce visual meaning.[38] These points of contact, which emerge into the space of the viewer, allow for an active cognitive repositioning of surface and subject, producing a multivalent

[34] N.G. BAKER, *The Evangelists in Insular culture, c. 600-c. 800 AD* (unpublished doctoral thesis, 2 vols., University of York, 2011); ID., "Engaging with the Divine: The evangelists as tools for contemplation", in: *Making Histories: Proceedings from the Sixth International Insular Arts Conference*, ed. J. HAWKES (Donnington, 2013), pp. 229-242; ID., "Crying over the evangelists: Compunction in the insular world", in: *The Art, Literature and Material Culture of the Middle Ages: Transition, Transformation and Taxonomy*, ed. M. BOULTON and J. HAWKES with M. HERMAN (Dublin, 2015), pp. 264-277.

[35] HAWKES, "Stones of the north", pp. 34-53, and EAD., "A sculptural legacy", pp. 124-135.

[36] HAWKES, "Stones of the north", p. 45.

[37] HAWKES, "Stones of the north", pp. 34-53, and EAD., "A sculptural legacy", pp. 124-135. See also R.N. BAILEY, *England's Earliest Sculptors* (Toronto, 1996) and *Theorizing Anglo-Saxon Stone Sculpture*, ed. C.E. KARKOV and F. ORTON (Morgantown, WV, 2003).

[38] BOULTON, "'The end of the world'", pp. 279-290. See also HAWKES, "Stones of the north", pp. 34-53.

viewing encounter that transcends space and plane between viewer and viewed object, and encouraging those looking at such surfaces to look beyond the fame, to look through it, to experience spaces that recede from the frame or penetrate out from it. In her discussion of such stone panels being in fact icons, Hawkes, citing Hans Belting, states that:

> "the act of viewing the image / icon allows the viewer to recall to memory the person or event depicted, and so to recall the Divine in His heavenly glory". Put another way, the icon [here understood to include stone sculpted panels] functioned as a portal through which the human viewer could gain proper understanding of the Divine through contemplation and remembrance.[39]

This statement, combining Belting's discussion of icons with Hawkes' reading of Anglo-Stone sculpture, is a perceptive acknowledgment of the sensory complexity of a medieval viewing encounter – that is to say, of a type of visual engagement that is bound up with perceiving the past and the future, while being immersed in the present.

While the discussion here has presented selected visual examples from Continental and Anglo-Saxon contexts that introduce the ways in which these images may be affected by the type of phenomenological, performative viewing encounter suggested throughout, there is no room to deal fully with analogous architectural examples that are found across Anglo-Saxon England. However, in closing, I would like to mention some examples which may (when viewed in conjunction with the decorative programmes and the liturgical smells and bells they housed) also act as transformative points of sensory encounter with the sacred for their viewer, despite the mostly fragmentary state in which they remain to be encountered by the modern viewer. Notably, some of the best preserved examples of such transformative surfaces occur on entrances or threshold spaces, that themselves produce potent liminal associations of crossing between one place and another, moving between the secular and the sacred. Such threshold spaces include the figural sculpture over the entrances of St Peter's Church at Wearmouth,[40] and St Mary's Church at Deerhurst,[41] both of

[39] HAWKES, "Stones of the north", pp. 47-48 and nn. 62 and 63. See also H. BELTING, *Likeness and Presence: A History of the Image before the Era of Art* (Chicago, 1994), pp. 10-11.

[40] TAYLOR and TAYLOR, *Anglo-Saxon Architecture*, pp. 338-349 and 432-446 for Jarrow and Wearmouth respectively; R. CRAMP, *Wearmouth and Jarrow: Monastic Sites*, 2 vols. (London, 2005-2006); and MCCLENDON, *Origins of Medieval Architecture*, pp. 59-84.

[41] TAYLOR and TAYLOR, *Architecture*, pp. 193-211.

which also present instances of animal head terminals and interlaced zoomorphs at their thresholds.[42] Other examples may include the reused spoliated sculpture and dedicatory plaque placed onto the facade of the church at Kirkdale;[43] the architectonic detailing of the walls of St Laurence's at Bradford-on-Avon;[44] the shifting shape of the lintel into the central chamber of Wilfrid's crypt at Ripon and the layout of the crypt at Hexham;[45] and the spoliated chancel arch at Escomb,[46] all of which would be appropriate candidates for this type of visual engagement / analysis.[47] Indeed, this list might usefully be expanded to include the apsidal columnar divisions and the various *porticus* spaces seen across Anglo-Saxon ecclesiastical architecture, which, like their more decorative sculptural and architectural counterparts listed above, powerfully engage with space, symbolism and institutional identity.

To conclude, I would like to turn to the words of the phenomenologist Merleau-Ponty, who stated that "[p]ainting does not imitate the world, but it is a world of its own".[48] If, in this case, we swap that most modern of art historical preoccupations, painting, for the visual lexicon of the Anglo-Saxon world, and step back to take another look at these now familiar surfaces and structures

[42] See R. GEM, E. HOWE and R. BRYANT, "The ninth-century polychrome decoration at St Mary's Church, Deerhurst, Gloucestershire", *The Antiquaries Journal* 88 (2008), pp. 109-164 and E. HOWE, *Painted Anglo-Saxon Sculpture in St Mary's, Deerhurst: Materials, Technique and Context* ([Deerhurst], 2011: *Deerhurst Lecture* 2010).

[43] TAYLOR and TAYLOR, *Architecture*, pp. 358-359; C.L.R. TUDOR, *A Brief Account of Kirkdale Church: With Plans, Elevations, Sections, Details, and Perspective Views* (London, 1876). See also M. BOULTON, "Embroidered stones: Considering the symbolism of Anglo-Saxon skeuomorphs and the Kirkdale grave-slab", in: *Art, Literature and Material Culture*, pp. 198-216.

[44] TAYLOR and TAYLOR, *Architecture*, pp. 86-89.

[45] TAYLOR and TAYLOR, *Architecture*, pp. 297-312 and 516-18 for Hexham and Ripon respectively. See also R.N. BAILEY, "St Wilfrid, Ripon and Hexham", in: *Studies in Insular Art and Archaeology*, ed. C. KARKOV and R. FARRELL (Oxford, OH, 1991: *American Early Medieval Studies* 1), pp. 3-24; ,ID., *St Wilfrid's Crypts at Ripon and Hexham: A Visitor's Guide* (Newcastle upon Tyne, 1993); ID., "Seventh-century work at Ripon and Hexham", in: *The Archaeology of Cathedrals*, ed. T. TATTON-BROWN and J. MUNBY (Oxford, 1996), pp. 9-18. For further reading around these spaces see *Wilfrid: Abbot, Bishop, Saint*, particularly HAWKES, "Stones of the north", pp. 124-135; E. CAMBRIDGE, "The sources and function of Wilfrid's Architecture at Ripon and Hexham", pp. 136-151; and P. BIDWELL, "Wilfrid and Hexham: The Anglo-Saxon crypt", pp. 152-162.

[46] TAYLOR and TAYLOR, *Architecture*, pp. 234-238.

[47] See, for example, TAYLOR and TAYLOR, *Architecture*, pp. 134-143; É. Ó CARRAGÁIN, "The term *porticus* and *imitatio Romae* in early Anglo-Saxon England", in: *Text and Gloss: Studies in Insular Learning and Literature Presented to Joseph Donovan Pheifer*, ed. H.C. O'BRIAIN *et al.* (Dublin, 1999), pp. 13-34, and HAWKES, "*Iuxta morem Romanorum*", pp. 66-99.

[48] M. MERLEAU-PONTY, *The World of Perception* (Abingdon, 2004), p. 96.

and their common perceptions, becoming better aware of how they may have been perceived in the medieval period and of the sensory perceptions they produce today, we may see not just a world, as suggested by Merleau-Ponty, but a world beyond the world, as frequently evoked by the art of the medieval.

Plant Life in the *Poetic Edda*

MICHAEL D. J. BINTLEY

> What an old, old simile that is,
> between man and timber![1]

In recent years, scholarship in early medieval studies and other allied fields has increasingly addressed the representation of relationships between humans and non-humans. The latter category has included actors of various kinds, including those we would most often think of as active (mammals, reptiles, birds, fish, insects, and so on), and those which we would be less accustomed to attribute any independent life at all in the modern world, such as human-made or naturally occurring objects and phenomena. Plant life, which has also received some attention, sits somewhere between these broad categories. Plants can move and grow, on the one hand, but on the other they cannot see or hear or walk in the same way as animals – or at least, we are not accustomed to think of them as doing so in the modern developed West. Instead, plant life appears either as an element of landscape, or as a backdrop for the more important things that humans and animals do, or in commodified form at the base of an ecological pyramid. Notwithstanding, literatures both ancient

[1] W. THACKERAY, *Vanity Fair*, ed. J. SUTHERLAND (Oxford, 2008), p. 147.

Sensory Perception in the Medieval West, ed. Simon C. THOMSON and Michael D.J. BINTLEY, *Utrecht Studies in Medieval Literacy*, 34 (Turnhout: Brepols, 2016), pp. 227-243.

BREPOLS PUBLISHERS DOI 10.1484/M.USML-EB.5.109513

and modern indicate human knowledge and understanding of plants as beings comparable with humans, with a similar capacity to endure pain, suffering, and loss, in both metaphorical and literal terms. This chapter will offer a case study of the ways in which trees and other plants are represented in Old Norse eddic poetry.[2] It will examine their presentation as beings who possess sensory and emotional qualities, starting with a discussion of the hardships of the central pillar of Norse cosmology, Yggdrasill, before considering the ways in which the suffering of trees is used as a means of portraying the suffering of humans, and concluding with some reflections on what this evidence suggests about interactions between humans and plants in early medieval Scandinavia.

The relationship between humans and trees has been subject to relatively frequent discussion in Norse scholarship. The most recent synthesis is by Clive Tolley, who presents a comprehensive analysis of this material in *Shamanism in Norse Myth and Magic*.[3] Studies of this relationship with a literary focus have otherwise been limited, and relatively few attempts have been made to see what the relationship between humans and trees in Old Norse poetry may have to say about how trees were understood as beings in themselves.[4] A recent study by Christopher Abram considers the implications of the widespread deforestation of early medieval Iceland, in contrast with the view of the natural world which seems apparent in poems such as *Sonatorrek* (*c.* 960) and *Vǫluspá* (*c.* 1000).[5] The contrast between Iceland's human-made environmental disaster and the representation of trees in these poems is of special interest, as Abram notes, because "these Old Norse poems do, now and then, bespeak a conception of the fundamental interconnectedness of the various aspects of the world ... that is something like the essence of ecological thinking".[6]

[2] M.D.J. BINTLEY, *Trees in the Religions of Early Medieval England* (Woodbridge, 2015); ID., "*Brungen of Bearwe*: Ploughing common furrows in Riddle 21, *The Dream of the Rood*, and the *Æcerbot* charm", in: *Trees and Timber in the Anglo-Saxon World*, ed. M.D.J. BINTLEY and M.G. SHAPLAND (Oxford, 2013), pp. 144-157; and ID., "Recasting the role of sacred trees in Anglo-Saxon spiritual history: The South Sandbach Cross 'Ancestors of Christ' panel in its cultural contexts", in: *Trees and Timber*, pp. 211-227.

[3] C. TOLLEY, *Shamanism in Norse Myth and Magic*, 2 vols. (Helsinki, 2009: *Folklore Fellows Communications* 296-297), esp. pp. 304-368; a comparative study considering elements of similar traditions in early medieval England is offered in BINTLEY, *Trees*, pp. 129-152. This chapter serves as the basis for the present discussion.

[4] All Heideggerian allusions intended.

[5] C. ABRAM, "Felling trees and feeling trees in medieval Iceland", in: *Nordic Naturecultures*, ed. C.C. THOMSON and C. OSCARSON (forthcoming). I remain indebted to Chris for sharing this chapter with me before publication.

[6] ABRAM, "Felling trees", forthcoming.

My discussion of plant life in eddic poetry will begin with *Vǫluspá* and *Grímnismál*, both of which Abram addresses in his study, though I reach a rather different conclusion about the representation of Yggdrasill. For all that he takes the appearance of plant life in these texts (and *Sonatorrek*) to be "heartening and surprising" in certain respects, Abram concludes that he does "not see how the foregoing will help us in the ecological struggles that face us in the twenty-first century".[7] It would be bold to say otherwise. Nevertheless, following my analysis of the sensory and emotional lives of plant life as it appears in the *Poetic Edda*, I will end on a more optimistic note. Whilst the recognition of what we would now call ecological thought in Old Norse literature may not directly influence contemporary ecological policy, there is still some value in contributing to an intellectual climate change, and this we can do by representing some of the earliest flowerings of these Northern European naturecultures.[8]

The Norse 'world-tree of eddic mythology', Yggdrasill, requires little introduction even to those who know relatively little about Norse mythology.[9] The Scandinavian world tree is thought to have had parallels amongst various other 'Germanic' peoples in the North Sea zone, including potentially the early medieval English, but also has independent cognates elsewhere throughout the world.[10] The fullest description of the tree, as Abram notes, appears in stanza 19 of *Vǫluspá*, in which the seeress tells us that:[11]

Ask veit ek standa,
heitir Yggdrasill,
hár baðmr, ausinn
hvítaauri.
Þaðan koma dǫggvar
þærs í dala falla.
Stendr æ yfir, grœnn,

[7] ABRAM, "Felling trees", forthcoming.

[8] For further discussion of 'naturecultures' see D. HARAWAY, *The Companion Species Manifesto* (Chicago, IL, 2003).

[9] R. SIMEK, *Dictionary of Northern Mythology*, trans. A. HALL (Cambridge, 1993), pp. 375-376.

[10] TOLLEY, *Shamanism in Norse Myth and Magic*, 1, p. 304; C. TOLLEY, "What is a world tree?", in: *Trees and Timber in the Anglo-Saxon World*, pp. 177-185; see also C. CUSACK, *The Sacred Tree: Ancient and Medieval Manifestations* (Newcastle, 2010), pp. 1-25.

[11] ABRAM, "Felling trees", forthcoming.

Urðar brunni.[12]

> I know that an ash tree stands, called Yggdrasill – a high tree, drenched with shining loam. From it come the dews that fall in the dales. The ash stands, eternally green,[13] over Urðr's well.

There is little suggestion in this description of Yggdrasill that the tree is especially vulnerable. On the contrary, its appearance here is as the central pillar of the universe, as the "nourisher of the world",[14] and as the "*miǫtvið mæran*" ("mighty measuring tree", *Vǫluspá* 2) whose shape and form define the cosmos.[15] Despite this, the tree exists within time, like the Norse gods, and is ultimately subject to the same incendiary destruction at Ragnarǫk (st. 45):

Skelfr Yggdrasils
askr standandi,
ymr it aldna tré,
en iǫtunn losnar.

> Yggdrasill shudders, the ash as it stands, the old tree groans, and the giant gets loose.

Though the shuddering and groaning of the tree is not necessarily the same as human fear and trembling, and Yggdrasill is not fully anthropomorphised, the terms used here are common to human experience. In a similar fashion, the great tree who appears in the Anglo-Saxon *Dream of the Rood*, preserved in the Vercelli book (*c.* 975) not long before *Vǫluspá* was composed (though much older in its origins), tells us that it resisted the temptation to "*bugan oððe berstan*" ("bend or burst", l. 36) against the wishes of Christ at the crucifix-

[12] All references to *Vǫluspá* from *The Poetic Edda*, 2, *Mythological Poems*, ed. and trans. U. DRONKE (Oxford, 1997), pp. 7-24. My translation of the following stanza is also based on Dronke's. All translations are my own unless otherwise indicated.

[13] Tolley presents compelling evidence that the tree is ever-green, rather than an evergreen, resolving at least one issue that Abram treats as a consequence of an Icelandic poet's (assumed) ignorance of plant life outside of Iceland; see TOLLEY, *Shamanism*, 1, pp. 313, 328-332; ABRAM, "Felling trees", forthcoming.

[14] TOLLEY, *Shamanism*, 2, p. 94.

[15] On the significance of Yggdrasill as a seat of judgment, see BINTLEY, *Trees*, pp. 70-88; also TOLLEY, *Shamanism*, 1, pp. 336-338. Dronke suggested that the lines of Yggdrasill "suggest a cycle: the laving at the tree's base promotes its growth, so that from its great height it can in its turn enrich the earth"; see DRONKE, *Mythological Poems*, p. 127.

ion.[16] Whilst a tangible connection with the suffering of the humanised tree in the *Dream* is one of the poem's most prominent features,[17] and whilst we may well be familiar with bowing to authority, human experience of bursting apart is for the most part quite limited, reminding us that there are certain experiences that trees are more likely to undergo than humans. In this respect, the experience of Yggdrasill in *Vǫluspá* at Ragnarǫk is described in terms not far removed from human experience.

The suffering of Yggdrasill appears in yet more humanised terms, however, in *Grímnismál*, as Abram notes, drawing on the recent work of botanist Matthew Hall in *Plants as Persons*.[18] Hall's assessment of the place of plants in most world religions indicates that they occupy a subordinate position to humans and other animals.[19] In the contexts of Western European thought, Hall lays responsibility for this at the hands of classical and Judaeo-Christian philosophy, though in many respects the two belong to the same entangled bank.[20] Hall suggests that Northern European heathenism, and particularly that of the 'Germanic' kind, appears to have allotted a privileged position to plant life that is less common elsewhere. He offers the following stanza from *Grímnismál* (st. 35) to indicate knowledge and understanding of the sensory and emotional suffering of plant life.[21]

Ascr Yggdrasils
drýgir erfiði,
meira, enn menn viti;
hiǫrtr bítr ofan,
enn á hliðo fúnar,
scerðir Níðhǫggr neðan.[22]

The ash of Yggdrasill endures greater suffering than men know: a stag bites from above, and on the side it rots, and Níðhǫggr bites it from below.

[16] References to *The Dream of the Rood* from *The Dream of the Rood*, ed. M. SWANTON (Exeter, 1996), pp. 93-101.

[17] For a similar example from Old English Exeter Book Riddle 21 see discussion in BINTLEY, "*Brungen of Bearwe*".

[18] ABRAM, "Felling trees", forthcoming; M. HALL, *Plants as Persons: A Philosophical Botany* (Albany, NY, 2011).

[19] HALL, *Plants*, pp. 1-15.

[20] HALL, *Plants*, pp. 17-71.

[21] HALL, *Plants*, pp. 119-135 (esp. 126-128).

[22] References to *Grímnismál* from *Edda: Die Lieder des Codex Regius nebst verwandten Denkmälern*, ed. G. NECKEL, rev. H. KUHN, fifth edn. (Heidelberg, 1983), pp. 57-68.

Abram sees this stanza as imbuing Yggdrasill with "still greater subjectivity", but takes these lines to suggest "that men are incapable of true empathy with the suffering world-tree. They may feel kindred with Yggdrasill, but they cannot share in its experiences".[23] This is an entirely legitimate reading of these lines, but seems to treat this stanza from *Grímnismál* in isolation. In the preceding stanza (st. 34), we are told that:

Ormar fleiri
liggia undir aski Yggdrasils,
en þat uf hyggi
hverr ósviðra apa;

More serpents lie under the ash of Yggdrasill than any fool can know.

These lines do not suggest that humans are incapable of counting the serpents that lie beneath Yggdrasill, but that most are unaware of them. The same trope appears in *Hávamál* (138) in Óðinn's description of the tree on which he hung himself, and though this tree is not necessarily Yggdrasill, it is once again a tree whose properties are unknown rather than unknowable.

Veit ek at ek hekk
vindga meiði á
nætr allar níu,
geiri undaðr
ok gefinn Óðni,
sjálfr sjálfum mér,
á þeim meiði
er manngi veit,
hvers hann af rótum renn.[24]

I know that I hung on the windy tree for nine full nights, wounded with a spear and dedicated to Óðinn – myself to myself – upon that tree that came from roots that no-one knows.

This once again suggests that the issue at hand is a lack of human awareness (in this case of the tree's origins), rather than the impossibility of understanding the depths to which a tree's roots reach, the number of serpents that lie

[23] ABRAM, "Felling trees", forthcoming.
[24] References to *Hávamál* from *Hávamál*, ed. D.A.H. EVANS (London, 1986), pp. 39-74.

beneath it, or indeed the nature of its suffering. Abram points out that the mythic discourse may enable humans to "engage with the nonhuman physical world in different ways because (ironically) it does not aim to tell stories of the 'real' world".[25] This assessment seems to me to be closer to the truth. It is not that humans are unable to engage with the suffering of Yggdrasill and other trees, but that by entering into this mythic discourse – in other words the realm of poetry and the imagination – we are permitted to sound the depths beneath the mundane fabric of the everyday, and participate in the sensory and emotional experience of non-humans.

Elsewhere in Old Norse poetry, relationships between humans and plant life are even more direct. Men and women of all ages are likened to trees or directly identified with trees via kennings.[26] This is especially prominent in kennings in skaldic poetry,[27] and also in works such as Egill Skallagrímsson's *Sonatorrek* (*Hard Loss of Sons*), in which Egill compares one (or possibly both) of his dead sons with trees, as both Abram and I have discussed in some detail.[28] Although my aim here is to discuss the evidence of eddic rather than skaldic verse, the fact that this tradition is found in skaldic poetry is significant. The metres and particularly the named attribution of most skaldic verses may be used in many cases to confirm its antiquity.[29] This is an important consideration because the evidence indicates that connections between the bodies of humans and plant life were a well-established part of poetic and mythic discourse before the Scandinavian conversions. At the same time, it is also worth remembering that Norse poetry had not developed in a vacuum, and that the influence of Christian ideas upon aspects of Norse heathenism is now well recognised.

Eddic poetry, whilst stemming from the same branch as skaldic verse, cannot be dated with the same confidence, and much may have reached its surviving form after the conversion period.[30] In any case, readers of eddic po-

[25] ABRAM, "Felling trees", forthcoming.

[26] BINTLEY, *Trees*, pp. 129-152.

[27] BINTLEY, *Trees*, pp. 134-136.

[28] M.D.J. BINTLEY, "Life-cyles of men and trees in *Sonatorrek*", *Opticon 1826* 6 (2009) <http://www.ucl.ac.uk/opticon1826/archive/Issue6/AH_Bintley.pdf> [accessed 23 July 2015]; BINTLEY, *Trees*, pp. 130-132; C. ABRAM, *Myths of the Pagan North: The Gods of the Norsemen* (London, 2011), pp. 108-121; ABRAM, "Felling trees", forthcoming.

[29] J. JESCH, "Poetry in the Viking Age", in: *The Viking World*, ed. S. BRINK, with N. PRICE (Abingdon, 2008), pp. 291-298, at pp. 295-296; also K.E. GADE, *The Structure of Old Norse* Drótkvætt *Poetry* (Ithaca, NY, 1995), pp. 1-28.

[30] ABRAM, *Myths*, pp. 16-20.

etry through its manuscript forms would have encountered this literature in a Christian context, albeit with obvious awareness of the pre-Christian culture in which it was rooted. For this reason, it is no less valuable to recognise the importance of relationships between humans and plants in biblical texts which could have been known to audiences of eddic poetry. In the Old Testament, individuals and groups of people are compared with a variety of plants, including vines,[31] figs and olives,[32] palms,[33]oaks,[34] cedars,[35] grass and green shoots,[36] and other undefined trees and plants.[37] Similar examples are also found in the New Testament, as we might well expect, given that it largely a product of the same tradition. In the New Testament, humans are aligned with fruit trees and branches,[38] and Christ himself appears as the true vine.[687] As I have previously argued, the abundance of vegetative symbolism present in Judaeo-Christian writing appears to have been well received in early medieval Scandinavia and England, and to have aided rather than hindered conversion. This process appears to have benefited from similarly prominent ideas about trees and other plant life in pre-Christian Germanic belief, which therefore did not pose an obstacle to conversion, but rather served to facilitate the transition from the older traditional belief system to the new faith.[39]

One of the most prominent connections between humans and trees in eddic poetry concerns tree anthropogony, in an episode found in *Vǫluspá* (st. 17-18), where three of the Æsir, led by Óðinn:

[31] The examples in these footnotes are illustrative, not comprehensive. Genesis 49:22; Psalms 128:3.

[32] Judges 9:6-15; Psalms 52:8; Psalms 128:3.

[33] Psalms 92:12-13; Song of Songs 7:7-8.

[34] Isaiah 61:1-3.

[35] Ezekiel 31:1-18.

[36] 2 Kings 19:26; Job 5:25; Job 8:11-12; Psalms 37:1-2; Psalms 92:6-7; Psalms 129:6-7; Isaiah 5:24; Isaiah 37:27; Isaiah 40:6-8; Isaiah 51:12; Isaiah 53:2.

[37] Numbers 13:20; Job 15:30; Job 15:33; Psalms 1:3; Psalms 37:35-36; Psalms 96:12; Psalms 144:12; Isaiah 7:2; Isaiah 56:3.

[38] Matthew 7:17-20; Matthew 12:33; Luke 3:9; Luke 6:43-44; Luke 13:6-9; Jude 1:12; Romans 11:11-24. [687] John 15:1-8.

[39] BINTLEY, *Trees*.

Fundo á landi
lítt megandi
Ask ok Emblo
ørlǫglausa.

Ǫnd þau né átto,
óð þau né hǫfðo,
lá né læti
né lito góða.
Ǫnd gaf Óðinn,
óð gaf Hœnir,
lá gaf Lóðurr
ok lito góða.

They found on the shore Ash and Elm, weak and futureless. They had neither breath nor spirit, nor flesh nor voice, nor fair appearances. Óðinn gave breath, Hoenir gave spirit, Lóðurr gave flesh and fair appearances.

Much the same account is also found in Snorri Sturluson's *Gylfaginning* in *c.* 1225. This is unsurprising, given that *Vǫluspá* was one of his primary sources, but Anders Hultgård has suggested that Snorri may have known another variant of this anthropogonic myth.[40] Another narrative which suggests tree anthropogony appears in *Hávamál*, where Óðinn gives "*tveim trémǫnnum*" ("two tree-men", *Hávamál* 49) clothes which transform them into warriors.[41] It is worth considering what these lines tell us about the perceived differences between humans and trees. What do humans have that trees do not, in the views of *Vǫluspá* and *Hávamál*? There is certainly no suggestion here that trees are unable to undergo sensory and emotional experience.

Plants in eddic poetry experience suffering and loss in the same way as humans – in both physiological and psychological terms. Let us now see the various representations of this experience in the *Poetic Edda*. We can begin on a positive note, considering comparisons between the burgeoning of an individual's prowess and the flourishing of plant life, which occurs frequently enough

[40] *Snorri Sturluson: Edda; Prologue and Gylfaginning*, ed. A. FAULKES, 2nd edn. (London, 2005), p. 13; A. HULTGÅRD, "The Askr and Embla myth in a comparative perspective", in: *Old Norse Religion in Long-Term Perspectives: Origins, Changes, and Interactions: An International Conference in Lund, Sweden, June 3-7, 2004,* ed. A. ANDRÉN, K. JENNBERT and C. RAUDVERE (Lund, 2006), pp. 58-62, at p. 59. See further discussion of this episode in BINTLEY, *Trees*, pp. 136-137; and TOLLEY, *Shamanism*, 1, pp. 346-349.

[41] See also BINTLEY, *Trees*, pp.137-138.

to suggest the existence of a common topos. As his fame increases in the hearts and minds of his peers, the hero Helgi (in the eleventh-century *Helgakviða Hundingsbana* I, 9), is directly identified with an elm tree:

> *Þá nam at vaxa*
> *fyr vina brióstí*
> *álmr ítrborinn,*
> *ynðis lióma;*
> *hann galt oc gaf*
> *gull verðungo,*
> *sparði eigi hilmir*
> *hodd blóðrekinn.*[42]
>
> Then that shining-born elm tree, with the gleam of contentment, began to grow in his friend's hearts; he paid and gave gold to the troop, that chief spared not the bloodstained hoard.

The explicit comparison here is between the flourishing of Helgi as an heroic figure, and the vitality of the elm, but in the mind of the poet Helgi is not like an elm, he *is* an elm. *Helgakviða Hundinsbana* II, by comparison, more obviously makes use of simile in describing Helgi, although on this occasion he is compared with ash, rather than elm (st. 38) – possibly evoking Askr or Yggdrasill.[43]

> *Svá bar Helgi*
> *af hildingom*
> *sem ítrscapaðr*
> *ascr af þyrni,*
> *eða sá dýrkálfr,*
> *dǫggo slunginn,*
> *er øfri ferr,*
> *ǫllom dýrom*
> *oc horn glóa*

[42] References to *Helgakviða Hundingsbana I* from *Edda*, ed. NECKEL, pp. 130-139.

[43] Although Larrington writes that there is "no doubt" that this treeish metaphorical vocabulary for humans stems from the anthropogonic myth found in *Vǫluspá*, it seems equally feasible that the reverse may be the case – that this myth emerged as an aetiological explanation for the association between humans and trees, rather than vice versa. See *The Poetic Edda*, trans. C. LARRINGTON (Oxford, 1996), p. 279.

við himinn siálfan.[44]

So was Helgi beside the chieftains like the bright-growing ash by the thorns, and the young stag, dew-drenched, who is greater than all other beasts, and whose antlers shine before heaven itself.

However, this idea is not limited solely to trees, and elsewhere we see the same imagery of flourishing plants employed in the same fashion. In *Guðrúnarkviða II*, we see Sigurðr portrayed as a leek. The implicit idea here is that his stature is such in comparison with the sons of Giuki that he is as a leek to blades of grass (st. 2):

Svá var Sigurðr
uf sonom Giúca,
sem væri grœnn laucr
ór grasi vaxinn.[45]

So was Sigurðr in comparison with the sons of Giúki, as if he were a green leek grown out of the grass ...

This vegetative imagery may also find comparison in the opening lines of *Beowulf*, which describe the flourishing of Beow (MS *Beowulf*), whose "*blæd wide sprang*" ("fame sprang wide", l. 18), as his prowess increased like a flourishing sheaf of cereal crop.[46] If this is the case, then perhaps the same idea may also be present in the following lines from *Fáfnismál*, where Fáfnir describes the increase of Sigurðr in much the same terms, though there is no direct suggestion that this passage is referring directly to the growth of plant life (st. 7):

Veit ec, ef þú vaxa næðir fyr þinna vina bríosti,
sæi maðr þic vreiðan vega;
nú ertu haptr oc hernuminn,
æ qveða bandingia bifaz.[47]

[44] References to *Helgakviða Hundingsbana II* from *Edda*, ed. NECKEL, pp. 150-161.
[45] References to *Guðrúnarkviða II* from *Edda*, ed. NECKEL, pp. 224-231.
[46] R. NORTH, *Heathen Gods in Old English Literature* (Cambridge, 1997), pp. 194.
[47] References to *Fáfnismál* from *Edda*, ed. NECKEL, pp. 180-188.

> I know, if you did manage to burgeon in the hearts of your friends, you would be seen to fight ferociously; now you are a prisoner, and a captive – they say that a prisoner is always trembling.

There is very little indication in any of these passages, however, of what these plants are experiencing on a sensory level. But then again, should we expect this here? We would not expect significantly more than this in a description of a human filled with pride.

The experience of suffering is what really offers the best bridge between the sensory lives of plants and humans, given that plants have bodies, and often have limbs, which are just as prone to the violence of harsh weapons. Descriptions of plants (predominantly trees) which have suffered physical pain and hardship are as abundant as we might expect from a culture which made significant use of underwood and timber to suit various practical purposes. It is important to remember that the authors of this poetry were intimately familiar with the processing of this material – the stripping of branches, the felling of trees, and the burning of timber – and were attempting to represent the suffering of human beings in the same way that they knew trees suffered. In the stanza immediately following the description of his gifts to tree-men in *Hávamál* (st. 49-50), Óðinn has the following to say about the fate of humans who are separated from their kinfolk:

> *Hrørnar þǫll,*
> *sú er stendr þorpi á;*
> *hlýrat henni bǫrkr né barr;*
> *svá er maðr,*
> *sá er manngi ann;*
> *hvat skal hann lengi lifa?*

> The withered fir-tree – that which stands on the mound – is protected by neither bark nor needles; so it is with a man who is loved by none; why should he live long?

The movement of this image is slightly more subtle than it may first appear. In stanza 49, we have been introduced to Óðinn's clothing of the tree-men, so when the fir tree first appears, it stands alone in the mind as a single tree separated from its kindred of fir trees. Exposed upon the mound, a formation that has obvious associations with death, this line presents a naturalistic image of a tree that has been weathered. The focus changes, however, as the next line focuses more closely on its branches and trunk, bereft of bark and needles, which we subsequently understand to be like a man who has been deprived of those who love him. Bound up in this stanza, then, may be two simultaneous images: first that of a [human / tree] separated from other [humans / trees]; and secondly that of a [human / tree] deprived of [loved ones / needles and bark]. The same idea is also found in *Hárbarðsljóð* (st. 22), although it is not developed to the same degree, and appears in lines which stem from the same gnomic impulse to explain the fortunes of humans in terms of the fate of trees:

Þat hefir eic, er af annarri scefr,
um sic er hverr í slíco.[48]

One oak gains what is cut from another – it's every man for himself in such matters.

These lines may have their origin in a more southerly climate than those cited above in *Hávamál*, given that they describe the fate of an oak, stripped of branches with no mention of needles, but the idea is much the same. Those trees which stand beside one that has been stripped of branches are likely to prosper from the increased availability of resources, just as one man profits from another's ruin.

More delicate and personal imagery, expressing the same sentiments in terms of personal experience, equate the experience of Guðrún with both deciduous and coniferous woodland trees. In *Hamðismál* (st. 5), she describes herself in the following terms following the death of Svanhildr, saying that:

Einstœð em ek orðin
sem ǫsp í holti,
fallin at frœndom
sem fura at kvisti,
vaðin at vilia
sem viðr at laufi
þá er in kvistskœða
kømr um dag varman.[49]

[48] References to *Hárbarðsljóð* from *Edda*, ed. NECKEL, pp. 78-87.

[49] References to *Hamðismál* from *The Poetic Edda*, 1, *Heroic Poems*, ed. and trans. U. DRONKE (Oxford, 1969), pp. 161-167.

> I stand alone, like an aspen in the forest, with my kindred cut away like the branches of a fir; deprived of happiness, like a tree of its leaves, when a girl cutting branches comes on a warm day.

This seems to be collapsing several ideas together at the same time. First, she is an aspen, presumably a northern European quaking aspen (*populus tremula*), a deciduous tree so-called because of its delicate leaves, which flutter in the slightest breeze, and thus an appropriate choice of tree to identify with an individual who fears for her future.[50] Secondly, Guðrún is a fir stripped of its branches, stripped of her kinsmen. Thirdly, she is a wood (an area of woodland rather than a single timber), stripped of leaves. The tragedy of this is only magnified by the domesticity of the image that follows: that of a girl who has come cutting branches in the woodlands (perhaps redolent of a valkyrie). The girl who appears in this simile is aware on at least some level that she is depriving trees of their 'kin-wood', but at the same time her humanness also results in an ontological void between her human experience and the suffering of the forest. In *Guðrúnakviða I* (st. 19) we see the same idea in play, albeit more briefly, when Gúðrun tells us that:

> *Ec þóttac oc*
> *þiódans reccom*
> *hverri hœrri*
> *Herians dísi;*
> *nú em ec svá lítil,*
> *sem lauf sé*
> *opt í iǫlstrom,*
> *at iǫfur dauðan.*[51]

> I thought myself, amongst the retinue of my lord, to be higher than all of Óðinn's women; now I am so small, just like a leaf amongst the bay willows at the death of the prince.

This is a far more delicate image than we have seen so far, which serves to emphasise her much-diminished status following the death of Sigurðr. She is

[50] Dronke offered an alternative view, that this image "expresses not only her loneliness, but her sense that she, the last of her heroic line, towers above other breeds of men"; see DRONKE, *Heroic Poems*, p. 227.

[51] References to *Guðrúnakviða I* from *Edda*, ed. NECKEL, pp. 202-206.

no tree, stripped of leaves, nor is she even a branch – she is no more than a leaf, tiny and vulnerable at the extremities of the tree.

In *Guðrúnarkviða II*, we see the poet drawing twice upon the vulnerability of trees as the Völsung cycle draws to a close with the death of Sigurðr. First, in stanza 12, Guðrún expresses her death-wish in both human and tree-ish terms, desiring to expose herself to the ravaging of wolfish teeth or crematory flames:

Nótt þótti mér
niðmyrcr vera,
er ec sárla satc
yfir Sigurði;
úlfar þóttomz
ǫllo betri,
ef þeir léti mic
lífi týna
eða brendi mic
sem birkinn við.

I thought that the night was as dark as the waning moon, as I sat grieving over Sigurðr; of all things it seemed best to me for the wolves to take my life, or if they burned me like birchwood.

This would not be much to speak of, were it not for the specificity of the image, which invites comparison between Guðrún's desire for death, and the death of Signý in the hall of Siggeirr, who suffers a similarly incendiary fate. Elsewhere, in stanza 40, we see Atli's understanding, through dreams, that his sons have been murdered by his wife, though unaware that they are soon to be fed to him as beer snacks.

Hugða ec hér í túni
teina fallna,
þá er ek vildigac
vaxna láta,
rifnir með rótom,
roðir í blóði,
bornir á becci,
beðit mic at tyggva.

> I thought that here in the meadow the saplings had fallen, those I had wished to grow tall, ripped up with their roots, reddened with blood, borne to the bench and bidden to me to taste.

These lines refer to Atli's fallen sons in terms that echo those found in *Sonatorrek*, where Egill Skallagrímsson laments the deaths of his sons Bǫðvarr and Gunnarr. The dream state in which Atli experiences the scene described here permits the full surrealism of this image, rather like Nebuchadnezzar's dream in the Book of Daniel, in which the king himself is figured as a cosmic tree that is felled and has its stump bound for seven years, foretelling the seven years of bestial madness that he will endure in the wilderness as a consequence of his hubris.[52] Once again, these lines in *Guðrúnarkviða II* focus on the viscerality of the trees' suffering and destruction. These trees have not been felled with an axe in such a way that their coppiced stumps might still sprout green shoots of spring. They have been torn up by their roots, which the dream-state allows to be reddened with blood. Alternatively this could potentially be an allusion to the bleeding to which some trees are particularly prone when pruned (especially when this takes place at the wrong time of year), or to the red flesh of a tree like the alder. The absurdity of the image is compounded by the serving of these saplings as food for a feast. Just as humans eating the wood of trees is against the 'natural' order of things, so too is the consumption of human flesh – perhaps especially that of one's own children!

In the course of this essay I have argued that the sensory and emotional life of plants is directly accessible through Old Norse eddic poetry. In *Vǫluspá* and *Grímnismál*, the world tree Yggdrasill endures great and terrible hardships which, although distanced from human experience, remain nevertheless accessible to us through mythic and poetic discourse. If Yggdrasill operates as a *figura* for trees and plant life in more general terms, this represents an essential understanding within the Norse world-view that the life of trees is directly comparable with that of humans on certain basic levels. This is borne out by the alignment of human and tree-ish bodies in skaldic and eddic poetry. As I have noted here and elsewhere, a full assessment of the skaldic evidence has yet to be attempted, although an interim assessment of the proliferation of tree-ish terms for humans points to a certain pre-Christian antiquity in this trope in Norse culture. This trope would nevertheless have been comfortably accommo-

[52] Daniel 4:1-37.

dated within the Christian tradition, since this has an abundant crop of descriptions that aligned humans and plant life.

In the second half of the essay I focussed primarily upon what the evidence of eddic poetry reveals about the way in which the experience of plant life sheds light on human experience. Generally speaking, this is in one of two ways. The first has relatively little to do with sensory experience in any direct sense – the growth and flourishing of plant-life parallels the increasing fame and prowess of great heroes. The second is more complex and revealing, however, and may have much to say both about the way in which the life of plants was understood in early medieval Scandinavia, and perhaps about the way in which humans have thought about plants outside of these temporal and geographical limits. In the preceding discussion I have attempted to provide a comprehensive survey of the way in which trees and other plant life are represented in eddic poetry. The majority of allusions to the experience of plants comes in comparison with human experience – and primarily human suffering. More often than not, when plants are mentioned they appear to be in a state of pain, loss, or fear; the fragility of human life is thus emphasised by the fragility of plant life. Their limbs, like ours, are vulnerable to violence and hostile flames. At the beginning of this essay, I agreed with Matthew Hall's ideas on ecology.[53] At the same time, a perhaps unsettling conclusion that can be drawn from this body of ancient evidence is that it asks us to notice the sensory and emotional experience of plants when both we – and they – are experiencing pain and suffering.

As we have seen, Abram suggests that recognising and representing those aspects of Norse poetry which represent the interconnectedness of the world is unlikely to have any direct measurable effect upon ecological approaches in the short term.[54] The present author also agrees with Timothy Morton that we are in the midst of the ecological crisis, rather than teetering on its brink.[55] However, as many have observed since the ecological movement began to gather force in the twentieth century, intellectual climate change does not take place overnight, and abrupt interventions into long-term processes can do more harm than good. Ecological thought and ecological criticism is an ongoing part of the ecological movement in itself. Whether directly or indirectly, this essay contributes to the intellectual *florilegium* that passes through the hands of those

[53] ABRAM, "Felling trees", forthcoming.
[54] ABRAM, "Felling trees", forthcoming.
[55] See discussion in T. MORTON, *The Ecological Thought* (Cambridge, MA, 2010).

engaged in ecological thinking. However small these offerings may seem, they are in keeping with the dictum of some champions of eco-theory to 'think globally, act locally'. They can thus be taken to represent this ethos in practice, with the conscious aim that these ideas will take root and flourish – "*as an ook comth of a litil spir*".[56]

[56] Geoffrey Chaucer, *Troilus and Criseyde*, II, line 1335, ed. in: *The Riverside Chaucer*, ed. L.D. Benson, 3rd edn. (Oxford, 2008), p. 507.

Index

A/Y Memorandum Book (MS York, North Yorkshire County Library, E20): 57
acoustics: 4, 53-73, 99-100
actors: 54-55, 57-58, 60-66, 73
Ælfric: 40-41, 97-98, 123, 145-146; *Homily on St Bartholomew's Day*: 136-137, 140; *Pastoral Epistle*: 156
Æsir: 234-235
aesthetics: 5, 111, 115, 160-161, 173-179, 215
Afghanistan: 173
Against a Wen: 132-135; *see also* charms
Ailward of Westoning: 190
Alcuin/Alcuinian: 10, 18, 25-26; *De ratione animae*: 25
Alexander's Letter to Aristotle: 116, 121
Alice Crithecreche: 193
anaesthetia: 134-135
Andreas: 18, 22-23
angels: 9, 55-56, 59, 70, 105, 120, 201
anthropogony: 234-235, 236 n.
antiquarianism: 207-208
Apollinaris, saint: 217-218, 220-221
apses: 218-222
architecture: 4, 24, 57, 60, 63-66, 69-70, 79, 124, 155, 207-226
Aristotle: 77, 79
art: 3-4, 35-36, 39, 49, 62-63, 111, 159-179, 205-206, 207-226
Arundel Psalter (MS London, British Library Arundel 60): 17, 22
ash tree: 229-232, 234-237
Askr and Embla: 234-236
aspens: 239-240
Assumption of the Virgin, The: 56
Atlantic Ocean: 10
Atli: 241-242
audiences: 2-5, 8, 10-11, 13, 36, 48, 53-55, 57-58, 60-66, 69-73, 97, 131, 133-135, 143-144, 146-149, 150-153, 157-158, 160, 204, 234
Augustine of Canterbury, saint: 137-138, 179, 208
Augustine of Hippo, saint: 24
aurality: 4, 14, 56, 63, 70, 72-73, 76-77, 88, 92, 95, 98, 99-100, 121-122, 142, 144, 150-151, 153, 200
Bald's Leechbook (MS London, British Library, Royal 12 D. XVII): 132
barbarism: 210
bark: 81, 238-239
beaks: 79-80, 163
Bede, saint, *Apocalypseos*: 171, 176; *De natura rerum*: 79; *Historia ecclesiastica*: 138, 208
Belshazzar: 19
belts: 161 n., 162-163
Benjamin, Walter: 35-37
Beowulf: 22-24, 32, 37, 102, 107-108, 111, 115-116, 117-118, 121-123, 237

Beowulf manuscript (MS London, British Library, Cotton Vitellius A. XV): 29, 100, 102, 107-108, 115-118
Bethlehem: 56
betrothal: 189, 193-194
birches: 241
bird calls: 8, 14, 20, 26, 77, 80-93, 96-98
birds: 4, 8, 11, 13-15, 17, 20-21, 23, 26, 75-98, 151, 157, 227
bishops: 137, 144-145, 192-193, 218
blemmyae: 128
Blickling Homilies (MS Princeton, W.H. Scheide Collection 71): 27, 34-36, 40-47
blindness: 76, 181-194, 210
blood: 115-116, 144, 155-156, 171, 176-177, 199, 236, 241-142
Bodleian Library: 28, 30-31
body, bodies: 2-3, 9, 13, 20, 22-25, 51, 106, 127, 155, 183-184, 191, 195-207, 209, 214-217, 222-223, 238, 242
body determinism: 196
Bohemia: 173
Book of Kells (MS Dublin, Trinity College Library, A. I. (58)): 212-213
bosses: 167-168, 173-174, 176
brains: 160-161
Brendan, saint: 10
British Library: 28-29, 38-39, 42, 47
brooches: 164-169, 171-174, 176
buckles: 161 n., 162-164, 167-169, 172-173
Bury Psalter (MS Rome, Vatican Library, Reg. lat. 12): 103-105
Byzantium: 183, 186, 189, 192, 217-218
cabochon: 164-166, 173-176
Cædmon's Hymn: 143
carbuncles: 136
catalogues: 28-33, 79, 126
cedars: 234
chalices: 5, 141-158
Charles the Bald: 191
charms, Old English: 5, 124-140
Chaucer, Geoffrey, *Troilus and Criseyde*: 243
Christ: 22, 53, 63, 101, 147, 154, 185, 202-204, 218-219, 222-223, 231, 234; blood of: 144, 155-156, 171, 176; wounds of: 101, 155
Christ and Satan: 114, 116-118
Christ in Judgement (or *Christ III*): 117-118
Church, the: 124, 137-138, 156
churches: 55, 57, 138, 155, 170, 207-226
church bells: 65
classification: 75-80, 97-98, 150, 153, 207-210
clergy: 55, 97, 153, 186, 192-193
cloisonné: 164-168, 171-177
Codex Amiatinus (MS Florence, Biblioteca Medicea-Laurenziana, Amiatino I): 104-105
Codex Justinianus: 173
cognition: 2, 13-21, 40, 195-207, 224
coins: 170
Common Germanic: 86-87, 97
consciousness: 40, 174, 212, 215-217, 219, 243
Consular Diptych of Areobindus: 211-212
conversion: 138, 179, 233-234
compensation: 181-184, 187-189, 194
Corpus Christi: 54; *see also* Christ
cosmology: 218-219, 228
courts, legal: 182
craft, craftsmen: 27, 38, 40, 42, 46-51, 53, 60, 148, 160-161 n., 171, 174, 177-178
creativity: 5, 106, 108, 110-122, 202-205
crosses: 30, 55, 147, 153, 175-178, 204-205, 218-219, 223-224
crows: 78 n., 88
Crucifixion: 55, 231
cuckoos: 12, 17, 20, 88

Cuthbert, saint: 145, 177
Daniel: 19, 22, 117-118
Daniel, Book of: 242
Dante Aligheri: 201
Day of Judgment: 176
De opificio Dei: *see* Lactantius
De ratione animae: *see* Alcuin
deafness: 76, 182-183, 185, death: 9, 21, 116, 139, 146, 188, 198-202, 204, 206, 238-241
decoration: *see* ornament
Deor: 22, 24
Descartes, René: 2, 196
desire: 17, 21, 23, 25-26, 63, 241
devil: *see* Satan
digitalisation: 4, 27-51, 65-66
direct sound: 67-69
disability: 76, 182-194
Disticha Catonis: 198
divine, divinity: 5, 20, 25, 105, 136, 145, 153, 169-170, 219, 222-224
doves: 82, 87
drama: 4, 53-73, 155
Dream of the Rood, The: 143, 177, 230-231
dróttkvætt: 203
ducks: 80, 86
eagle owls: 90-93
eagles: 14-15, 82, 86, 133
early reflections: 67-69
ears: 3, 17, 69, 75, 92-93, 125-128, 144, 184-185, 192-193
Ecgbert, Count: 192, 194
ecological pyramids: 227-228
ecology: 79, 227-243
eddic poetry: 170, 197-198, 202-204, 227-243
Edictus Langobardorum: 187-189
editing: 38, 107-111
Egill Skallagrímsson, *Sonatorrek*: 228-229, 233, 241-242
Einarr Skúlason, *Geisli*: 203-204
Elene: 22
Elijah, prophet: 219
Elizabethan: 54, 73
elms: 234-236
embodiment: 2, 5, 39-40, 48-51, 178, 195-206, 212, 214-216
Escomb: 225
Etymologiae: *see* Isidore of Seville
evolution: 77 n., 78-79
exegesis: 9, 176, 209, 212, 219
Exeter Book (MS Exeter, Cathedral Library, 3501): 10, 32, 100, 106-107, 112-115, 117-118, 120, 144, 157
Exeter Book riddles: 106-107, 123-158; Riddle 12: 130; Riddle 25: 129-130; Riddle 48: 141-158; Riddle 59: 141-158; Riddle 86: 126-129
Exodus: 117-121
eyes: 3, 17, 125-126, 128, 130-131, 142, 144, 148, 150, 153-154, 160, 162-163, 181-194, 201, 216-217
Eyrbyggja saga: 22
Ezra, prophet: 105
fabric: 160, 163
Fáfnir: 237
Fáfnismál: 237
Faversham, Kent: 161 n., 164-165
feasting: 57, 64-65, 138-139, 242
figs: 234
filigree: 164-168, 173-174
fire, firelight: 1, 22, 163-164, 176
firs: 238-240
fish: 227, 241
fishermen: 10
Fitzwilliam Museum: 49
folk-taxonomy: 77-79, 83-84, 97-98
food: 76, 138, 242
forest: *see* woodland
Fouquet, *The Martyrdom of St. Apollonia*: 58, 71
freeman: 187-188
gannets: 14, 78 n.

garlic: 127-128, 130, 139
garnets: 164-168, 171-178
gates: 60, 199, 203, 219
geese: 81, 86
Geisli: *see* Einarr Skúlason
Giles, saint: 22
gender: 188-189, 191
Genesis: 107, 117-120
Gerald of Wales: 186, 192
Giuki: 237
Gloria: 56
God: 7-9, 12-13, 19, 24-25, 56, 59, 64-65, 102, 119-120, 126, 137-138, 142, 150-151, 156, 198, 201, 203-204
gods: 138-139, 170, 198, 202, 204, 230
gold: 9, 13, 26, 141-143, 146, 148-149, 154-157, 159-179, 236
goldsmiths: 161 n., 174
Good Friday: 60
goose: *see* geese
grass: 234, 237
graves: 9, 13, 169, 204
Greek: 23, 25, 32, 97 n., 125-126
Gregory the Great, Pope: 123, 137-140
Gregory's *Pastoral Care*, Alfred's translation of: 153-154
Grendel: 23, 115-116
Grímnismál: 26, 197, 229, 231-232, 242
Guðrúnarkviða I: 240
Guðrúnarkviða II: 237, 240, 242
guilds: 53, 59-61, 73, 183
Guthlac, saint: 19
Guthlac A: 112-114, 117-118
Guthlac B: 19, 117-118
Gylfaginning: *see* Snorri Sturluson
halls: 10-11, 14, 24, 72, 142-143, 170, 203-204, 241
haloes: 104-105, 223
Hárbarðsljóð: 239
Harold Godwinson, king: 192
Hávarðar saga Ísfirðings: 24
Hastings, Battle of: 192
Hávamál: 197-198, 232, 235, 238-239
hearing: 1, 3, 5, 14, 17, 22, 48, 53-73, 75-76, 88, 98, 99-100, 115, 122, 126, 150-153, 156-157, 182, 185, 199, 227
heart: 9, 13-15, 17, 19, 22, 152, 166-167, 200-201, 235-237
heathenism: 9, 21-26, 137-138, 148, 157, 231, 233
heaven: 8-10, 15, 17-18, 20-21, 56, 59, 64-66, 70, 101-102, 142, 156, 201-205, 217-219, 221-222, 236-237
Helgakviða Hundingsbana I: 235-236
Helgakviða Hundingsbana II: 236
Heliand: 19
hell: 64, 199-203, 205
hens, chickens: 82-83, 132-134
Heorot: 24
Hera, goddess: 25
herbs: 136-139
Hexham: 225
history of science: 76
Holderness, East Yorkshire: 175-176
Holy Thursday: 60
Homer, *Iliad*: 25
Homiletic Fragment II: 19
homilies: 30-31, 34-36, 40-47, 108, 136-137, 140
horror: 15, 127-129, 190, 201
horror vacui: 161
Hrothgar: 22, 24, 115-116
Hugsvinnsmál: 198
humiliation: *see* shame
hypermediacy: 38-39
hypnosis: 134-135
Ice Age: 92
iconography: 154, 168, 178, 210, 217-219, 222-224
icons, computer: 38
icons, religious: 223-224
idols: 147-148, 157
idiocy: 110-111
Iliad: see Homer

illusions: 23, 63
illustrations: 28-29, 31, 49, 100, 104-105
impulse: 17, 23
incipits: 56
incompetence: 110-111, 113, 118
India: 171, 173
Indo-European: 82, 83 n., 85-87, 93, 96
inscription: 105 n., 149, 154-156, 191
insects: 227
interdisciplinarity: 4, 65
interlace: 168, 224-225
internet: 36-38
Isidore of Seville, *Etymologiae*: 79, 89 n., 94 n., 97 n., 123-126, 130-132, 137, 139, 216-217
James, saint: 219
jaws: 163, 191
Jesus: *see* Christ
jewellery: 163, 171-173
jewels: 173, 177, 217-220, 222-223
John, Book of: 10, 131-132, 234 n.
John, Revelation of: *see* Revelation, Book of
John, saint: 219
jokes: 129-130
Jorvik Viking Centre: 1
Juliana: 113
Junius 11 (MS Oxford, Bodleian Library, Junius 11): 30, 100, 107, 113-114, 116-121
Justinian, *Digest*: 184
kerfs: 41-42
Kiernan, Kevin, *Electronic Beowulf*: 32-33
kings: 185 n., 187, 189, 192, 203-204, 242
Lacnunga (MS London, British Library, Harley 585): 132
Lactantius, *De opificio Dei*: 20-21, 24-26
Last Judgement, The: 59, 66
laws, law codes: 124, 173, 181-194
leaves: 133-133, 239-240
leeks: 237
legislation: *see* laws
Leo VI, Emperor of Byzantium, Novels: 189-190
Leofric of Exeter: 30, 144
Leviticus, Book of: 88-89, 192
Lex Alamannorum: 185 n., 187
libraries: 27-51, 144
Lichfield Gospels: *see* St Chad Gospels
light: 1, 16, 59, 106, 131-132, 153-154, 163-164, 167-171, 174, 176, 178-179, 185-186, 199-201, 203-204, 216
limbs: 126-127, 163, 176, 183, 238, 243
Lindisfarne Gospels (MS London, British Library, Cotton Nero D. IV): 10, 29, 104-105, 216
linguistic determinism: 196
linguistics: 2, 4, 97, 146, 157, 196, 203, 206
literacy: 75-76, 108
little owls: 90, 92
liturgy: 5, 56-57, 65, 141-158, 224
Liutprand, king: 189
ljóðaháttr: 197
Lokasenna: 197
Lombards: 187-189, 193-194
long-eared owls: 90-93
looking: *see* sight
love: 8-9, 17, 238-239
lyres: 11
Macclesfield Psalter: 49
magic: 131
manuscripts discussed: MS Arras, Médiathèque, 860 (530): 101; MS Cambridge, Corpus Christi College, 57: 115; MS Dublin, Trinity College Library, A. I. (58): *see* Book of Kells; MS Durham, Dean & Chapter Library, B. IV.12: 101-102; MS Exeter, Cathedral Library, 3501: *see* Exeter Book; MS Florence, Biblioteca Medicea-Laurenziana, Amiatino I: *see* Codex Amiatinus; MS Lich-

field, Cathedral Library: *see* St Chad Gospels; MS London, British Library, Additional 40165.A.1: 109; MS London, British Library, Arundel 60: *see* Arundel Psalter; MS London, British Library, Cotton Nero D. IV: *see* Lindisfarne Gospels; MS London, British Library, Cotton Vitellius A. XV: *see* Beowulf manuscript; MS London, British Library, Harley 585: *see* Lacnunga; MS London, British Library, Royal 4 A. XIV: 132-133; MS London, British Library, Royal 12 D. XVII: *see* Bald's Leechbook; MS Oxford, Bodleian Library, Junius 11: *see* Junius 11; MS Paris, Bibliothèque Nationale, MS. gr. 139: *see* Paris Psalter; MS Princeton, W.H. Scheide Collection 71: *see* Blickling Homilies; MS Rome, Vatican Library, Reg. lat. 12: *see* Bury Psalter; MS Vercelli, Biblioteca Capitolare, CXVII: *see* Vercelli Book; MS Würzburg, M.p.th.f.79: 109; MS York, North Yorkshire County Library, E20: *see* A/Y Memorandum Book
manuscripts: binding of: 31, 40-47, 49; circulation of: 30-31, 40-42, 45-46; courses on: 48-51; gutter of: 42; production and design of: 3, 27, 34-35, 41-46, 99-122
Martyrdom of St. Apollonia, The: *see* Fouquet
Mary, mother of Christ: 55-56
Matthew, saint: 104-105
mediation: 4, 38, 48, 99-100, 123-124, 126, 128, 132, 155, 159-160, 178
meditation: 101-102, 135
medicine: 124, 132-137, 139, 181-182
medical professionals: 182
Medina del Campo: 60
Mellitus, Bishop: 137-138, 140
metal: 5, 106, 159-179, 222-223; *see also* gold, silver
metaphor: 25, 188, 196, 200-202, 228
mimesis: 203-206
mind: 2, 5, 7-26, 130, 133-134, 196-199, 202, 212-214, 216-217, 223, 236
mind's eye: 152-154, 219
mistle thrushes: 93-98
monsters: 115-116, 128
mortality: 24-25, 199, 201, 204
mosaic: 123, 217-219, 222
Moses, prophet: 219
mounds: 238
mountains: 22, 90, 119-120, 219-220
museums, museology: 1, 49, 159-160
music: 55-57, 63-65, 68-72, 157
musicians: 72
mutilation: 181-194
Nebuchadnezzar: 242
needles, fir: 238-239
needles, sewing: 41
Neo-Platonism: 25-26
Netherlands: 59-60
neurology: 159
niello: 154, 164
Njǫrðr: 202
non-humans: 204, 227-243
notation: 55-57
Nowell Codex: *see* Beowulf manuscript
oaks: 26, 50, 234, 239
oars: 13
object oriented ontology: 39-40
obscenity: 129-130
ocean: *see* sea
oculus: 219
Óðinn: 26, 198, 232, 234-235, 238, 240
Óláfr, saint: 203-204
Old English: 4-5, 32, 37, 79, 87, 100, 102, 107, 109, 111, 114-115, 121-122, 127, 143-144
Old High German: 89-90, 97
olives: 234
one-eyed: 126-128, 130, 181-194

onions: 129-130, 139
online resources: 28-35, 38, 43, 48-49
Orderic Vitalis: 185 n., 191-192
ornament: 160-174, 177-178, 222
ornithology: 75-98; *see also* birds
ostriches: 97
otherworldly: 201-202, 206
owls: 85, 88-93
oxen: 139
pageant wagons: 53, 59-66, 70-71, 73
pageants: 53-73
palaeography: 33-34, 48, 50, 101, 106-111, 114
palms: 234
parables: 10
Paris Psalter (MS Paris, Bibliothèque Nationale, MS. gr. 139): 19, 144, 146, 148
Parker Library: 28-30, 42
partial-sightedness: 76, 187
Passion of Christ: 60, 155
Passion of Saint Christopher: 102, 121
Pater Noster: 135-137
patronage: 160-161
Pavia: 193
pendants: 171-176
peregrinatio: 9-10
performance: 4-5, 40-41, 53-73, 99-100, 107, 109-111, 136, 151-152, 154-155, 157-158, 191, 194
performance space: 60, 64-66, 69
performative: 209, 215-219, 222, 224
peripheral vision: 191, 194
perspective: 39-40, 135, 143-144, 147, 150-151, 189
perspective, artistic representation of: 209-211, 214
phenomenology: 2, 5, 198-199, 206, 208-226
Phoenix, The: 114-115, 120
phylogeny: 78-79
pillars: 228-230
pipers: 84
pitch: 55
plants: 228-243
Plato: 24
Pliny the Elder, *Historia Naturalis*: 79, 170
polyphony: 55-57
pommels: 173
prayer: 101-102, 131-132, 136-137, 149, 154-155
Priory Hill, Dover, Kent: 172-173, 176
Prittlewell, Essex: 161 n.
Proverbs, Book of: 75-76, 98
Psalter: 17, 19, 22, 29, 49, 55, 103-105, 144, 146-148
psalms: 144, 147, 152, 157
Psalms, Book of: 234; Psalm 18: 143; Psalm 48: 9; Psalm 113: 144, 148-149, 157; Psalm 115: 144, 146-148, 157
psychology: 159, 184, 209, 235
public space: 4-5, 53-63, 65-67, 69-73, 149, 159-160, 164, 208, 210-212, 223-225
punctuation: 111-114, 120
punctures: 43-45, 101
punishments: 181-194, 201-202
quire signatures: 34-35, 45-46
Ragnarǫk: 230-231
Rothari of the Lombards, Edict: *see Edictus Langobardorum*
ravens: 26, 201
reading: 3, 37-38, 55, 63, 75-76, 94, 102, 106, 109, 112-115, 119, 128-130, 135, 143-146, 149, 152, 154-157, 186, 190, 201, 209, 212, 234
reception: 22, 64-66, 76, 99-100, 105, 121, 187 n., 234
remediation: 4, 38, 48
Renaissance: 210-211
repetition: 17, 50, 75, 107, 108, 113, 126, 130, 135-36, 145, 149, 167, 187, 199
Revelation, Book of: 75, 156, 176, 199, 219

reverberant sound: 67-68
rhetoric: 24, 197-198, 201
Rhine: 10
riddles: *see* Exeter Book riddles
rings: 11, 141-143, 148, 151-152, 165, 167, 173-174, 176
Ripon: 225
Robert of Courcy: 191
romanitas: 208-209
Rome, Romans: 138-139, 169-171, 173, 184, 208, 217
roots: 232-233, 241-242
roots (linguistic): 80-87, 93-94, 96-97
Rothbury Cross: 223
rumination: 144, 149
Ruthwell Cross: 223
sacred space: 152, 155, 208
Sant'Apollinare in Classe, Ravenna: 217-222
Satan: 9, 138, 212
scaffolds: 57-58, 61-62, 70-72
Scandinavia: 1, 170, 228-229, 233-234, 243
scribal colophons: 101-102, 105-106
scribes: 3, 5, 27, 45, 48, 95, 99-122
sculpture: 4, 60, 159, 195, 208, 223-225
sea: 7-26, 87, 94 199, 229
Seafarer, The: 4, 7-26
seafaring: 7-26
seaxes: 173
seeing: *see* sight
semantics: 13, 75-98, 119-121, 148, 194
sensory impairment: 5, 181-194
serpents: 232-233
shackles: 13
shame: 129-30, 183-184, 189
shepherds: 22, 56
Shepherds, The: 56
ships: 13, 15, 22
Siggeirr: 241
sight: 5, 21, 39, 48, 54, 76, 99, 142, 146, 150-152, 154, 157, 183, 185-190, 194, 199
sight impairment: 183, 185, 187
Signý: 241
sign language: 185
Sigurðr: 237, 240-241
silence: 54-55, 99-100, 142, 144, 148-152, 154, 185
silver: 148, 154, 156, 164, 166-167, 170-172, 178
singing: 12, 14, 54-58, 66, 70, 79, 83, 93-94, 96, 136-137, 144, 151-152
Skáldskaparmál: *see* Snorri Sturluson
slaves, slavery: 184, 187-188
slavishness: 95, 108
smell: 1, 3-4, 27, 39, 48-51, 76, 106, 185-186, 224
snakes: *see* serpents
Snorri Sturluson, *Gylfaginning*: 23, 235; *Skáldskaparmál*: 203
social elites: 169, 191, 193-194
Sólarljóð: 5, 195-206
song thrushes: 93-98
soul: 9, 19-21, 24-26, 142, 152, 154-156, 197-198, 200-201, 204, 216-217
sound: 4-5, 22, 39, 48, 53-73, 76, 80, 83-85, 88, 96, 98, 134-135, 146, 148, 150-152, 160, 199-200, 203
soundscapes: 63-65
space: 3-5, 41, 62-64, 66-68, 72, 119-120, 149-150, 152, 155, 157, 160-161, 166, 173, 208, 210-212, 214-215, 217-219, 222-225
sparrows: 97
species: 75-98
speech: 63, 65, 68, 70, 72, 119-120, 125, 142, 144, 149-154, 157, 182
speech impediment: 183, 185
St Chad Gospels (MS Lichfield, Cathedral Library, St Chad Gospels): 37
St Laurence's church, Bradford-on-Avon: 225
St Mary's church, Deerhurst: 224-225

St Peter's church, Wearmouth: 224
starlings: 93-94, 97
stone, stones: 85, 168, 171-176, 208, 217, 219, 222-224
Stonegate, York: 66, 69-73
streets: 53-73
stupidity: 185
Sulis-Minerva: 138-139
sun, sunlight: 1, 163, 195-206
Sutton Hoo, Essex: 162-164, 167
Svanhildr: 239
swords: 169, 173, 191
Symphosius, *Aenigmata*: 127
syncretism: 138-139, 197-198, 204
Tabor, mount: 219
Tacitus: 138
tactility: *see* touch
talionic revenge: 188
Tassilo Chalice: 154-155
taste: 3, 17, 48, 76, 241
tawny owls: 90-92
taxonomy: 77-80, 88, 91-98, 147
tears: 55, 102, 187
theology: 18, 24-26, 141, 144, 157, 201
Theophanes: 192
Thietmar of Merseburg: 186 n., 192-193
thinking: *see* thought
Thomas Becket, saint: 190
thought, thinking: 5, 15, 19, 21, 23-26, 101-102, 110, 119, 121, 130, 142, 147, 150, 153-154, 193, 196-197, 214, 229, 231, 240-241, 243
thoughtless, unthinking: 109, 114
thrushes: 93-98
thunder: 64
timber: *see* wood
tongues: 142, 144, 148, 164, 200
tools: 50-51, 54, 73, 101-102, 121-122, 134, 169-170, 196, 203, 223 n.
touch: 1, 27, 48-51, 76, 184-186, 216
tumour: 133-134, 139
Transfiguration: 218-219
trees: 5, 138, 227-243
Triumph of Archduchess Isabella, The: *see* Van Alsloot
Vafþrúðnismál: 197
Vainglory: 10
valkyries: 240
Valladolid: 60
Van Alsloot, *The Triumph of Archduchess Isabella*: 59, 66
Vercelli Book (MS Vercelli, Biblioteca Capitolare, CXVII): 100, 108, 117-118, 230
verses, manuscript presentation of: 111-121
viewing: 4, 27, 30, 37-38, 42, 48, 58, 61, 143, 154-155, 159-179, 183, 190-191, 199, 207-226
vines: 234
violence: 20, 183, 188-189, 194, 238, 243
Virgin Mary: *see* Mary, mother of Christ
Visio Philiberti: 197
visions: 18, 157, 177, 190-191, 194, 198-206, 215-216
volume: 55, 64
Vǫluspá: 170, 236
wagons: *see* pageant wagons
Wanderer, The: 13-14, 22-23
water: 18, 79, 82, 133, 177, 199-200, 203
waves: 11-15, 23
wealth: 9, 13, 53, 169, 171, 178, 198
weapons: 157, 170, 171-172, 191, 238
whales: 18
Widukind: 192
Wikipedia: 37
Wilfrid, saint: 225
William of Auvergne: 192
William of York, saint: 190
willows: 240
windows: 32, 57, 59, 62, 66, 69-70
wine: 10-11, 15, 155-156
winter: 9, 11
Wipert: 190

wire: 166-167, 174
wolves: 24, 132-133, 240-241
Wonders of the East: 121, 128
wood: 54, 59-60, 66, 70-71, 73, 82, 156, 200, 227, 238, 240, 242
woodland: 20, 90, 228, 239-240
world: 2-5, 9-10, 15, 28, 38, 50, 78-79, 123-126, 128, 130-132, 135-137, 139-140, 149, 152, 159, 198, 201-203, 226, 228-229, 233
world tree: *see* Yggdrasill
world view, Christian: 131, 136, 140
world view, non-Christian: 242
worship: 55, 137-139, 155, 170
writing: 33, 49-50, 76, 99-122, 132, 136, 140, 145-146, 154, 186, 195
Wulfstan: 145
Yggdrasill: 228-233, 236, 242
York: 1, 53-73
York Minster: 57
York Mystery Plays: 53-73
YouTube: 37 n., 49
Zion, mount: 119-120
zoom, zoom function: 28, 30, 37-39, 42
zoomorphs, zoomorphism: 148, 151, 161-164, 178, 225